Surveying the Covid-19 Pandemic and Its Implications

Surveying the Covid-19 Pandemic and Its Implications

Urban Health, Data Technology and Political Economy

ZAHEER ALLAM, PHD, MBA, MA
Live+Smart Research Lab
School of Architecture and Built Environment
Deakin University, Geelong
Victoria, Australia

ELSEVIER

Elsevier
Radarweg 29, PO Box 211, 1000 AE Amsterdam, Netherlands
The Boulevard, Langford Lane, Kidlington, Oxford OX5 1GB, United Kingdom
50 Hampshire Street, 5th Floor, Cambridge, MA 02139, United States

Library of Congress Cataloging-in-Publication Data
A catalog record for this book is available from the Library of Congress

British Library Cataloguing-in-Publication Data
A catalogue record for this book is available from the British Library

ISBN: 978-0-12-824313-8

Publisher: Joe Hayton
Acquisitions Editor: Brian Romer
Editorial Project Manager: Alice Grant
Production Project Manager: Kiruthika Govindaraju
Cover designer: Alan Studholme

Typeset by TNQ Technologies

Foreword

Can we assess in real time the consequences of public health responses to COVID-19, and beyond COVID-19, can African nations be better prepared to withstand future pandemics?

The spread of the novel COVID-19 virus has caught the world by surprise, and as such, many uncertainties remain on the most effective solutions to apply in order to slow down the propagation of the virus. Authorities are making decisions about mitigation, confinement, isolation, quarantine, and health-care system capabilities. Individuals, depending on the country, culture, social-economic context, age, and season, are also making decisions concerning the pandemic.

Five Asian countries—Japan, South Korea, Hong Kong, Singapore, and Taiwan—have had only 831 deaths combined by 5 May, despite their proximity to China, a phenomenon referred to as the "New Asian Miracle." These countries are part of a region that has grappled with other acute respiratory infections such as SARS and MERS, also caused by types of human coronaviruses. Their effective responsiveness to the novel coronavirus is attributed to the experience gained from managing similar outbreaks in the past.

African countries who registered cases well into February have also been early responders. Almost all countries have instituted partial or full lockdown, limiting movement both externally and internally. Nigeria was the first to report the SARS-CoV-2 genome sequence from Africa on 4 March. South Africa is now leading the continent in testing per capita (4342 tests/million people as of 5 May). At the beginning of April, Kenya had converted existing factories into mask production. Almost all African countries, from Egypt to South Africa, are building affordable ventilators and using digital and emerging technologies for tracking and other economic activities.

On one hand, South Korea, Taiwan, and Rwanda responded to the public health threat early and have focused on testing, tracking, and isolating. On the other hand, Japan and Senegal have concentrated resources on testing and treating the infected, with Senegal showing an impressive recovery rate. At the same time, the economic stopgap and stimulus responses appeared to be critical if a public health response is to succeed. Finally, decisive political leadership is critical to accelerating containment and recovery.

So, what can other countries do in the immediate future to avert the effects of COVID-19? How can they prepare for future shocks of the same magnitude, whether it be a public health crisis or a natural disaster?

Several important lessons gleaned from interventions taken by various governments point out to the need of establishing a holistic and Pan-African data-driven decision-making approach to assist government agencies with emergency and health foresight. Understanding how various public health measures affect the progression of the current pandemic taking into account the specific country context is essential. Ultimately, understanding the interplay between urban health, data technology, and political economy to not only better design policy measures in the case of emergency response but also to approach health foresight in a more holistic way when dealing with new emerging infections must be a priority.

Dr. Youssef H. Travaly

ABOUT

Youssef Travaly is the Vice-President for the African Institute of Mathematical Science (AIMS) Global Network and the former President of AIMS Senegal. He leads the Next Einstein Forum (NEF), an initiative of AIMS. Youssef is a senior executive with 20+ years of experience working in the US, in Europe and in Africa with universities, research institutions, private sector and regional organizations, national and international NGOs, both at a strategic and operational level, in science, innovation, design of public policies, including innovative products policies.

Contents

CHAPTER 1

The First 50 days of COVID-19: A Detailed Chronological Timeline and Extensive Review of Literature Documenting the Pandemic

INTRODUCTION

The COVID-19 pandemic took the world by surprise and unfolded extremely rapidly. It began relatively slower, and only a little is documented on its actual first case, with claims as from November, while others links it to on December 1. Besides not knowing when it began, there was also very little known on the many issues about the virus, including its mode of transmission, its incubation time, and the medication the vaccination, among many other elements. Even to date, at the time of writing, there still remain some gray areas about the virus including its origin and whether it could have permanent impacts on patients, and whether it is possible for patients to develop immunity, among many other areas that are still being looked into. Following these uncertainties, there had been numerous health policies with a number of those being rendered ineffective as more knowledge about the virus is revealed. For instance, at the beginning, the World Health Organization (WHO) advised that masks should only be worn by health professionals or patients while in hospital, but later on, after it established that there were possibilities of human-to-human transmission, it became apparent that everyone need to wear a mask while in public to prevent transmitting or contracting the virus.

However, while the impacts of the virus in the first 50 days were still relatively smaller, and the spread as per the available information was still slower, there were already 44 confirmed cases reported in China, Wuhan region (41 cases), Thailand (2 cases), and Japan (1 case). From the 41 reported cases in Wuhan, 2 people had succumbed to the unknown disease, whereas 12 are said to have recovered and discharged. Interestingly, on this pandemic, though it took health official approximately 38 days to identify that they were dealing with a new kind of coronavirus, an artificial intelligence (AI)—powered algorithm developed by BlueDot, a Canadian startup tech company, provided early warnings that the world might be experiencing a new virus outbreak (Bowles, 2020). The warning came 7 days earlier before the Chinese scientist identified the virus (Huang et al., 2020), and 9 days before they notified the WHO, which then made the official announcement to the world (WHO, 2020e). This early warning supports that computer predictions could be relied upon in predicting future pandemics before they arise, hence saving allowing for early preparations the challenges of future pandemic.

In these first 50 days of the COVID-19 pandemic, despite the virus having spread to two more countries outside China, most of the global community were not particularly worried, as the perception was that only those who had come into contact with the Wuhan seafood market had the highest probability of being infected. Therefore, even with the help of technologies like that of BlueDot, the countries that were seen to be at risk of the 2019-nCoV outbreak (the temporary name previously given to the virus) were those neighboring China and those directly linked to Wuhan via airlines. For this reason, some of the countries that were flagged to be at risk included Taiwan, Australia, United Arab Emirates, Hong Kong, Japan, and Thailand. This chapter documents the outbreak over the first 50 days through the sections in the following.

Surveying the Covid-19 Pandemic and Its Implications. https://doi.org/10.1016/B978-0-12-824313-8.00001-2

DAY 1—DECEMBER 1, 2019

The earliest date of symptoms for COVID-19, according to a study performed by Huang et al. (2020) and published in the Lancet journal, was December 1, 2019. However, there are other sources (Bryner, 2020; Davidson, 2020) claiming that individuals with similar symptoms may have presented themselves to hospital as early as November. According to the report, by South China Morning Post (Ma, 2020), the first person who presented similar cases was a male patient of 55-year old from the province of Hubei. However, Chinese doctors only came to realize that they were dealing with a new and serious virus late December, when similar symptoms continued to increase every day, and mostly originating from Wuhan. According to the article in Lancet, the first patient, and whom they insist may be the first case, was reported on December 1, 2019, and whom did not have direct link with the Wuhan Seafood Market that has been associated with the origin of the virus. This finding interestingly matches with Ma (2020) who also argues that the November 2019 case was not from Wuhan. The story as to the origin of the virus has fueled much political and social divides and is expected to evolve as further efforts are poured into understanding this crisis.

DAY 8—DECEMBER 8, 2019

The number of new patients voluntarily presenting themselves to hospital continued to increase (Bryner, 2020). Hospitals report new one to five cases with similar symptoms on average each day. However, this being a new virus, some sources quoted December 8 as the first day where the first patient in the city of Wuhan sought medical help for pneumonia-like symptoms. At this time, the European Centre for Disease Prevention and Control (ECDC, 2020c) contended that many dimensions, which were known today, like the need for social distancing, human-to-human infections, lack of vaccine or cure, and many such issues, were unknown, and the precautionary measures taken then were routinely delivered. Also, during these early stages of the onset of the virus, there was no clear evidence of how many people were affected. For this reason, information from Chinese authorities (Wuhan City Health Committee, 2020) and those of the WHO (WHO, 2020a) stated that the December 8, 2019, marked the onset of the first 41 cases that were tested and which were later confirmed positive with COVID-19, then known as "2019-nCoV."

DAY 29—DECEMBER 29, 2019

As hospitals continued to receive more patients with unknown "pneumonia-like symptoms," fear of the outbreak is already spreading, especially among the social media (WeChat) use within China, more so Wuhan (Secon, 2020). Li et al. (2020) explained that during the period beginning December 1, 2019, the recurrence of the words "SARS" and "shortness of breath" in the social media started to increase, and by December 29, it had peaked. Meanwhile, in the hospitals, doctors were observed to concede that there might be a new virus of unknown etymology in Wuhan, presenting symptoms of acute respiratory syndrome. The reporting is affirmed by availability of the first four cases officially confirmed. All the four cases were linked to the Huanan (Southern China) Seafood Wholesale Market, which has been highly linked to have been the source of the virus. While only four cases had been pointed, by this date, Bryner (2020) reports that already, over 180 people in Wuhan had been infected, but since doctors had not earmarked them as suspected cases noting that there were no suspicion of this "unknown" disease. The 180 cases were only identified after doctors cross-verified records. The suspicion after reporting the four cases was that they were not suffering from SARS (severe acute respiratory syndrome), which was still in surveillance since it broke in 2003. With the possibility of an unknown outbreak, at this time, the concern was to establish the transmissibility, severity, and other issues that may be related to this new virus (Adhikari et al., 2020).

DAY 31—DECEMBER 31, 2019

The situation unfolded rapidly on this day. First, the Chinese officially reported to the WHO of the possibility of a new virus with symptoms of pneumonia, but of unknown etymology. The information to WHO officials based in China was that this disease had been detected in Wuhan, from the Hubei Province. By the time of this reporting, the ECDC supported that Wuhan Municipal Health Commission was already handling 27 pneumonia cases with 7 of those in critical conditions (ECDC, 2020b). While reporting, the officials did not have the information about how the disease was transmitted, and in some sources (WHO, 2020e), they have ruled out human-to-human infection. While that is the case, all patients with the said symptoms who had been received so far in hospitals in Wuhan were placed under quarantine, as work to establish and identify the type of the virus and its origin began (Safi, 2020).

While this marked the first official day that the COVID-19 pandemic gained and attracted attention from the international body (WHO), and the Centers for Disease Control and Prevention (CDC), as noted in the previous dates, different cases had been reported. With ambiguity on this, there are contradictory figures from different sources denoting cases with varying dates. But the following days succeeding the event, reporting has been taken over by international organization and by the WHO, leading to more coordinated and reliable figures.

DAY 32—JANUARY 1, 2020

On January 1, 2020, the Wuhan's Huanan Seafood Wholesale Market was indefinitely closed following its associated link with the virus outbreak (Juan, 2020). The role and link of the market in this story was not only made by the Wuhan Municipal officials but also by the USCDC (Patel and Jernigan, 2020). While workers in the market, under the watchful eyes of the police, proceeded to close their businesses, health officials were collecting samples from surfaces in the market and sealing them in plastic bags to be analyzed further. The closure included banning of live animals from this market and any other wet markets (WHO, 2020e). Sale of wild animals to restaurants, via online markets or in any other such market, was also banned. Besides preventing further spread of the virus, the other intention of the closure of the market was to allow for environmental sanitation and disinfection of the same. There were also some levels of public awareness performed, especially to farmers who reared animals, where emphasis on sanitation was being stressed upon (WHO, 2020c).

Outside the market, Chinese social media were amassed with different messages pointing to the fact that Wuhan, an industrial city of over 11 million people, was experiencing an outbreak of an unknown disease. According to Safi (2020), the fears being spread in those social media platforms were catalyzed by leakage of some medical documents from a hospital in Wuhan showing that some people with the virus had been reportedly transferred there. Since uncertainties revolved around the virus, panic was building up around the perception that SARS backer-emerged. Following the spread of this fear, eight individuals accused of spreading rumors were arrested and imprisoned by the Public Security Bureau (Tardáguila and Chen, 2020).

Outside China, its neighbors were starting to take caution. Taiwan was reported to immediately take the issue seriously and demanded the screening for any signs of pneumonia-like or flu symptoms for all individuals coming from China.

Until this date, the number of those reported to have shown the signs of the disease in question still remains unknown, but consensus builds around the number of cases to be 41 (Zhao et al., 2020).

DAY 38—JANUARY 7, 2020

After rigorous probes, tests, analysis, and other medical practices, the Chinese authorities made a global announcement (Huang et al., 2020) that they have successfully identified the virus as a novel coronavirus, similar to the one associated with SARS and the middle east respiratory syndrome (MARS). Prior to this ground breaking discovery, the officials had 2 days earlier, on January 5, ruled out that the virus they were dealing with was either SARS or MARS, hence concluding that it was indeed a new type of virus. Upon its successful identification, it was tentatively named as "2019-nCoV." The identification came after Chinese scientists successfully isolated the virus from one of the patients quarantined in a hospital in Wuhan (Huang et al., 2020). According to an article by Singhal (2020), the identified virus had greater than 95% (>95%) homology with the bat coronavirus and was also greater than 70% similarity with the virus responsible for causing SARS (SARS-CoV).

As the identification occurred, it was also reported that the samples previously collected from the Wuhan market tested positive, thus confirming the fears that the virus could have originated from there.

Even after identification of the virus, it was still not clear of how it could be transmitted. But the executive director of the WHO's Health Emergencies Programme, Dr. Mike Ryan, argued that the virus being a respiratory pathogen could possibly be transmitted from human to human (WHO, 2020e). At this stage, it is reported that approximately 44 people had contracted the disease and were still under quarantine as reported earlier.

Beyond China, as report by the WHO (WHO, 2020a), neighboring countries were stepping up their health precautions. For instance, Japan began to institute comprehensive screening of all travelers coming from Wuhan, and anyone with signs of fever or flu were placed under quarantine. In the United States, the country's CDC created a 2019-nCoV incident management structure that would help the country as it prepares for upcoming cases.

DAY 42—JANUARY 11, 2020

On January 9, 2020, Chinese officials reported to the WHO that they have finally identified the virus, and subsequently, the WHO made the official announcement (WHO, 2020e) of the same to the world. On January 11, the Chinese health officials share unfortunate news that a 61-year-old man who had been admitted in one of the hospitals in Wuhan had died. From the report (Ravelo and Jerving, 2020), the man had other underlying health conditions such as chronic liver disease and abdominal tumors, but the cause of his death was attributed to 2019-nCoV. By the time of his death, he was reported to have suffered from issues such as respiratory failure and severe pneumonia, septic shock, and multiple organ failure. He was also observed to have suffered from severe acid-based metabolism disorder and cirrhosis. His hospital treatment included antiinfection, ventilator-assisted breathing, life support, and other treatments, but with no positive results. His death was marked as the first known death from this new virus.

In regard to new cases, health officials did not record any other case except the 44 cases that had been received up to January 3. They also expressed that according to an epidemiological survey (WHO, 2020e), there was no clear evidence that the disease could be transmitted from human to human. However, they affirmed that all the cases in hospital were of people who had been exposed to the Wuhan Seafood market.

On this day, the first 2019-nCoV virus genome sequence was deposited in the GENBNK (the NIH database that where all public genetic sequences are stored) and shared with virologist.org (an online hub for prepublication of data, where the public can freely access for public health–related activities and research) and also uploaded to the platform "Global Initiative on Sharing All Influenza Data" (GISAID) (ECDC, 2020b), through a collaboration of a number of organizations including the Shanghai Public Health Clinic Centre, the Central Hospital of Wuhan, Huazhong University of Science and Technology, and Wuhan Center for Disease Control and Prevention among others. All this happened before the information on discovery of the genome sequence was officially shared with the WHO. However, the details were to be shared with the WHO the following day together with other viral sequences that were to be shared with GISAID (Holmes, 2020). In parallel, Chinese Health officials were considering to temporarily close down the Chinese laboratory that was the first to share the coronavirus genome with the world. The laboratory was closed on the following day (hJanuary 12) (Pinghui, 2020).

DAY 43—JANUARY 12, 2020

The WHO was briefed of the availability of the first viral genome sequence of coronavirus, and other five other genomes, which were subsequently deposited in the GISAID platform (Holmes, 2020). A lab in China, which was first to share genome, publicly closed down "for rectification" as ordered in the previous day, but still there was no clarification of what this "rectification" was supposed to mean. In addition, on this closure, as reported by Pinghui (2020), the laboratory was not given notice as to why they were asked to be closed down, even after relentless permission applications to reopen without any success. But it is assumed the "rectification" here is all about the lab releasing their genome sequence publicly before the officials could publish theirs. Despite this bad blood between the laboratory and the officials from the Shanghai Public Health Clinic Centre and other agencies involved in establishing and depositing the viral genome sequencing, the information is said to be critical in assisting scientists from different parts of the globe in the development of the testing and diagnostic kits and also in search for vaccine and cure for the disease.

Another major happening of the day is the publishing of interim guidelines by the WHO on issues pertaining to travel advice, testing in laboratories and medical investigations. These targeted to help countries across the globe to prepare for any eventuality that may arise from the nCoV spread. The guidelines also targeted to urge the travellers, especially from or in Wuhan to practice extra health caution. Also, the guidelines insisted on the need for countries not to impose any travel restrictions on the international travelers (Schnirring, 2020).

DAY 44—JANUARY 13, 2020

While no new cases were reported in Wuhan, or in any other parts of China, beyond its border, Thailand confirmed their first case, which was also thought to be the first international 2019-nCoV one. This first case was a woman, noted to have frequented local fresh market in Wuhan, but did not visit the condemned Huanan South China Seafood Market. The 61-year-old Chinese citizen was intercepted at the Bangkok airport by the thermal surveillance scanners that detected her high temperature (fever). The identification of this case occurred on January 8, where she was hospitalized immediately and samples were taken from her, but the healthy officials delayed reporting the case until January 13. When the samples were subjected to a number of medical tests such aa the reverse transcriptase polymerase chain reaction test and subjected to genetic sequencing, they came back positive for the 2019-nCoV. During the travel, she and five family members were in a tour group of 16 members who traveled directly from Wuhan to Bangkok. Before the tests were done, the woman reported to have had experienced fever, chills, sore throat, and headaches. Of all those in her company, no one had shown any similar signs (Schnirring, 2020); thus, she is the only one who was isolated.

With the patient having insisted she did not visit the suspected seafood market in Wuhan, the hypothesis of the origin of the virus was put into disarray, and the WHO insisted that the scope for the investigation of the source of the virus needs to be extended beyond the seafood market to other local markets that are observed to have also been involved in selling of live animals, including bats, which have been linked with the origin of the virus. Another issue that came up from the history of this patient is the incubation period of the virus. According to her, her last visit to the markets was on January 5. Therefore, since then, to the time she was detected to have symptoms, a number of days had passed. This also led to further question of the incubation period of the 2019-nCoV.

Following the identification of the first case outside China, a research group (BlueDot developed an AI-based system to track the virus spread as from December 30, 2019 (Bowles, 2020)) from Toronto embarked to map out top destinations that would be at high risk following the airline travel history from Wuhan. From the research, those flagged as top destinations included Thailand, Hong Kong, Japan, Taiwan, Australia, and the United Arab Emirates.

Following the confirmation in Thailand, health officials from the country declared that they were tracing and monitoring over 182 contacts that may have interacted with the woman patient (WHO, 2020b).

DAY 47—JANUARY 16, 2020

From January 13, a number of happenings have been reported. On January 14, for instance, following the first confirmation outside China, Wuhan embarked on a concerted effort of screening all passengers traveling out of the city either via the air, the rail, or buses. The screening was performed at the points of departure (airports, railway stations, ferry terminals, and bus stations) through the help of 35 infrared thermometers that were installed in those key points (WHO, 2020d). On this day still, the WHO, after consultation with Chinese officials, reported that there were no clear evidences to conclude that the 2019-nCoV virus could be transmitted from person to person, but the option could not be excluded (WHO, 2020e). But, while that was going on, of the 41 quarantined cases, 2 of the cases were confirmed to be a married couple, thus watering down the argument that the virus could not involve human-to-human transmission.

On January 15, a major event happened in Wuhan, China, where a 69-year-old man died from the virus (Siu et al., 2020). Like the first reported death, this man also had some other underlying health conditions such as myocarditis, abnormal renal function, and multiple organ failure (Ravelo and Jerving, 2020). Outside China, Japan confirmed their first case, a man in his 30s who had lived in Wuhan and traveled back to Japan on January 6. While in Wuhan, he reported to have developed a high fever (January 3) (Sim, 2020), but it was only days later, in Japan that he was confirmed to be coronavirus positive, as reported by the Japanese Ministry of Health, Labor and Welfare (Gan, 2020). The man, who had not visited the Huanan seafood market, was taken in hospital in Japan as from January 10 where he stayed up to January 15, where, though he tested positive, he recovered and was dismissed from hospital.

On January 16, Vietnam isolated two Chinese travelers coming from the Chinese city, and though they had not been found positive, this was done as a preventive measure following the news of the spread of the virus outside China.

In Germany, a team of researchers from German Centre for Infection Research (DZIF), Berlin, are noted to have successfully developed a prototype of the first diagnostic test that could help in identifying the coronavirus. The laboratory assay was approved and published by the WHO as a guideline for diagnostic detection, and it became the first test kit in the world (Drosten, 2020).

DAY 48—JANUARY 17, 2020

A second case was reported in Thailand. This time, it was a 74-year-old woman who had traveled from Wuhan and arrived at Bangkok Suvarnabhumi Airport on January 13. Upon arrival and screening, she was found to have fever and was isolated into a local medical institute where the coronavirus testing was performed and come back positive (The Government of the Hong Kong Specia Administrative Region, 2020). The confirmation of the case was made by the Ministry of Public health of Thailand. Following this case, Thailand was put on a high alert, since in the following weeks was the beginning of the Lunar New Year Holidays, and during such times, millions of Chinese travelers usually travel to the country. The alert involved intensifying surveillance in all the country's (four) airports, especially in respect to flights coming from Wuhan. But amid such alerts, the country's top officials insisted that there was no outbreak of the virus (Promchertchoo, 2020).

In the United States, the USCDC was noted to have dispatched a team of a 100 people to three of its airports in San Francisco (SFO), New York (JFK), and Los Angeles (LAX) to complement the existing staff in conducting screening for all individuals entering the country from Wuhan, China. The medical team would cooperate with officials from Homeland Security and Customs and Border Protection (CBP) to ensure total compliance with the screening requirements (USCDC, 2020).

In regard to new infections, the Medical Research Council (MRC) Centre for Global Infectious Disease Analysis (MRC GIDA) at Imperial College argued that it had made some estimations, which showed that cases in Wuhan would likely have increased to almost 1700 (Imai et al., 2020). They argued that such numbers could be ascertained if pneumonia or related cases within Wuhan and other connected cities within China could be investigated. The calculations were based on flight and population data, following the fact that cases in Thailand and Japan had already been detected, and there were possibilities that there could be new cases not yet reported in other destinations that had originated from Wuhan since the period that the coronavirus was reported.

However, despite availability of those estimates, a summary report capturing happenings up to January 17 was published by ECDC (2020a) highlighting that the number of confirmed cases after successful laboratory testing still remained at 44 (41 in Wuhan, China, 2 in Thailand, and 1 in Japan). Of these, 2 had died, 12 had been discharged from hospital, and 5 were reported as severe cases. After the confirmation of the 44 cases, health officials to this date had managed to trace, identify, and monitor 763 close contacts. Of those, 644 were given a clean bill of health, whereas 119 were still under close medical observation, although none of them had tested positive to the virus (Wuhan Municipal Health Commission, 2020).

REFERENCES

Adhikari SP, Meng S, Wu Y-J, et al. (2020) Epidemiology, Causes, Clinical Manifestation and Diagnosis, Prevention and Control of Coronavirus Disease (COVID-19) During the Early Outbreak Period: a Scoping Review. Infectious Diseases of Poverty 9: 29.

Bowles J. (2020) How Canadian AI Start-up BlueDot Spotted Coronavirus Before Anyone Else Had a Clue. Available at: https://diginomica.com/how-canadian-ai-start-bluedot-spotted-coronavirus-anyone-else-had-clue.

Bryner J. (2020) 1st Known Case of Coronavirus Traced Back to November in China. Available at: https://www.livescience.com/first-case-coronavirus-found.html.

Davidson H. (2020) First Covid-19 Case Happened in November, China Government Record Show – report. Available at: https://www.theguardian.com/world/2020/mar/13/first-covid-19-case-happened-in-november-china-government-records-show-report.

Drosten C. (2020) Researchers Develop First Diagnostic Test for Novel Coronavirus in China. Available at: https://www.dzif.de/en/researchers-develop-first-diagnostic-test-novel-coronavirus-china.

ECDC. (2020a) Cluster of Pneumonia Cases Caused by a Novel Coronavirus, Wuhan, China. Available at: https://www.ecdc.europa.eu/sites/default/files/documents/Risk%20assessment%20-%20pneumonia%20Wuhan%20China%2017%20Jan%202020.pdf.

ECDC. (2020b) Event Background COVID-19. Available at: https://www.ecdc.europa.eu/en/novel-coronavirus/event-background-2019.

ECDC. (2020c) Update: Cluster of Pneumonia Cases Associated With Novel Coronavirus – Wuhan, China - 2019. Available at: https://www.ecdc.europa.eu/en/news-events/update-cluster-pneumonia-cases-associated-novel-coronavirus-wuhan-china-2019.

Gan N. (2020) China's New SARS-like Virus Has Spread to Japan, But we Still Know Very Little About it. Available at: https://edition.cnn.com/2020/01/15/asia/wuhan-virus-questions-intl-hnk/index.html.

Holmes E. (2020) Novel 2019 Coronavirus Genome. Available at: http://virological.org/t/novel-2019-coronavirus-genome/319.

Huang C, Wang Y, Li X, et al. (2020) Clinical Features of Patients Infected With 2019 Novel Coronavirus in Wuhan, China. The Lancet 395: 497–506.

Imai N, Dorigatti I, Cori A, et al. (2020) Report 1: Estimating the Potential Total Number of Novel Coronavirus Cases in Wuhan City, China. London, UK: Imperial College London COVID-19 Reseponse Team, 1–5.

Juan D. (2020) Wuhan Wet Market Closes Amid Pneumonia Outbreak. Available at: https://www.chinadaily.com.cn/a/202001/01/WS5e0c6a49a310cf3e35581e30.html.

Li Q, Guan X, Wu P, et al. (2020) Early Transmission Dynamics in Wuhan, China, of Novel Coronavirus–Infected Pneumonia. 382: 1199–1207.

Ma J. (2020) Coronavirus: China's First Confirmed Covid-19 Case Traced Back to November 17. Available at: https://www.scmp.com/news/china/society/article/3074991/coronavirus-chinas-first-confirmed-covid-19-case-traced-back.

Patel A and Jernigan DB. (2020) Initial Public Health Response and Interim Clinical Guidance for the 2019 Novel Coronavirus Outbreak — United States, December 31, 2019–February 4, 2020. Morbidity and Mortality Weekly Report (MMWR) 69: 140–146.

Pinghui Z. (2020) Chinese Laboratory That First Shared Coronavirus Genome With World Ordered to Close for 'Rectification', Hindering its Covid-19 Research. Available at: https://sg.news.yahoo.com/chinese-laboratory-first-shared-coronavirus-145827147.html.

Promchertchoo P. (2020) Wuhan Virus: 2 More Cases Confirmed in Thailand. Available at: https://www.channelnewsasia.com/news/asia/wuhan-virus-china-two-more-cases-found-thailand-12301606.

Ravelo JL and Jerving S. (2020) COVID-19 – a Timeline of the Coronavirus Outbreak. Available at: https://www.devex.com/news/covid-19-a-timeline-of-the-coronavirus-outbreak-96396.

Safi M. (2020) 100 Days That Changed The World. Available at: https://www.theguardian.com/world/ng-interactive/2020/apr/08/coronavirus-100-days-that-changed-the-world.

Schnirring L. (2020) China Release Genetic Data on New Coronavirus, Now Deadly. Available at: https://www.cidrap.umn.edu/news-perspective/2020/01/china-releases-genetic-data-new-coronavirus-now-deadly.

Secon H. (2020) Chinese Social-Media Platform WeChat Saw Spikes in the Terms 'SARS,' 'Coronavirus,' and 'Shortness of Breath,' Weeks Before the First Cases Were Confirmed, a Study Suggests. Available at: https://www.pulselive.co.ke/bi/tech/chinese-social-media-platform-wechat-saw-spikes-in-the-terms-sars-coronavirus-and/x8mhrmx.

Sim W. (2020) Japan Confirms First Case of Infection From Wuhan Coronavirus; Vietnam Quarantines Two Tourists. Available at: https://www.straitstimes.com/asia/east-asia/japan-confirms-first-case-of-infection-with-new-china-coronavirus.

Singhal T. (2020) A Review of Coronavirus Disease-2019 (COVID-19). Indian Journal of Pediatrics 87: 281–286.

Siu T, Tham E and Lee SY. (2020) China Says Second Person Dies in Wuhan Pneumonia Outbreak. Available at: https://www.reuters.com/article/us-china-health-pneumonia-idUSKBN1ZG01B.

Tardáguila C and Chen S. (2020) China Arrested 8 for Spreading 'Hoaxes' About What Is Now Known as Coronavirus. What Happened to Them? Available at: https://www.poynter.org/fact-checking/2020/the-2019-coronavirus-virus-lands-in-the-u-s-after-killing-17-and-taking-eight-to-prison/.

The Government of the Hong Kong Specia Administrative Region. (2020) CHP Closely Monitors Additional Confirmed. Available at: https://www.info.gov.hk/gia/general/202001/17/P2020011700960.htm.

USCDC. (2020) Public Health Screening to Begin at 3 U.S. Airports for 2019 Novel Coronavirus ("2019-nCoV"). Available at: https://www.cdc.gov/media/releases/2020/p0117-coronavirus-screening.html.

WHO. (2020a) Emergencies Preparedness, Response: Novel Coronavirus – China. Available at: https://www.who.int/csr/don/12-january-2020-novel-coronavirus-china/en/.

WHO. (2020b) Novel Coronavirus – Thailand (ex-China). Available at: https://www.who.int/csr/don/14-january-2020-novel-coronavirus-thailand/en/.

WHO. (2020c) Novel Coronavirus (2019-nCoV) Situation Report-4. World Health Organization.

WHO. (2020d) Novel Coronavirus (2019-nCoV) Situation Report- 1. Available at: https://www.who.int/docs/default-source/coronaviruse/situation-reports/20200121-sitrep-1-2019-ncov.pdf?sfvrsn=20a99c10_4.

WHO. (2020e) WHO Timeline – COVID-19. Available at: https://www.who.int/news-room/detail/08-04-2020-who-timeline—covid-19.

Wuhan City Health Committee. (2020) Wuhan Municipal Health Commission on Unexplained Viral Pneumonia. Available at: http://wjw.wuhan.gov.cn/front/web/showDetail/2020011109035.

Wuhan Municipal Health Commission WCHC. (2020) Wuhan Municipal Health Commission on Pneumonia Infect by New Coronavirus. Available at: http://wjw.wuhan.gov.cn/front/web/showDetail/2020011609057.

Zhao S, Musa SS, Lin Q, et al. (2020) Estimating the Unreported Number of Novel Coronavirus (2019-nCoV) Cases in China in the First Half of January 2020: A Data-Driven Modelling Analysis of the Early Outbreak. 9: 388.

CHAPTER 2

The Second 50 days: A Detailed Chronological Timeline and Extensive Review of Literature Documenting the COVID-19 Pandemic From Day 50 to Day 100

INTRODUCTION

During the first 50 days, most attention was geared on the identification of the virus and trying to predict whether it had the potential to impact other parts of China and other parts of the globe and whether it could be passed from one person to another. However, during the second 50 days, it became apparent to the entire global community that the world at large was dealing with a very serious, contagious, and deadly disease. The reality check came right on the 51st day when China reported an additional 237 confirmed cases in a single day, and South Korea confirmed their first case. From then onwards, there was no turning back on the number of cases that were being reported, and by the 100th day (March 9, 2020), the number of confirmed cases across the globe had increased to 109,577 and the deaths as a result of the disease, which the WHO and other organization collectively renamed to "COVID-19" on the 73rd day amounted to 3809. By then, the virus had spread to 104 countries and territories. In addition, the number of confirmed cases reported in those regions had increased to 28,673 and 3 of those had unfortunately died (WHO, 2020c). Within these 100 days, the disease had transformed from being classified as just a mere novel coronavirus to being classified as a "Public Health Emergency of International Concern" (PHEIC).

Initially, the virus was spreading rapidly in China but in less than 100 days, the epicenter had shifted to Europe. At the start of the 51st day, Europe was safe and free from this virus, but by the 100th day, as will be shown later, the entire region was affected, both in terms of the spread of the virus, and the daily increase in numbers of people who were dying. During the same period, measures such as border restrictions, nationwide lockdowns, and banning of transportation in or out of different countries became widespread. As those measures started to increase, the harsh reality of the impact of the disease started to show on economies, social lives, and across health sectors, with basic equipment started to become scarce. Schools closed down, sports activities became untenable, and political push and pulls started to crop out.

During this eventful time (day 50 till day 100), there were also flashes of global oneness as people, governments, and professionals from different parts collaborated to offer support to financial and in-kind assistance. There was also a wave of collaboration toward research, especially for vaccine developments. Different foundations and philanthropists also advanced support, especially to vulnerable economies and countries. This period also exposed the shortcomings in decision making and weaknesses in healthcare in some countries, and regions, and even more, the vulnerability of the human race in itself, especially when dealing with an invisible enemy like this virus. This also proved that human beings are closely linked, needing social interaction and migration flows—synonymous to the 21st century, as most of the cases were imported to different countries by travelers flying from one area to the other. The following sections further document the unfolding of the pandemic during the second 50 days (day 50 to day 100).

DAY 51—JANUARY 20, 2020

On this day, the number of confirmed cases increased by almost sevenfold from the previously recorded cases as reported by WHO (WHO, 2020w). In China, the cases increased to a high of 278, while Japan with one

Surveying the Covid-19 Pandemic and Its Implications. https://doi.org/10.1016/B978-0-12-824313-8.00002-4

case and Thailand with two had no new cases. Nevertheless, the Republic of Korea became the third region, outside China to confirm 2019-nCov case, while the United States became the fourth with a single case reported. The total number of cases was 282, and all of them were in one way or the other linked to Wuhan City. At this point, all the three outside China were exported from Wuhan.

Of the 278 cases reported in China, 258 cases were all confirmed from the Hubei Province, while 14 were reported from Guangdong Province. The others came from Shanghai Municipality (1 case) and Beijing Municipality (5 cases) (WHO, 2020w). In terms of severity, the situational report by the WHO indicated that 51 cases were severe while 12 were in critical condition. Unfortunately, during the same period, a number of six fatalities had also been reported from Wuhan City. Besides, 60 cases of the 278 all occurred on the 20th of January (WHO, 2020w).

In the United States, the confirmed case involved a man in his 30s who had traveled from Wuhan on the 15th of January. The arrival of this man was 2 days earlier before the directive on passenger screening was applied in the three US airports. Of importance is that by the time of his arrival, he had not shown any signs of the disease, but, after being consulted by a medical professional and informing the latter that he had traveled from Wuhan, he was tested and it came out positive. His confirmation sparked the process of contact tracing and the monitoring of anyone whom he may have interacted with (Rabin, 2020).

The increase in the number of cases, especially outside Wuhan raised the suspicion that the virus had the potential to be transmitted from person to person, thus explaining why there were increased efforts to conduct contract tracing in all the countries and regions that cases were confirmed. In addition, this increased the investigation on the mode through which the virus was being transmitted so that it could be contained before it spread further to other countries.

In South Korea, following the confirmation, health authorities are reported to have increased and strengthened their surveillance. Although such practices had begun as early as the 3rd of January, the confirmation increased their efforts, with options for screening and quarantine being introduced for all travelers coming from Wuhan (WHO, 2020w).

DAY 53—JANUARY 22, 2020

The new developments in regard to 2019-nCoV, where an expanding number of geographies are confirming coronavirus cases prompted an emergency meeting of members of the WHO to determine whether they would advise the WHO Director-General to declare the virus outbreak a public health emergency of international concern (WHO, 2020ao). After the meeting, it was apparent that the decision would be deferred until another day. While that was happening, the Republic of North Korea made a bold decision of closing all its borders to foreign travelers to protect its citizens from the virus (Sang-Hun, 2020). This decision had severe economic implications though, as most North Koreans depended on tourists, especially from China. In particular, during that period when most Chinese were preparing to travel for the Lunar New Year celebration, tourism in North Korea was to experience severe losses.

In China, authorities reported that 314 confirmed cases in the mainland. Subsequently, the number of deaths from complications related to the disease rose to a high of 6 (WHO, 2020y). Following this, the Wuhan authorities ordered for a "temporary" closure of all airports, long-distant bus stations, ferry terminals, and rail stations within the borders of the city to prevent anyone to travel outside the city. This directive was to take effect as from the following day at 10 a.m., but for air flights and trains, the order was to be implemented right then (Xu, 2020).

Internationally, Macau and Hong Kong reported its first cases. In Hong Kong, the patient was a 39-year-old male living in Wuhan, who had not visited any wet market or come into contact with any wild animals. He also reported that according to his recollection, he had not had any contact with any individual with any sigh of pneumonia. His case was confirmed in Queen Elizabeth Hospital after he had been taken following fever and nasal congestion. Later, he was transferred to Princess Margaret Hospital for isolation treatment (Dongwang, 2020). The patient in Macau is a 52-year-old businesswoman from Wuhan who traveled to Zhuhai, Macau via a high-speed rail from Wuhan. She passed through the screening checkpoints but did not show any symptoms and was allowed to continue. However, 3 days later, she presented herself to the hospital after experiencing a cough, and it is then that she was confirmed to be positive. A week before traveling to Macau, she reported to have experienced a dry cough and sore throat, but she did not consider it to be coronavirus. As she did not have any sign of the virus, she was accompanied by two friends to the hospital, who were quarantined for medical surveillance after she was found positive (Lum and Chung, 2020).

Thailand also confirmed two more cases to push the number in the country to four. One of the patients was a Chinese male tourist aged 68, who was intercepted at

Suvarnabhumi Airport, Bangkok on January 19, and whose test results came back on 22nd (Promchertchoo, 2020). The other one is a 73-year-old Thai woman who had arrived back from Wuhan. Despite these cases, health officials from Thailand ruled out human-to-human infections but asked people to be on high alert, but not to panic as the national healthcare was ready and equipped to handle current and future cases.

DAY 54—JANUARY 23, 2020

Finally, the city of Wuhan was placed on locked down, with no inbound or outbound travel allowed "until further notice." Movement within the city however was allowed, but very restricted. This decision though critical affected the normalcy of more than 11 million people who resided in the city. Neighboring cities within Hubei Province like Huanggang and Ezhou, Xiantao, Chibi, and Lichuan are seen to take lead from Wuhan, as they also declare lockdown (BBC News, 2020). In Huanggang, the officials also shut down businesses such as cinemas, exhibitions, cafes, and theaters in addition to suspending transportation services. Xiantao also prohibits any form of gathering within the city. Overall, the lockdown in these different cities (14 so far) left around 41 million cutoffs from the rest of the world for an unknown time duration (Kindred and Hawken, 2020). Other popular places within China that have been prohibited include the Forbidden Land, Great Wall, and Disneyland China. However, the intention of the lockdown, from a medical perspective is justified and focused on reducing the cases after it has been realized that the virus is spread via human-to-human interaction.

Internationally, more countries have been added to the list of those reporting coronavirus cases outside China. These include Singapore, which reported the case of a 66-year old man who resided in Wuhan but had traveled to the country on January 20. Following his confirmation, two suspected cases were quarantined await their test results (Garda, 2020a). Vietnam also confirmed its first two cases that include a Chinese man aged 66 years old and his son aged 28 years old. The case of these two proves beyond doubt the possibility of human-to-human infection as the father is the one who had traveled from Wuhan on January 13. He landed in Hanoi, Vietnam's capital city, where his son, who had been in the country for several months, met him. The father developed symptoms as from January 17, and the son followed suit on January 20, where after going to the hospital, they underwent tests and confirmed to be positive on the 23rd (Garda, 2020b).

According to a report by the WHO (WHO, 2020r) on the virus update as of January 23, cases outside China in countries such as Thailand, Japan, Hong Kong, Taipei Municipality, United States of America, Republic of Korea, Singapore, and Macau all had been imported from Wuhan, China. Thus far then, the total number reported globally was 581 cases, of which, 571 have all been confirmed in China. Of the total confirmed cases in China, 17 had unfortunately succumbed to the virus. On another news, the WHO failed to declare the virus as a PHEIC, by arguing that the situation in Wuhan and other regions that had confirmed cases of 2019-nCoV did not yet meet the threshold for such a declaration (WHO, 2020an).

DAY 55—JANUARY 24, 2020

Even after enforcing lockdowns on some cities, the number of confirmed cases in Mainland China increased to 830, with 177 individuals in critical condition and the number of deaths increased by nine people to reach 26, with one of the death, outside the Hubei province, in Heilongjiang province (News, 2020). Following this, travel restrictions in countries were extended to more cities to try and prevent the spread of the virus even further. In addition to those measures, authorities in China started the race to build two hospitals in 10 days and 13 days, respectively. The first one is a 1000-bed capacity hospital, while the second one will have the capacity of 1300 beds (Quito, 2020). The two hospitals are both dedicated to catering for the increasing number of coronavirus cases, since projections, and the realization that virus could not only be passed from human to human but also take up to 14 days to incubate before the symptoms could be detected. The revelation about the symptom-free for several days was made by a team of Chinese researchers (Huang et al., 2020), and they warned that this could be serious, as an individual could infect numerous others before showing signs himself.

Internationally, the number of reported cases started to increase with more countries reporting their first cases. In Europe, the first such country is France, which reported the first three confirmed cases -announced by the Health Minister Agnes Buzyn, who also feared that cases in the country were likely to rise in no time (CNBC, 2020). Malaysia also confirmed its first three cases, all related to a 66-year-old man who had been confirmed as positive in Singapore the previous day (Sipalan, 2020). Elsewhere, Nepal also reported a positive case of a student studying in China but had returned home tested positive to the virus (Reuters,

2020g). Besides those new cases, there were others in countries that had already been affected. These include the United States that reported the second case in Illinois of a patient who had a travel history with Wuhan. She had returned to the United States on January 13 and later after developing the symptoms of the disease. After tests, she was confirmed positive and was immediately isolated in the hospital (USCDC, 2020b). The other cases were reported in Hong Kong, which confirmed three more cases bringing its country total to five individuals with the disease (The Government of the Hong Kong Specia Administrative Region, 2020). Singapore also confirmed two more cases (Khalik and Goh, 2020), while Thailand reported a new case to bring its country tally to five positive cases (Bangkok Post and Reuters, 2020). Japan (Reuters, 2020e) and South Korea (Medical Express, 2020) also reported a case each meaning that each had two cases reported in the respective countries.

DAY 56—JANUARY 25, 2020

From the WHO's 2019-nCoV situation report of January 25, 2020 (WHO, 2020s), the number of laboratory-confirmed 2019-nCoV cases increased by more than 50% from the previously announced 830–1320 globally. Of these, 1287 were reported from Mainland China while 5 were confirmed in Hong Kong Special Administrative Region (SAR), 2 in Macau SAR, and 3 from Taipei. Of 1287, 237 reported to have been severely ill. The remaining 23 cases were reported from different regions outside China, where 21 of those had traveled from Wuhan City to the destination where they were later confirmed. Besides the confirmed cases, the number of deaths as a result of the 2019-nCoV increased to 41, all reported in China, with 39 of those happening in Hubei province, while two were reported in Hebei and Heilongjiang provinces. In summary, from the previous day, the total number of new confirmed coronavirus cases reported increased by a total of 474 cases, and the deaths increased by 15. In Hong Kong, following the spread of the virus, the response was strengthened, including prohibiting air travel to or from any part of Wuhan City (Chung et al., 2020).

Of the newly reported deaths, one was a medical professional (a doctor) who had been in the frontline in fighting the coronavirus since its confirmation. The 62-year-old professional who worked at a hospital in Wuhan, Hubei province, was noted to have died from the disease, which he may have contracted from the numerous patients that were being brought into his hospital (Standaert, 2020). His death further affirmed the claim that the virus was transmittable from human to human, and hence the need for extra caution and the use of personal protective equipment (PPE).

On this date, Australia joined the list of countries that had confirmed cases (Murphy, 2020). One was confirmed in Victoria, while the other three in New South Wales. The case in Victoria was the first to be confirmed and regarded as a Chinese man in his 50s who had traveled from Wuhan to Melbourne on January 19. After developing some symptoms, he was reported to have presented himself to a medical center where he was immediately isolated, and the testing started, where he was confirmed to be positive the following day (Daoud, 2020). This confirmation prompted the contact tracing of his family members whom he had reported to have spent time with since he arrived in the country, and anyone else, including the passengers in his flight that he may have interacted with. After this confirmation that happened in the morning hours, later that day, three more cases were confirmed in New South Wales as noted earlier (Doherty, 2020).

Canada also confirms its first case of a man who had traveled from Wuhan to Toronto a week ago but presented himself to the hospital on January 23 after developing respiratory symptoms. Specimens from him underwent testing in a Lab in Ontario, and they came back positive (Sunnybrook, 2020). Besides these new countries, others outside China with previous cases also started confirming new ones. Japan had one new case (Reuters, 2020f), Thailand added two new cases (CNA, 2020k), Malaysia added three new cases (New Straits Times, 2020) while Singapore reported one new case, reaching a total of four cases reported in the country (Ministry of Health Singapore, 2020). In Sri Lanka, two female individuals, one local and one of Chinese descent were admitted to the hospital after they were suspected to be infected with the virus (Daily Mirror Online, 2020).

DAY 57—JANUARY 26, 2020

For the past 24 h, the number of laboratory 2019-nCoV cases increased by a total of 694 globally bringing the global confirmed cases to a total of 2014. China leads with the number confirmed therein reaching 1985, with 324 of these in critical condition (WHO, 2020t). Of 1985, 2 were reported in Macau (Macau News, 2020)—bringing their total to 5 reported cases, 5 in Hong Kong (Chung et al., 2020), and 3 in Taipei. The number of those who died within the same period increased by 15, pushing the total of those who have succumbed to the virus to 56 (52 reported in Hubei province, and 4 outside that region). Outside China's boundaries, 29 more cases were reported within the 24 h since the last update, but there was no new country with reported new cases.

Of the 29 international cases, United States, as confirmed by the Centre for Disease Control (CDC), reported three new cases; two from California and one in Arizona, thus pushing the country's total to five cases (NBC Los Angeles, 2020). The new cases are all from people who had reported a travel history to Wuhan. In Thailand, the Deputy Prime Minister announced that the country, within the last 24 h, tested 8 suspected cases, where 5 cases were noted to be negative and allowed to go home, while 3 were confirmed to be positive, and hence isolated in the hospital under the watchful eyes of the Ministry of Public health. The latter also reported that 84 contacts were also investigated with 45 receiving a clean bill of health while 39 were still retained for further investigation to make sure they were freed from the virus (PPTV Online, 2020). In Africa, the first suspected case in the continent was being investigated in Ivory Coast. The suspect is a 34-year-old woman, who had returned in the country from Beijing, and was admitted for testing after showing flu-like symptoms (BBC News, 2020a,b).

Following the increasing number of cases, it was reported that China's National Health Commission recommended that its health officials could, in some cases, make use of HIV drugs to treat the coronavirus. Elsewhere, scientists drawn from different parts of the globe started working on drugs and vaccines that could prevent, and where possible treat the virus. From those seen to be on the forefront were health officials and scientists from China's CDC (Jeong-ho et al., 2020). On this day still, China was noted to have officially banned the trade of wild animals within its borders (Ellis-Petersen, 2020).

DAY 58—JANUARY 27, 2020

The number of cases globally keeps increasing exponentially. According to the situational report by WHO (WHO, 2020x), in the past 24 h, the number of laboratory-confirmed cases has increased by approximately 2798, of which 461 have been marked as severely ill. Over the same period, the number of deaths has climbed to 80. There are also 5794 people who are quarantined in different hospitals in China awaiting their test results. In China alone, the number of positively confirmed cases increased by 2741, with all the severe cases and deaths being reported there (WHO, 2020x). Outside of China, the number of laboratory-confirmed cases also increased substantially (by 39 individuals) over the 24 h period from 11 different countries. The ages of those confirmed outside China, according to the report range from 2 to 74 years, but the median age was marked at 45 years. Of those 3,927 were reported to have a travel history to China, more specifically Wuhan, where the epicenter of the 2019-nCoV was at the time (WHO, 2020x).

Of the international landscape, three countries had their first cases. These include Cambodia where a Chinese man, who traveled from Wuhan together with his family on January 23, developed symptoms of the disease on January 25, and his tests came positive on 27th. Following that confirmation, all Chinese en route to Thailand from Cambodia were subjected to mandatory thermal health scans for any sign or symptoms of the virus (Penh, 2020). The other country reporting a first case is Germany where a man from Starnberg district (Saey, 2020), who had been infected by a Chinese woman who had not shown any sign (asymptomatic) but tested positive days later (Rothe et al., 2020). She had traveled to Germany on January 20 for a business trip and left to her country on January 22. On her way back, she developed the symptoms and was confirmed on January 26 while in Shanghai (Joseph, 2020). This case opened the dilemma on this virus even further and demonstrated the danger that it poses, especially in regard to transmission. On this note, it is worth noting that it had been argued that the incubation period could range between 2 and 14 days (Backer et al., 2020). Sri Lanka is the other country with a first confirmed case of a Chinese woman in her 40s that had traveled to the country on 19th and experienced the symptoms on January 25. She was later confirmed positive following hospital tests (Reuters, 2020k).

In the United States, following increased intelligence that the virus may spread even further, the government, through the CDC, announced that it would be extending its screening to 17 more airports to ensure that every passenger coming from China is comprehensively screened. In addition, the State Department raised its travel advisory to "level 4" for Wuhan, thus restricting American nationals from traveling to Wuhan as long as the virus is live (White House, 2020).

On the same date, the Bill & Melinda Gates Foundation committed to offer $10 million to fight the coronavirus outbreak in China and also to allow African countries to prepare for the outbreak (Bill & Melinda Gates Foundation, 2020).

With increasing pressure, the Mayor of Wuhan offered to resign following his observation that the response to the 2019-nCoV was very slow, especially following inadequate information sharing to the public (Yan, 2020).

DAY 60—JANUARY 29, 2020

On January 28, the total number of confirmed cases globally increased to 4593 after China reported 1771 new cases, with 18 more reported from 14 other countries. The number of severely ill increased to 976, while those who had died from the disease increased to 106 from the previously reported number of 80. In China also, the number of those suspected and hence isolated in hospital increased to 6973 (WHO, 2020ai).

Outside China, 18 cases were reported in Thailand with six cases, Singapore two, Japan three, Germany three (all coworkers with the first case reported the previous day), France reported four new cases, with one observed to be critical (WHO, 2020ai).

The following day, on 29th, more people continue to be admitted in hospitals, with new laboratory-confirmed cases. Since the previous reporting, the cases had increased by new 1472 cases globally, with China confirming 1460 of those cases. The number of those admitted as critically ill over the past 24 h also increased by a total of 263, to push the total of all severely ill to 1239 cases. In addition, over the same period, the number of deaths increased to 132 deaths from the previous 106 reported deaths. Until January 29, all the reported deaths had occurred in China (WHO, 2020u). However, the number of countries that have fallen victim to the virus increased in the course of 1 day by 2, which includes United Arab Emirates (UAE) and Finland (Ravelo and Jerving, 2020). In UAE, which is also the first country in the Middle East to report a positive case has first had four first cases, who, unfortunately, were members of the same family of the Chinese descent, but were all in stable condition (Aljazeera, 2020e). The case in Finland is of a Chinese female tourist aged 32 years old who had traveled from Wuhan 5 days before presenting herself for treatment in a hospital in Finland. After rigorous testing, she was confirmed to be positive. Following her confirmation, Finland officials reported that they were tracing 15 people who may have been exposed after interacting with her (Yle, 2020).

As the number of cases in China continues to surge and also those in other countries, Japan and United States became the first countries to evacuate their citizens from Wuhan, which had already been placed under lockdown from January 23, 2020.

Airlines from different parts of the world had begun suspending flights to China. These include those from North America (United States), some from Europe (Germany, France, UK), and also from some Asian countries (Pham, 2020). Reducing flights except for essential services is big news, especially on the economic front—including of those airline companies. While that was happening, Chinese president Xi Jinping and WHO's Director Tedros Adhanom agree that the WHO should send experts to help in matters 2019-nCoV (Ravelo and Jerving, 2020). In China, despite the huge health crisis the country was in, the police engaged in arresting those accused of spreading false information. Thus far, some quarters support that the Chinese were seen as not only fighting the virus, but also freedom of speech.

DAY 61—JANUARY 30, 2020

The major occurrence of the day was the official declaration by the WHO that 2019-nCoV is now classified as a PHEIC (WHO, 2020z). The WHO also proposed an interim name for the disease to be "2019-nCoV" and awaited the official direction on the same from the International Committee on Taxonomy of Viruses. While this was expected, with the WHO seen to be delaying the decision every time they met, the announcement triggered unprecedented reactions from different parts of the World (Cohen, 2020). For Instance, the United States a key player in funding WHO immediately issued a level 4 travel advisory for all of China (U.S. Department of State, 2020a). In other words, it banned all travels from the virus' epicenter (China at the time). For many countries, especially in developing and least-developed economies, where health systems are relatively "weak," the announcement was astounding, as it meant that they had no option but to prepare for the worst. Another country that did not wait for the dust to settle to close its border with China is Russia. Those wishing to travel in or out of Russia only had 1 day as the closure was to start the following day (Ellyatt, 2020). During the declaration, it was also revealed that the Foreign Ministry of Russia had also suspended (temporarily) the issuing of electronic visas to Chinese nationals (Ellyatt, 2020).

The decision for closing borders to restrict traveling—hence the propagation of the virus, by different countries and international businesses like airlines is understandable. In fact, the initial lead comes from China itself, which until now had placed over 60 million of its population in different cities under lockdown in an attempt to stop the spread of the virus (Wang and Wee, 2020). However, the virus was seen to have already started overwhelming the country's health system. For instance, despite the lockdown, for the past 24 h, since the last official reporting, the number of those confirmed to be virus positive had increased by a total of 1739 to push the total numbers in China to 7736 confirmed cases, with 1370 of these in severe conditions. In addition, the number of those suspected to have the virus increased to 12,167. In the course of the 24 h also, the country reported 38 more deaths from the virus, pushing the total to 170 (WHO, 2020z).

Outside of China, the virus spread to four more countries (India (Unnithan, 2020), Philippines (Gregorio, 2020), and Italy) each confirming a single case, and Italy confirming two cases. In addition, to the already affected countries, the number has also increased, pushing the international numbers to 82 confirmed cases from the previous reported 68 cases. In particular, the spread of the virus is seen to be more active in the Asian region, with countries such as Japan (NHK, 2020), Vietnam, Singapore (CNA, 2020l), Malaysia (Harun, 2020), South Korea (Yonhap, 2020b), India, Philippines, and Tibet being all impacted. The virus is also seen to be gain ground in Europe with three countries already starting to see a gradual increase in confirmed cases. In North America, things are seen to be contained with only the United States reporting an additional case. However, as the transmission is now believed to be person to person (USCDC, 2020a), countries geared up to ensure that the situation is handled even more carefully.

DAY 62—JANUARY 31, 2020

In the wake of the declaration of the virus as a PHEIC, more countries were seen to close their borders and others applying travel restrictions for persons coming from China. Such decisions were taken in countries such as Mongolia and Hong Kong, amid criticism that such a move was discriminatory to Mainland China, which was already facing an upward hill from the immense impacts of the virus. However, on this, it is the Medical Union of Hong Kong that was increasing the pressure to ensure that the closure of borders was effected (Chang, 2020). Singapore also took a similar approach and instituted a total ban on all Chinese and other foreigners who may have been in China for the previous 14 days (Xinghui, 2020). On this still, the United States strengthened its protective measures from only restricting people from China from coming into the country, to banning any entry of foreign visitors who in the course of the past 14 days from the date of this ban had set foot in China. The ban followed the country's declaration that the 2019-nCoV is a public health emergency domestically (HSS, 2020). In the United States, staff from the US Department of Health and Human Service were reported to have complained that they were not adequately prepared, equipped, and trained to handle such cases, especially in quarantine areas (Cockrane et al., 2020).

In regard to the spread of the disease, over the past 24 h, things have not improved and have become even more worrying. For instance, despite countries like Russia and the United Kingdom increasing efforts, including instituting travel advisory, and reducing flights to only for essential services, they also had cases confirmed. In the United Kingdom, the cases are two family members who had traveled back to the country and were now in hospital in England. Following this, the UK officials announced that they would be evacuating at least 150 British and EU citizens trapped in China, and quarantine them for 14 days to ensure that their health status is being monitored (Aljazeera, 2020f). In Russia, the first two cases were confirmed after tests were done on people who were already in quarantine in different parts of the country. The affected individuals are Chinese citizens (Reuters, 2020i). Italy also became another EU member that was reporting its first case. This came days after the Italians were reported to have shown sympathy to the Chinese after they were reported to have started xenophobic experiences across the globe following the emergence of the virus in China (Giuffrida and Willsher, 2020). The confirmation was of two Chinese Citizens (a couple) who were on a tourist expedition in Rome. Following the confirmation, the government declared a state of emergency in the country and immediately announced a ban on all flights between Italy and China (The Local, 2020).

Those new cases, when collated with those from other regions, bring the total reported globally in a space of 1 day to 2008. Therefore, the total number globally has increased to 9826, with 9720 of these confirmed in China and 106 outside China. The suspected cases also increased to 15,238, with those severely ill increasing to 1527—all reported in China. The total number of deaths has also increased to 213 from the previous count of 170 (WHO, 2020aa).

DAY 64—FEBRUARY 2, 2020

The world began the month of February with the cases in China from 2019-nCoV having exceeded the global total of those reported of SARS-nCoV1 in 2002–03. This is true despite the identification and confirmation time for 2019-nCov being only 9 days while SARS-CoV took months. On February 1, the number of those confirmed to be positive globally increased by 2128, pushing the total tally to 11,953. China was still the epicenter with 11,821 cases reported, with those reported outside the country increasing by 26 new cases to reach 132 cases, with four new countries reporting their first cases. Unfortunately, the number of those succumbing from the virus was also increasing, with new 46 deaths reported in a span of 24 h, rendering a total of 259 deaths, all from China (WHO, 2020ab).

Internationally, the reality of the virus spread had started to become severe in countries like the United States, which reported its eighth case, and Australia also reported three new cases and Japan 3 more cases. Others included Singapore, Vietnam, and South Korea. In Europe, Spain became the latest victim of the virus with the first case reported.

On February 2, more bad news was reported globally. Over the past 24 h, the number of cases had increased by over 2604, with 315 reported to be severely ill (WHO, 2020ac). The most unfortunate report is the death of 45 more people (305 total deaths), with the first death outside China reported in the Philippines (Government of Philippines, 2020). The death though was a 44 years old Chinese man who had traveled to Philippines a week earlier and he, together with his partner, had tested positive on January 30 (Luna, 2020). Following this death, the Philippines immediately imposed a travel ban for all foreigners traveling from not only China but also Hong Kong and Macao. For the residents coming back, they had to undergo a mandatory 14 days quarantine in designated places (Government of Philippines, 2020). On this date still, though the number of countries with the 2019-nCoV cases did not increase, some of the 23 (outside China) already affected reported new cases (14 new cases in total) (WHO, 2020ac).

In terms of response to the outbreaks, nations across the globe were seen to have continued to sympathize with China, with medical donations originating from all parts of the globe (Barrett, 2020). However, the Chinese citizens, though appreciative, were not happy with how the local Red Cross was distributing and delivering the donations to where they were urgently required (Yuan, 2020). Health workers were pleading for more PPE, but the agency was seen to drag its effort, with only 200,000 PPE distributed, out of over 2 million donated (Yuan, 2020). On other news, Canada sent official requests to officials in Hubei to allow the evacuation of 543 Canadians from Wuhan unsuccessfully. In America, despite reporting new cases, homeland security was assuring its citizens that there was no need for panic, as according to them, the coronavirus was "a low risk to the US" (Sgueglia, 2020).

In Sport, following the spread of the virus, the much-awaited Formula "E" race originally scheduled for March 20, 2020, in China was canceled (BBC Sport, 2020), to prevent further spread of the virus.

DAY 65—FEBRUARY 3, 2020

Amid the unprecedented challenges that China had been facing, it was able to achieve one of its objectives of constructing a coronavirus hospital (Huoshenshan Hospital in Wuhan) in a record time of 10 days. On February 3, the hospital was opened and immediately started receiving 2019-nCoV patients. Its opening was timely as the country had already confirmed approximately 17,238 cases, with 2831 reported in the past 24 h. Similarly, 186 new severe cases that would greatly benefit from the hospital had been reported within the same period. The deaths in the country in the same period had increased by 57 people bringing the total deaths to 362. Globally, 7 new cases were reported, but no new country had been affected (WHO, 2020aj). To stop the disease, China started clinical trials of the *"remdesivir drug,"* an antiviral drug by the company "Gilead" that was also previously tested against Ebola in 2015 (Parsey, 2020).

In regard to responses from different quarters, the WHO developed a prototype "2019-nCoV kit," similar to those used in cases of outbreaks of high threat pathogens, to be mass produced in the coming days (WHO, 2020aj). In Hong Kong, health workers went to strike to pressurize their government to institute a total ban on entry or exit of people from mainland China, to prevent further spread of the virus (Law, 2020). In Wuhan, to ensure that there is no bottleneck in the supply and delivery of medical supplies, the responsibility is shouldered on the People's Liberation Army Ground Forces, who immediately conceded that there were some hiccups in delivery and distribution of donations in the previous day, but they would rectify that going forward (Chan, 2020). While that was happening, over 4000 passengers en route Vietnam from Guangzhou aboard the *"World Dream,"* cruise ship—which left China on January 19—were all quarantined after the tests: four of them coming back positive (Leng and Huifeng, 2020). Other responses of the day included the WHO partnering with social media giants to control the spread of misinformation on the 2019-nCoV spread, which the agency mentioned was complicating the efforts being taken to contain the spread and avert more deaths (Zhou et al., 2020).

Economically, things were worsening in China with its stock markets plunging after resuming economic activities following the Lunar New Year break. The Shanghai Stock Exchange plunged by 7.72% while the Shenzhen Stock Exchange plunged by 8.45%, almost hitting the daily maximum permitted plunge of 10% (Farrer, 2020). Similarly, the country's currency (the Yuan) weakened against the dollar trading at 6.9249 and closing at 7.0257 (Jiao, 2020). Globally, the World Bank released a statement indicating that it was working toward providing financial support to countries being impacted by the coronavirus, especially to help them strengthen their surveillance and response systems (The World Bank, 2020a).

DAY 66—FEBRUARY 4, 2020

The spread of the virus and its impact continued to be felt especially in mainland China, where, in a period of 1 month, the country lost approximately 425 individuals to the virus, with the rate of death seen to be increasing significantly each day with the number of new confirmed cases. In addition, as the incubation period of the assumed 14 days come to an end since the first cases were reported, the number of infections is seen to keep on rising. For instance, on this day alone, the number of cases in China has increased by a total of 3241 to reach 20,471, with 2788 of these labeled as critically ill (WHO, 2020v). Globally, the numbers have increased to 159 after six more cases were reported in five Asian countries. In Europe, the number of those reporting new cases increases after Belgium reported its first case, which pushed the total laboratory-confirmed cases in the European Union to 24 (The Brussels Times, 2020).

Globally, the responses to the spread of the virus are intensifying with each country doing the best they can. For instance, in the United States, the country's Food and Drug Administration issued an Emergence Use Authorization to allow the emergency use of CDC diagnostic tests in all CDC labs across the country to help in the control of the virus (FDA, 2020). Besides this, the country sent a consignment of PPEs to help China continue with the fight against the virus (U.S. Embassy in Georgia, 2020). Elsewhere, to reduce the increasing spread, Taiwan instituted a prohibition on all foreign travelers from entering its borders if they have been in China in the past 14 days (Chung, 2020). In South Korea, due to panic as more cases are being reported, individuals have been hoarding urgently needed masks, resulting to shortage, thus prompting the government to impose penalties, fines (up to $42,000), and jail terms (up to 2 years) for all those found hoarding these stocks (Choi, 2020).

On the economic front, the impact and fear of the 2019-nCoV continue to be felt. For instance, in South Korea, Hyundai Motor Company halted its production line following disruption in its supply chain, as most of the necessary parts are sourced from China, which was on lockdown and with transportation grounded (Johnson, 2020). However, surprisingly, the stock market around the world gained some strength, including in China that had previously plunged to a point of almost being suspended (Jiao, 2020). The Chinese stock market rebounded after the People's Bank of China (PBC) released approximately US$71 billion into the country's financial system to increase liquidity (BBC, 2020a).

Socially, the Chinese still face some form of racism and xenophobic treatment, especially in western countries. In addition, they perceive the decisions by different countries to ban Chinese nationals, and also foreigners who had traveled to China in the past 14 days as another form of discrimination.

DAY 67—FEBRUARY 5, 2020

The persistence of the health workers in Hong Kong was seen to reap positive results, as already, 10 out of all 13 main border crossing points to mainland China were suspended (CNA, 2020h). In addition, the authorities in the country announced that anyone coming from mainland China would have no option than to undergo a mandatory 14 days quarantine (CNA, 2020a). Hong Kong was not the only one taking the precautionary measures. In the United States, the evacuation of its citizen from China was underway, with the second round completed on February 5. Similarly, a number of other airplanes with more citizens were on the way and from China and were expected in California, Texas, and Nebraska (CDC, 2020b). In addition to this, all volunteers (139 individuals) associated with US Peace Corps were also evacuated from China (Peace Corps, 2020). France and UK were also reported to have advised that the only travels that would be allowed to China are those being classified as unavoidable, involving essentials only.

Those measures that countries continue to institute are warranted, especially if health reports from different regions were to be used as the baseline. For instance, in the past 24 h, China alone had reported 3893 new cases, with 66 deaths. Outside China, the number of deaths reached 191 after 32 new cases were reported in a span of 24 h (WHO, 2020ak). In Japan, a cruise ship, the "*Diamond Princess,*" carrying 3500 passengers recorded 10 positive cases, forcing the entire vessel into quarantine, with plans to test all the passengers initiated (WHO, 2020ak). The reported cases of the day include one of an infant, only 30 hours old (Churchill et al., 2020)-raising fears that the virus could be transmitted vertically (transmitted while still in the womb), and another one only 6-month-old in Singapore (Chee, 2020).

In addition, the devastation of the virus on the Chinese economy by now became more apparent; hence, countries are trying to avoid similar impacts. On this, among the response strategies that have been instituted in the past 24 h include shipping of diagnostic test kits by US CDC to all its labs across the United States to ensure that testing of all suspected cases is fast-tracked (Sun, 2020). Globally, the World Health Organization launched a financial kitty of $675 million aimed at helping in preparedness and response to 2019-nCOV (WHO, 2020aq). These funds would be advanced to states with weaker health systems to allow them to respond effectively to the virus, and also prevent further spread of the same. In China, efforts to overcome the diseases increased with the Wuhan Institute of Virology acquiring a patent for the Gilead's *Remdesivir drug*, that health workers had started to use as a potential cure to the virus and administered to patients (Associated Press, 2020).

DAY 69—FEBRUARY 7, 2020

The situation in China continued to worsen as the number of new cases reported each day exceeds 3000, and deaths over 50 each day. For instance, on February 6, new cases reported were 3697 (WHO, 2020ad), while the next day (February 7), the number of new cases was 3151 (WHO, 2020ae). In each of these days, 73 people lost their lives from the virus, including an American who died on February 6 in Wuhan (Hopkins, 2020). One of the deaths that sparked a lot of concern, and anger is that of the Chinese doctor—Li Wenliang, who, along with other 7 individuals, had been arrested, on January 6, for whistleblowing on the coronavirus situation in China (Xiong et al., 2020). Following his death, the government received massive criticism via different social media, including Twitter and Weibo, but, in Weibo, Chinese officials acted to censor messages referring to the case (Tan, 2020). Overall, the global tally had increased to 31,481 confirmed cases as of February 7 with 4821 of these severely ill. This number included 41 cases confirmed in Japan, who had come from the *Diamond Princess* cruise ship, where 10 others had been reported the previous day. The confirmation of these pushed the total confirmed cases in Japan to 46 (Sim, 2020).

Following those increased numbers, a number of interventions were initiated, especially on February 6. For instance, in China, security and health officials resulted in extreme measures that included door-to-door searching for all sick individuals, who were round-up and taken to designated quarantine centers (Qin et al., 2020). While that was happening, Japan extended a $10 million aid to the WHO as a contribution toward the 2019-nCoV outbreak, especially aimed for countries with weak health systems (Schnirring, 2020). On the same date, the WHO revealed plans of hosting a global research and innovation forum a week from now (February 11–12) that would converge scientists, public health agencies, and ministries of health and funders, to discuss ways in which research and action on the 2019-nCoV could be accelerated (WHO, 2020av). The other financial aid that came in to help strengthen the fight against the virus included a US$100 million pledge by the United States to China after talks between US President Donald Trump and Chinese President Xi Jingping, where President Trump also praised China for the efforts in fighting the virus (Pompeo, 2020).

On the economic front, the virus has continued to impact different businesses, especially the airline industry that has seen an unprecedented grounding—with only a few flights mainly for repatriation and shipment of health equipment. In view of this, an airshow scheduled in Singapore after some of the participants like the Lockheed Martin Corporation (CNA, 2020g) and Raytheon Technologies Corporation desisted, fearing the 2019-nCoV, was canceled (Reuters, 2020a). In other cases, Burberry, the British luxury fashion store closed a third store in China (Chalmers, 2020), a move that was also taken by VF Corporation (American Footware and Apparel company), which announced that its subsidiary: "Vans," would reduce its stores in China by 60% (Linnane, 2020), while Honda closed three of its manufacturing plants based in Wuhan, China, until February 13 (CNA, 2020e). On the oil market, Russia is reported to have rejected the Organization of the Petroleum Exporting Countries (OPEC) plans to cut oil production as a measure to respond to the virus outbreak (Faucon and Said, 2020), which has seen a reduction of demand for oil in China. However, cutting the production, OPEC would somehow help stabilize the oil prices that have plummeted since the 2019-nCoV outbreak started to escalate (Reed, 2020). While those were happening, the Asian Development Bank (ADB) approved a US$2 million financial package to support response capacity effort against the virus (ADB, 2020b). The funds target to boost coronavirus response capacity in the republics of China, Thailand, Vietnam, Myanmar, Lao, and Cambodia.

DAY 71—FEBRUARY 9, 2020

As the 2019-nCoV spread continues to gain momentum, with no clear end, either in China where it started or globally, concerted efforts across the globe continued relentlessly. In China, with the confirmed cases increasing from 34,598, and deaths increasing from 723 deaths—as recorded on February 8 (WHO, 2020af)—to 37,251 confirmed cases and 812 reported deaths on February 9 (WHO, 2020ag) respectively, the government reinforced measures. For instance, on February 8, the country's president, Xi Jingping is reported to have led other government officials in visiting hospitals and treatment centers in Beijing, to get first-hand information on how the prevention and control measures were being implemented, especially at the primary level (Xinhua, 2020c). He was also keen to observe how basic and important daily supplies were delivered and distributed, especially following earlier mismanaged cases, as reported earlier, by Red Cross China. While that was happening, the second hospital, Leishenshan Hospital, with a bed capacity of 1500 beds was opened and immediately started serving the 2019-nCoV patients. The opening of this hospital came was timely, as following the widespread of the virus, buildings across Wuhan were being converted into hospitals to accommodate the increasing number of patients (Daly et al., 2020). In addition to these interventions, on 9th, the government of China allocated US$ 10 billion (Newey, 2020) to the coronavirus fund to help boost efforts in place to contain the virus, which had already claimed more people than those killed by SARS-nCoV (774 globally) in 2002–03 (Safi et al., 2020). These funds add to the US$ 28.66 million that had been issued by the National Development Reform Commission for the same purpose of responding to the outbreak (Xinhua News Agency, 2020).

Outside China, the number of confirmed cases is also increasing—288 cases reported on 8th to 307 (19 new) cases on 9th. Of these, 6 cases were confirmed in Japan, coming from those quarantined after the Diamond Princess Cruise ship incidence (Japan Time, 2020). The others were reported from other parts of Asia and Europe (Spain and the UK). On 8th, five new cases were reported in France, involving British nationals who were staying in a skiing resort (BBC, 2020b).

As the spread continued, the situation at economic and social fronts was becoming dire. For instance, on 8th, Apple extended the suspension of its stores all across China (Feiner, 2020), while Hyundai Motor Company closed its largest factory citing lack of parts (The Straits Times, 2020a). This came a day after it had closed 3 of its plants in China. On other news, following the two previous incidences involving cruise ships, the Norwegian Cruise Line banned temporarily passport holders from China, Hong Kong, and Macau, and any other travelers who may have visited those three countries in the past 30 days (Lovelace and Feuer, 2020). This came as countries such as Kuwait (Gulf Insider, 2020), Qatar (The Straits Times, 2020d), South Korea, and Israel (CNA, 2020b) issued a travel advisory to their citizens, urging them to consider delaying travel plans to those affected regions.

DAY 72—FEBRUARY 10, 2020

On the previous day, a team of health experts that the WHO had promised to send to China, to assist in containing the 2019-nCoV outbreak, had arrived (Nebehay, 2020). Their arrival coincided with the country recorded a new death toll high of 97 people in a single day, pushing the total death count to 907. These deaths now surpass the total recorded (858) in 2012 following the Middle East Respiratory Syndrome (MERS) outbreak (WHO, 2020ah; Ravelo and Jerving, 2020). In addition, the number of confirmed cases in China has reached 40,235 (40,554 globally) in the country, with 6484 of those in dire need of urgent attention. Globally, according to the WHO (WHO, 2020ah), the number of countries affected by the disease outside China remains 24 with 319 total confirmed cases, with 12 on these recorded within a period of 24 h from countries like Singapore, which now has a total of 45 cases, UAE (Middle East Monitor, 2020), the United Kingdom whose total confirmed cases have reached 8 (BBC, 2020h), the United States, which confirmed one new case to bring its country tally to 13 confirmed cases (Edwards, 2020b), and Malaysia, which by now has 18 confirmed cases (Yusof, 2020).

Despite those cases, there are numerous response efforts globally. To begin with, the WHO reached an agreement with "Foundation for Innovative New Diagnostics" that aimed at strengthening the diagnostic systems capacity in countries that may not be sufficiently equipped to combat the outbreak (Development Aid, 2020b). At the same time, it was established that globally, approximately 168 laboratories have been found to have the prerequisite capacity to diagnose the virus, thus increasing the optimism of speeding up the testing processes (Japan Times, 2020). That news came right on time when, the United Kingdom had already issued a warning that the 2019-nCoV was not to be taken lightly as it constituted "a serious and imminent threat to public health" (Perma.cc record, 2020), and on its part, it would take even sterner measures, including forced quarantine to safeguard its public from the spread.

However, the strain on governments by the outbreak and the uncertainties it caused were becoming clear. For instance, the US government released a budget proposal for the year 2020/2021 (FY21) to reduce the country's financial support to the WHO and Global Health Programs. This concerns a $65 million reduction proposal for the WHO and also a 34% decrease to Global Health Programs (Hansler, 2020). Such proposed reduction would greatly impact the operations of these organizations, while, they are pressed upon following the increasing impacts of the virus on the global sphere. In China, the impacts of the outbreak on its citizens incited them to travel to work in cities that were not yet under lockdown, despite calls by most companies for employees to stay and work from home. In Russia, as the fear of 2019-nCoV continued, requiring all foreign travelers to quarantine for 14 days, there was no special treatment even for the diplomats—as was the case of a Chinese diplomat forced into quarantine just like anyone else (The Moscow Times, 2020).

DAY 73—FEBRUARY 11, 2020

Seventy-three days since the virus broke in China, the WHO officially assigned the virus the name SARS-CoV2 and the disease it caused as "COVID-19" (WHO, 2020q). In addition, the organization, just like the United Kingdom, officially agreed that this outbreak was a "very grave threat to the rest of the world," but also contended that a vaccine for the same would take at least 18 months to be developed (The Straits Times, 2020b). These happenings occurred when a high-level delegation of global research and innovation were holding their forum in Geneva and were tasked with the responsibility of coming up with a roadmap for identifying research priorities on the disease (WHO, 2020o). On other fronts, Shenzhen University in China launched a COVID-19 test kit, taking only 22 minutes to detect coronavirus antibodies from serum or plasma test samples (University, 2020). The kit was successfully developed following a joint collaboration between Shenzhen University, Shenzhen Tianshen Medical Devices Co., Ltd., and Third People's Hospital (Jiemian, 2020a). The availability of this test kit was deemed as a plus to the fight against COVID-19, which have—at the time, already proven to be catastrophic.

The earlier response interventions occurred the same day when the global tally of the confirmed case reported increased to 43,103 cases with 7333 of those reported to be in critical condition. In China, the confirmed cases were 42,708, while those reported in other countries increased by 76 to reach 395 (WHO, 2020q). Of these, 65 cases were reported in Japan, from the group of 3700 passengers that had docked from *Diamond Princess* Cruise ship (Chappell, 2020). Following those new cases, the number of confirmed cases in Japan increased to 135, making it the second most affected country after China. The number of deaths reached 1018, with all, except one, reported in China. On this day, most of the cases reported were from Asia with countries like Thailand, Singapore, Vietnam, and Hong Kong (Lokkei et al., 2020) recording new cases. Outside this region, only Germany confirmed two new cases, pushing its total confirmed cases to 16 (Nienaber and Reese, 2020). In Vietnam, the newest victim was a 3-month-old girl (Hai, 2020). In the United States, the first batch of 195 people evacuated from China and was placed under a mandatory 14 days quarantine was released from the "March Air Reserve Base," which served as a quarantine facility, with none of them confirming positive to the disease (Waldrop, 2020).

The COVID-19 confirmation cases coming from the cruise ship were startling, such that, another cruise ship, the *MS Westerdam*, that was stranded at sea for days—having been denied entry in places like Guam, Philippines, Taiwan, and Japan—is also denied docking rights by Thailand. The ship carrying 1455 passengers and 802 crews was destined for Yokohama, Japan from Singapore (Bangkok Post, 2020), but, at the time, it had to wait longer, before it could dock "somewhere."

DAY 75—FEBRUARY 13, 2020

After being stranded on the sea for days, finally, Cambodia agreed to allow the *MS Westerdam* Cruise ship to dock in its port (CNA, 2020c). This is one day after Japan had denied it entry. As it docked, the situation from *Diamond Princess* Cruise ship had worsened after 39 more cases were confirmed, increasing the number reported from there to 175. On the same day (February 12), the WHO's initiated forum in Geneva concluded a raft of recommendations. First, they agreed that there was a need for simpler diagnostic tools allowing for quicker testing. They also emphasized the need for the acceleration vaccine search and therapeutics, plus the adoption of best practices in infection prevention (WHO, 2020k). In the United States, the fight against COVID-19 experienced setbacks after it was discovered that the testing kits distributed by the CDC to different places returned "inconclusive" results (Grady, 2020). While that was happening, a new case was reported in the country (US), rendering a total case count of 14 and the following day, the 15th case was confirmed, pertaining to a male patient in quarantine in a military base in Texas who had traveled from Wuhan.

On February 13, positive cases continued to increase, including on the international scene, with most (44 new cases) of these coming from the *Diamond Princess* Cruise ship, raising its cases to 218. In addition to these, four more cases were reported in mainland Japan, and unfortunately, the country recorded its first death from the virus (CNA, 2020f). Singapore recorded eight new cases, while Hong Kong had three new cases. Vietnam and Malaysia confirmed a case each. Vietnam, besides its new case, placed an entire rural community of about 10,000 people under quarantine for 20 days in Vinh Phuc, located 44 km from Hanoi (Nguyen, 2020). The measure was taken noting that 16 cases reported in the country were from this area. In China, as from the February 13, there was a change in diagnostic criteria, where new cases reported henceforth included laboratory-confirmed cases as well as those confirmed via clinical diagnosis like radiology (WHO, 2020l). Following this new development, the number of new cases skyrocketed to 14,840 cases against the 1826 laboratory-confirmed new cases that the WHO had reported during their daily briefing. Despite this new development, the WHO and other countries continued to report only laboratory-confirmed cases. The new number of deaths on 13th increased by 254, to push the total deaths globally to 1368 (WHO, 2020l).

As more cases continued to be discovered, the same way were the interventions being initiated. For instance, in China, a local pharmacy was placed under investigation for flaunting a directive requiring that all medical equipment would not be sold at a price above 15% its stock price. The pharmacy was reported to have sold 44,000 single-use masks for US$ 0.143 instead of US$ 0.086, which coincided with the 15% provision. If found culpable, it was to be charged a fine of US$6110.54 for exploiting the public in times of crisis (Surging News, 2020). On the following day, health officials in Hubei released approximately 1.3 million masks to pharmacies and requested them to sell to the public at price not exceeding US$ 0.287 (BJnews, 2020). In the United States, the government proposed an immigration ban that would bar anyone from entering the country during this period (Zere, 2020). In Europe, health ministers met in Brussels for an emergency health meeting following the increasing number of cases in the region, and their goal was to forge a common approach that would see them prevent the spread of the virus in the region (DW, 2020b).

DAY 79—FEBRUARY 17, 2020

For the past 4 days, a number of things have transpired in regard to the COVID-19 spread and its impacts globally. On February 14, the first African case was confirmed in Egypt, involving a foreigner of undisclosed nationality (Aljazeera, 2020b). The number of cases confirmed from the ill-fated *Diamond Princess* Cruise ship continued to rise, with the number reaching 454 by February 17 (McCurry and Ratcliffe, 2020). In Malaysia, on 15th, an American woman who flew from Cambodia after disembarking from the *MS Westerdam* Cruise ship was confirmed positive together with the other two—not from the ship (Global News, 2020). On 16th, Taiwan reported the first death from COVID-19 of a man in his 60s (CNA, 2020j). Another death was reported in France, which is also a first to have occurred outside the Asian region (Peltier, 2020). Besides those, as is evident from the WHO's situational report number 28 (WHO, 2020m), the number of confirmed cases has reached 71,429, with 70,635 of those reported in China, and 794 coming from 25 other countries. The number of total deaths also increased with those reported in China accumulating to 1772, and 3 reported outside China. Of the confirmed cases in China, 1716 cases involved health workers who had been in the frontline against the disease, and unfortunately, 6 of those had died. However, amid all those problems, deaths, and increased cases, a report (Wu and McGoogan, 2020) released by Chinese health officials supported that COVID-19 is less deadly as compared with both SARS and MERS, thus giving hope to the world, but on the same, the WHO Director-General advanced that despite that information, there were still gaps that remained and efforts should not be diluted in the fight against this outbreak (WHO, 2020at).

To contain further spread, and following the reported case of people returning to work in China, the government extended areas covered by lockdowns and travel restriction, thus, overall, cutting off approximately 760 million (Zhong and Mozur, 2020). This came as the WHO Director-General hinted that there were possibilities that COVID-19 would reach pandemic levels (WHO, 2020p). Banks in China, including the Guangzhou branch of the country's central Bank and the PBC banks, took the fight against the disease further by announcing plans of destroying all used banknotes collected from hospitals, wet markets, and buses (Yeping, 2020). The rest of the money collected from areas not directly linked to the outbreak were to be quarantined for 7 days before being released back into the banking system (France-Presse, 2020a). This came as further investigations through which the virus could be transmitted continued to be explored. In the United States, the government announced plans to evacuate its citizens who were quarantined in the

Diamond Princess Cruise ship, but at that moment, only those who had tested positive would be airlifted, where they received treatment in Japan (U.S. Department of State, 2020b). On 17th, this procedure was enacted where 328 individuals were airlifted, which included 14 confirmed cases were airlifted back to the United States, where they were quarantined for 14 days.

Although interventions to save lives were going on, the economic situations in different countries, and of different companies were deteriorating. A pointer to this is the disclaimer by Apple to its investors that their expected revenue targets for the first quarter of the year (March) would not be achieved following the impact of the widespread outbreak of COVID-19 (Apple, 2020). In Hong Kong, the public had panicked following the increased cases, and they ended up being trapped in panic-buying. This caused a shortage of essential products, causing some unprecedented cases like the theft of HK$ 1600 worth of toilet papers by armed robbers (Frew, 2020). In Singapore, the Prime Minister was quoted to warn citizens that the country was heading to a recession, as the impact of the disease had taken a toll on the economy, especially that there was no clear indication as to when the pandemic was to be over (Lee, 2020).

DAY 81—FEBRUARY 19, 2020

This will remain a historical day to the *443* passengers, who were part of those quarantined on the *Diamond Princess* Cruise ship for 14 days as they come out alive and free from the coronavirus. By the end of the 2 weeks quarantine, 621 people confirmed positive (BBC, 2020f). In addition, the fate of another large group that had not yet been tested from the same ship, but had shared a cabin with the positive cases, was still unknown, and they had to wait until their test reports are brought back. Of those who remained, over a 100 were American citizens working for the government, through the country's CDC, mentioning that they would not be welcomed back home until they complete a mandatory 14 days quarantine (CDC, 2020c). According to the statement, even those who will risk flying to America before the expiry of this quarantine period will still be put under mandatory quarantine, and test negative before being cleared and free. That statement came only a day after the government, through the Department of State and Department of Health and Human Services had repatriated 328 Americans who had also disembarked from the same cruise ship (U.S. Department of State, 2020b).

The day was also historical for passengers who had disembarked from the *MS Westerdam* Cruise ship after Cambodia announced that all of them, except the American woman who had tested positive, were negative (Julie, 2020). As highlighted earlier, these passengers had been denied access by more than five countries fearing that they would be positive.

The events surrounding that cruise ship only highlight how the virus had strained different governments, and each was doing whatever seemed right at the moment to safeguard the majority of the population that were safe from the virus. Such is the case also observed in Russia, which announced a total ban on Chinese citizens on its soil as from February 18 (Reuters, 2020b). This tension between Russia and China may have been triggered by the happenings in China where, earlier on the day (February 18), it revoked press credentials of three journalists attached to the Wall Street Journal (The Wall Street Journal, 2020) following an article their employer had published earlier referring to China as "the real sick man of Asia." The decision by Russia could alternatively have been triggered by the unfortunate death of Liu Zhiming from COVID-19, who until his demise, was the director of the Wuchang Hospital in Wuhan (Griffiths, 2020).

The death of Zhiming, was among the 2005 others witnessed in China as of February 19. The number of cases in the country increased by 1752 to push the country's total to 74,280 (WHO, 2020d). Globally, there were 120 new cases reported, pushing cases outside China to 924, which included two first cases reported in Iran. Later during the day, these two patients died. The other cases were reported in Japan, with 79 coming from the Diamond Princess Cruise ship, and 20 others reported in South Korea. In Hong Kong, a 70-year-old woman who had been admitted in hospital from the disease succumbed, pushing the number of deaths in the country to 2 (Cheung and Lum, 2020).

Following the increasing cases in Japan, authorities were forced to cancel one of the biggest social events (Napponbashi Street Festa) that was to be held in Osaka (Loo, 2020). The event, which entails anime cosplay, was set to attract over 200,000 people, but unfortunately, due to the current local and global health landscape, canceling it is the only best option (Baseel, 2020). In China, a survey conducted on the plight of those living with HIV during this period where the world is engulfed in COVID-19 outbreak established that a third were in dire need of treatment, and the situation caused by the lockdown and restricted movements was worsening their cases.

DAY 83—FEBRUARY 21, 2020

On 20th, another doctor, a 29-year-old respiratory specialist from Wuhan succumbed to COVID-19 disease, a day after the director of Wuchang Hospital had died. His death came when two others were reported involving two passengers aboard Diamond Princess, where also 13 more cases were confirmed bringing the total confirmed cases from the cruise ship to 634 (Mizumoto et al., 2020). On this, while the decision to quarantine the ship was for the best interest of everyone, including the Republic of Japan, the decision was highly criticized, especially in regard to how the quarantine was managed (BBC, 2020f). According to different quarters, the exponential escalation of positive cases on the cruise ship would have been avoided, and this incident opened the question as to how quarantine facilities elsewhere were being handled, and whether that was the best option that could have been adopted. Elsewhere, the situation in the Republic of South Korea was seen to be worsening since the past 2 days, with 53 new cases reported on 20th and 100 more cases reported on 21st, bringing the country's tally to 204, marking the country as the second most affected after China (Culbertson, 2020). The spike in spread in this country is attributed to a secret church service that had taken place, where "patient 31" who had attended church service was believed to have caused the explosion of cases (Shin and Yi, 2020). On the same date (February 21), the country also reported a second death from the disease.

In Italy, things had also started to hasten, where 17 new cases were reported, with the death of one of the patients: a man aged 78 years old. Following this incident, the country was quick to close down public spaces including schools and prohibiting public gatherings in 10 of its towns, especially in the northern part of the country, where the outbreak seemed to be gaining traction (Winsor and Schumaker, 2020) (Aljazeera, 2020a). The situation in Iran was also worsening, having reported 18 confirmed cases in a span of 3 days, which also resulted in the death of four individuals. Another country that was seeing an increase in the number of confirmed cases was the United States, which also reported 20 new cases in a span of 24 hours, bringing the country's total to 35 (Johnson). The country's *Association of Public Health Laboratories (APHL)* feared that despite this change in the number of confirmed cases in the outbreak, the country only had testing capacities in only three states: California, Nebraska, and Illinois (Thomson Reuters, 2020).

In total, including the mentioned cases, the confirmed cases globally during the past 2 days increased by 1569, bringing the global total confirmed cases to 75,748. Out of those, 1073 were reported outside China in 27 countries, where 8 deaths had occurred since the beginning of the outbreak. Deaths in China had already reached 2121 (WHO, 2020a). On the reporting, earlier, officials in China mentioned that they would be including the confirmed cases from the clinical test (radiology), but on 21st, it was announced that they would no longer use this but will rely only on laboratory-confirmed cases to report the number of cases in the country, just like the other countries were doing (WHO, 2020a). In the same country, it was reported that among the confirmed cases to date, 500 were from five prisons, showing that the spread was extensive and could be experienced in the type of establishment. Elsewhere, Israel and Lebanon are said to have recorded their first positive cases of COVID-19, with the patient in Israel having come from Diamond Princess.

DAY 85—FEBRUARY 23, 2020

On this day, the situation and attention of the outbreak were seen to have shifted, somehow from China to countries like South Korea, Iran, and Italy, where the number of cases and deaths seemed to be increasing. On the previous day (February 22), these three countries reported two more deaths, with total deaths in Italy, South Korea, and Iran climbing to two, four, and six, respectively (France 24, 2020). On 23rd, two more deaths occurred in both Iran and South Korea, and more people died in Italy (Reuters, 2020l). These unfolding events prompted a number of issues that would impact these countries going forward. For instance, in Iran, all schools, universities, and other learning institutions were suspended, and the institutions closed indefinitely, in 14 provinces (Aljazeera, 2020d). In South Korea, the country's alert level was raised to the red—the highest level (BBC, 2020g), allowing the government to take stringent measures like restricting public transportation, calling for lockdowns, imposing mandatory and force quarantine, and denying or banning foreign travels from any country. While that was happening, the number of confirmed cases increased to 602 after 169 people tested positive (The Straits Times, 2020f) with more expected to be reported, and this prompted the government to designate Daegu and Cheongdo counties as its temporary "special care zones" to handle all reported cases (CNA, 2020i). All soldiers in the country were also prohibited from taking leave or leaving the barracks (Junga, 2020).

In Italy, the government also announced national emergency measures to contain the spread, which was the fastest besides those in Asia. On February 23 alone, the country had confirmed 73 new cases, which increased its total to 152 confirmed cases (Guidelli, 2020). Elsewhere in Europe, the United Kingdom confirmed four new cases evacuated from Diamond Princess, which in total have had 691 confirmed cases out of the 3700 passengers that had boarded the cruise ship (BBC, 2020c).

The situation of the three mentioned countries did not only worse locally, but externally, their neighbors and even foes from afar were rethinking the imposition of bans. For instance, Iran's neighbors like Afghanistan, Armenia, Pakistan, and Turkey all closed their borders with Iran. Italy also received similar treatments from Austria, which temporarily halted train services from, or into, Italy, fearing that the COVID-19 virus could be exported to its soil (DW, 2020a). It also received restrictions from the United States after the CDC issued a level 1 warning for it and for Iran. The United States had, on the previous day, issued a level 2 warning for Japan and South Korea (CDC, 2020a). The case for Japan was not only related to the increasing numbers of confirmed cases, but also, because it is accused (it also apologized for the same (France-Presse, 2020b)) of having allowed 23 passengers to disembark the Diamond Princess Cruise ship before being tested, and their status ascertained (France-Presse, 2020b).

South Korea was also distanced not only from the United States but from other countries like Singapore and Israel. For Israel, besides issuing a travel advisory to the country, it denied landing permits to 130 South Korean nationals who were aboard a flight from Seoul (Harkov, 2020).

In Africa, the WHO conducted a survey on the preparedness of different African countries, and on February 22, it reported that the overall readiness level on the continent was at 66% (WHO, 2020au). The agency thus recommended urgent interventions on the continent to allow different countries to strengthen their capacities in all medical areas to be able to handle the outbreak, though the continent was considered as safe at that moment. Following this report, the African Union Commission called for an emergency meeting with health ministers to deliberate on those findings, and to craft preparedness plans (AU, 2020).

DAY 86—FEBRUARY 24, 2020

Amid the increase in cases across the globe, there is some good news coming from China, which over the past few days has seen some cities outside Hubei province ease restrictions, including those on transportation. The news, coming from a report (WHO, 2020al) compiled by a group of experts—who had been in the country for the past 2 weeks, on a fact-finding mission regarding COVID-19, and read by Dr. Bruce Aylward indicated that the cases in the country were falling (WHO, 2020n). True to this report, the average confirmed cases dropped from a high of 3000 cases a day to an average of 400, with those reported on the 24th accounting for 415 cases. However, the report advised that the country should continue being vigilant as there was no cure for the disease found yet, and the number of deaths arising from the disease in China was relatively high.

While China was improving, the situation in other countries was becoming serious and demanding. In the Middle East, a day after countries distanced themselves from Iran to avoid the spread of the disease, five of them (Afghanistan, Bahrain, Iraq, Kuwait, and Oman) confirmed their first case, all linked to a traveler from Iran. At the same time, Iran confirmed 18 more cases, and four deaths, taking the total deaths in the country to 12 (ANSA, 2020). In Asia, countries like Hong Kong, Taiwan, and Singapore were still confirming new cases, but South Korea was worse, with 231 new cases in a day, raising its confirmed total to 833 cases (The Straits Times, 2020e). However, observation showed that Europe was slowly becoming a new epicenter. In particular, the situation in Italy was becoming very serious, as its confirmed cases increased to 229 overnight after 74 new cases drawn from six administrative regions were reported (ANSA, 2020). It also reported four more deaths pushing its country's total to seven. In North America, new cases were reported in the United States, which confirmed 18 new ones (Salo, 2020) and in Canada, which reported a single case (The Canadian Press, 2020). In total, the global cases had reached 79,331 with a bulk (77,262 cases) of these being in China (WHO, 2020n).

On the economic scene, the impacts of the widespread of the disease were evident, especially in the global stock market that was reported to have plunged by 3.6%; the lowest reported in 2 years (Mclean et al., 2020). The situation in Italy and South Korea were linked to this drop. The economic demand prompted by the COVID-19 outbreak also led the Trump administration to request Congress for a $2.5 billion package to help the country further prepare to combat the disease (Office of the President, 2020). The Asian Development Bank also contemplated postponing its 53rd annual meeting that was slated on May 2–5 following events in South Korea, which seemed to be worsening.

Politically, the outbreak has seen numerous activities postponed globally with the latest one being the postponement of the 13th session of National People's Congress scheduled for March 3, and one that is deemed as one of the most significant political meetings in China for the members of the party (Xinhua, 2020a). The US CDC escalated its travel bans with South Korea, Iran, and Italy after it issued travel advisory warning levels to 3 (for South Korea) and 2 (for the other two countries) (CDC, 2020a). A similar action taken previously preoccupated China, which warned its nationals from traveling to the United States, in fear of discrimination and unfair treatment (The Straits Times, 2020c).

DAY 87—FEBRUARY 25, 2020

The number of cases globally increased to 80,239, with China reporting 518 new cases and 390 reported outside China, with more four countries (Algeria, Austria, Croatia, Switzerland) reporting their first cases all related to travelers who had come from Italy (WHO, 2020e). The Algerian case is the second on the African continent with both cases involving foreigners. In Italy, 94 more cases were reported—bringing the country's total to 323, with 4 additional deaths, rendering a death toll of 11 (Bocci, 2020). In Iran, the situation was still critical with 34 new cases confirmed, pushing the total tally to 95, and among the new cases is Mahmoud Sadeghi, a member of Parliament (MP) (Alfaisal, 2020) and Deputy Minister for Health; Iraj Harirchi, who was part of the committee leading the country's COVID-19 taskforce (Aljazeera, 2020c). The country also lost a total of 16 patients to this disease (Reuters, 2020d) and was also associated with numerous other confirmed cases in other countries. For instance, Iraq confirmed five cases, all imported from Iran, Kuwait had four, while Oman confirmed 2 new cases returning from Iran. South Korea, another country facing an uphill task in relation to COVID-19 outbreak, reported 144 more cases, reaching 977 cases. It also had four deaths, raising the total deaths in the country to 11 (Maresca, 2020).

The cases from cruise ships have not ceased, with reports from the Diamond Princess indicating that a fourth patient associated with the ship succumbed to the COVID-19 disease (CNA, 2020d). In addition, on the same day, another cruise ship, *MSC Meraviglia*, which had been at sea, requested permission to dock and disembark passengers, but the request was denied by both Jamaica and the Cayman Islands (Gajanan and Mansoor, 2020).

In the United States, the request sent by the Office of the President requesting for funds to fight COVID-19 was received by Congress and the US senators were briefed on the same (Taylor, 2020). The CDC warned of signs that the spread of COVID-19 in the country was imminent, thus urging people to be vigilant and ready (Edwards, 2020a). This warning prompted the city of San Francisco to declare a state of emergency over the outbreak, becoming the first one to do so in the United States (Axelrod, 2020).

In China, as people prepared to get back to work, after the outbreak in the country was reported to be declining, the State Council offered some relief to the small-scale traders in the province of Hubei, by introducing a 3-month tax exemption measures (Jiemian, 2020c). Other stimulus packages were advanced to migrant workers and university students as a way of helping everyone get back to their previous normal self (Jiemian, 2020b). At the same time, to ensure that the second wave of outbreak was not experienced, Shenzhen introduced a legislative intervention that would see a ban on the consumption of some nonaquatic animals (Shenzen China, 2020).

DAY 91—FEBRUARY 29, 2020

February 26 was an eventful day, with diverse news from different spheres. Europe was becoming the epicenter with countries like Georgia, Greece, Macedonia, Norway, and Romania all reporting their first cases. Unsurprisingly, all these cases except for Georgia (traveler was from Iran) were linked to travelers coming from Italy, which by then had over 50,000 people in a forced lockdown (Giuffrida and Cochrane, 2020). This explains why most people were moving out of the country to other European countries, but unfortunately, as they move out, they also imported the disease. In Italy, 132 new cases were reported in the day, taking the confirmed cases to a high of 455. In Asia, South Korea confirmed a total of 284 new cases with its total tally reaching 1261 cases and 12 deaths (WHO, 2020b). Most of these were linked to "patient 31" who had attended the secret church service as noted earlier. Besides these cases, other new ones were reported in different parts of the world, and for the first time since the first case was identified, cases outside China (459) surpassed those reported in China (412). Such news prompted a new awakening regarding how countries responded to the virus. For instance, in the United States, President Trump appointed Vice President Mike Pence to lead the fight against COVID-19 (Shear et al., 2020). In Germany, the health minister declared that the country was "at the beginning of an epidemic" (AP, 2020), thus demanding that everyone should be ready to take their part to fight it. In Asia, the ADB approved another $2 million (first one was approved on February 7) to assist Asian and Pacific countries to prepare, and boost their resilience against the outbreak (ADB, 2020a). In Europe, the European Commission requested member states to review their preparedness plans and inform the commission accordingly. In addition, it informed its members of the decision for a joint procurement procedure that would allow them to access essential medical supplies with ease (Commission, 2020).

On 27th and 28th, more countries in Europe (Denmark, Estonia, The Netherlands, Iceland, Lithuania, New Zealand, and Monaco) reported their first cases, and as had been the trend, all those were from travelers from Italy. This happened as the situation in Italy continued to deteriorate as the number of deaths increased to 21 while confirmed cases reached a total of 888 (Ministry of Health Italy, 2020a). In Iran, the number of legislators reported to have contracted the disease increased to four, as the number of confirmed cases continued to swell, same with the number of deaths—which had reached a high of 34 (Al Arabiya, 2020). In addition, one of the country's Vice President, Masoumeh Ebtekar was also infected with the disease, the same as the mayor of Tehran (Reuters AFP, 2020). The other country that was still high pressed by COVID-19 was South Korea, which, by the end of day—on February 28, had reported a total of 2337 (The Straits Times, 2020g) and 16 deaths (Yonhap, 2020a). That said, globally, these 2 days were dramatic, with the number of new cases outside China increasing exponentially to 6009 cases, of which, 1318 cases were reported in a single day. The number of deaths outside China also increased to 86, while in China the total deaths were 2838. Globally, all the confirmed cases reported since the onset of the coronavirus were 85,403, with 79, 394 of those in China alone (WHO, 2020b). Elsewhere, in Mongolia, the president and some officials who had accompanied him to China, voluntarily submitted themselves to a 14-day quarantine (Nikkei, 2020).

Following the increasing global health challenge, the WHO Director-General urged countries to be decisive and aggressive in containing the virus, to avoid being overwhelmed. This was mentioned as the WHO raised the global risk of the spread of the disease to "very high," but the organization was not yet ready to declare COVID-19 as a pandemic (Branswell, 2020). The WHO had also sent a team of experts in Iran to help contain the outbreak, as already, 97 cases in 11 countries had been exported from there as people fled the outbreak (WHO, 2020as). In acknowledgment of the challenge of exported cases, the organization updated its guidance on travel advisories and retracted from its earlier stand that it was against any form of travel restriction (WHO, 2020ap). This time around, it was advised that where necessary, countries could impose some form of temporary restrictions to ensure it does not suffer from imported cases.

Amid those advices, more countries reported new cases on 29th including Ecuador, Ireland, Luxembourg, and Qatar, all from imported cases. On the same day, numerous other cases were reported in different countries, especially, Italy with 239 new cases and 8 deaths, Iran with 205 cases and 9 new deaths, Spain with 26 new cases, China with 427 new cases and 47 deaths, and many other countries adding to the list (WHO, 2020b). The United States reported its first death involving a man in his 50s (William Wan et al., 2020), including the increasing number of confirmed cases prompting Washington State to declare a state of emergency (Selsky, 2020). Indeed, the situation on this day evidently confirmed that the world was headed to a "tight corner" health-wise. To put this in perspective, the number of those who contracted the disease globally—at that time, totaled 87,137 and the number of deaths worldwide had reached a high of 2977. The number of countries already affected by the virus had also risen to 59, as reported by the WHO (WHO, 2020f). The situation on other spheres globally, concerning the economy, sports, politics, and social activities seemed to have been suspended as everyone, and every effort was geared on overcoming the widespread outbreak of this disease.

DAY 94—MARCH 3, 2020

The beginning of March is seen to have picked from where the other one ended—unprecedented increase in the number of confirmed cases, and more countries being affected. On March 1, the day ended with 1806 new cases having reported: 206 in China, and 1600 cases in other countries. In addition, by the end of the day, 6 more countries (Armenia, Czechia, Dominican Republic, Luxembourg, Iceland, and Indonesia) had reported new cases, bringing the total number of countries battling the disease to 65. The number of those who had died also increased to 3043, with 66 deaths reported in a span of only 24 h (WHO, 2020g). On March 2, the cases continued to increase, especially outside of China, to 90,869 cases, of which 1922 were reported within 24 h 69 more deaths were reported on this day, with 38 of these happening outside China (WHO, 2020h). In addition, 8 more countries (Andorra, Jordan, Latvia, Morocco, Portugal, Senegal, Tunisia, and Saudi Arabia) reported their first cases, bringing the total affected to

72 countries besides China. Of the new countries, 3 were from Africa, thus pushing the number of countries affected on the continent thus far to six. The same unfortunate trends were observed on the third of March where 4 new countries, including 2 from South America (Argentina and Chile) joined the list of those affected by COVID-19 disease. A total of 86 people lost their lives on this date, and 2223 new confirmed cases were reported globally (WHO, 2020i).

Among the countries that were highly impacted included Iran, which had over 2336 confirmed cases (BBC, 2020d), including 23 Member of Parliaments (Fazeli, 2020). The country also lost 77 people in less than a month since the disease was reported in the country. Italy was overwhelmed, where by March 3 it had lost 80 people and over 2500 were hospitalized (FQ, 2020). Just like the reports by the end of February, the situation in South Korea was growing from worst to worst, with over 5000 confirmed cases, and 36 deaths (Xinhua, 2020b). Besides this, the situation in all over Europe was becoming dire, as already, almost every member country was affected.

While those things were happening, there was a myriad of interventions that were being initiated, both at the local and international levels to contain the disease. For instance, on March 1, the United Nations (UN) was reported to have given part of its Central Emergency Response Fund amounting to $15 million to the WHO and United Nations Children's Fund (UNICEF) to support their efforts in less-abled countries in responding to the impacts of COVID-19 (UNICEF, 2020). On the following day, the US Government committed $37 million of the $100 pledged earlier (on February 7) from the Emergency Reserve Fund set aside for Contagious Infectious Diseases through US Agency for International Development to allow to the financing of countries affected, or at high risk of being affected (development Aid, 2020a). On 3rd, another financial support ($12 billion) was committed by the World Bank aimed for the same purpose of combating COVID-19 (The World Bank, 2020b). Such funds were aimed as precautionary measures and prove helpful, especially as the WHO, on March 3, estimated that the world would require approximately 89 million medical masks, 76 million medical gloves, and over 1.6 million eye goggles each month, besides other PPEs required to combat the disease. The WHO estimated that such a demand would only be satisfied if the manufacturing sector was able to increase its capacity by at least 40% of the status at the time (WHO, 2020am).

Other interventions taken especially on local scenes include the declaration of state of emergency in Florida after two positive cases were reported in the state (Folley, 2020). In the United States still, the Central Bank reduced the country's benchmark interest rate by 50% to a range between 1% and 1.25%; the first of such action since the 2008 recession (Timiraos, 2020). In Iran, the government advanced a temporary amnesty to at least 54,000 prisoners to protect them from being infected and to reduce the outbreak, which may be worse when reported in prisons (BBC, 2020d).

DAY 96—MARCH 5, 2020

In the last 48 hours, the attention on COVID-19 disease shifted to Europe and North America. Within this short period, the United States recorded an increase in confirmed cases in the country to 228 and the number of deaths reaching 14. Following this, more states including Maryland and California declared states of emergencies over COVID-19 (Office of the Governor, 2020a). The events also prompted a tumble in mortgage rates, which plunged to a record low of 3.29% (Gopal, 2020). While this was going on, the government received a boost, after Congress overwhelmingly passed $8.3 billion emergency coronavirus bill (Emma and Scholtes, 2020), which now awaited the input of the senate before being sent to President Trump for signature.

Besides the United States, Italy was another country that saw an unprecedented increase in the country's confirmed cases that reached 3850, and the number of deaths to 148 (Ministry of Health Italy, 2020b). France reported 92 new cases—including an Assembly member, Jean-Luc Reitzer, being one of those infected (MSN, 2020). Germany saw its cases increase to 349 after 87 more people were confirmed. In Spain, the numbers were increased to 234, with those in the United Kingdom increasing to 116, and with its first death (BBC, 2020i). Around and beyond these countries, more cases were reported during this period, where globally 98,192 people were confirmed positive, of which 17,481 were drawn from 88 countries outside China (WHO, 2020j).

As Iran continued to experience more challenges, including the death of Hossein Sheikholeslam, former MP, and Iran's former ambassador to Syria. These prompted the WHO to send experts to assist in containing the disease, where it was reported that despite this, it rejected a humanitarian aid offer from the US government (Smith, 2020).

The disease had now caused disruption in many sectors including the education sector globally where over 290.5 million students were affected, with at least 13 countries already having closed down schools indefinitely (UN, 2020). On the economic front, the IMF projected that the global growth in 2020 will be lower than the previous year's levels, and to ease the strain that countries, especially emerging markets and low-income ones, the institution proposed financial packages. This included a $50 billion loan facility dubbed, rapid-disbursing emergency financial facility that those countries could access to fight COVID-19. Of that, $10 billion was specifically set aside for least-developed economies without interest (IMF, 2020).

DAY 99—MARCH 8, 2020

For the first time since the onset of COVID-19 outbreak, the province of Hubei announced no new cases on March 6, while the number of new cases and deaths in the entire country continued to reduce—being, 143 new cases reported and 30 deaths. Indeed, some of the new cases being received in different parts of China were now imported from other countries, with 4 out of the 143 reported imported by people who traveled from Italy (Beijing Municipal Health Commission, 2020). While cases here were decreasing, elsewhere, the number was exponentially increasing. For instance, in France, on March 6 alone, there were 190 new cases, while Germany reported 290 cases in the same period. Italy reported the largest daily increase of 778 new cases, while the Netherlands confirmed 44 more cases. Spain had 104 new cases, Switzerland 123 new cases while the United States recorded 148 new cases and 19 deaths. The new cases were reported across the globe, and in total, on 6th, there were 3735 new cases, of which 3633 cases were reported in 93 countries excluding China. The same trends were observed on 7th, but in Iran, of the 21 people that died that day, was a first time sitting MP, Fatemeh Rahbar (France-Presse, 2020c). Besides cases of deaths, 1076 people were also confirmed to be infected, thus pushing the total tally in the country to 5823 cases, with 145 deaths. In Africa, Egypt, with the highest number of confirmed cases, reported 33 more cases—associated to a Nile cruise ship (Reuters, 2020c), and on 8th, it reported the first death, which was also the first in the continent of Africa (Africanews, 2020).

In response to these increasing cases, the United Kingdom released $59.9 million from its international development fund toward the development of a vaccine and rapid diagnostic test kits (Worley, 2020). This aid came in a time that the virus started spreading rapidly in the least developed economies especially in Africa and the development of those kits were welcomed. As this was unfolding, the WHO reported that globally, there were more than 200 clinical trials already registered, and these were fashioned to offer diverse therapeutic treatments to combat the disease. Such trials also included traditional Chinese medicine (WHO, 2020ar). On the local scene, following the earlier ban in Shenzhen, China enforced a country-wide ban on the eating of wild animals, which are suspected to have been the source of the virus causing COVID-19 (Westcott and Deng, 2020). In the United States, New York (Office of the Governor, 2020b) and eight other states declared a state of emergency as of March 8 (Impelli, 2020) as the CDC performed over 5861 coronavirus tests (Samuels and Hellmann, 2020). In France, the government banned any form of public gathering that would attract more than 1000 people. Italy placed the state of Lombardy and 14 others in the north under lockdown, cutting off a population of over 16 million people (BBC, 2020e).

Further, following imported cases, Saudi Arabia suspended both air and water travels with its neighbors and others, including UAE, Kuwait, Egypt, Italy, Syria, S. Korea, Bahrain, and Lebanon (Reuters, 2020j). Similar actions were taken by Qatar, which closed its borders to deny 14 additional countries from accessing it (Reuters, 2020h). Thailand took the cue and demanded that individuals coming from South Korea, Italy, and Iran undergo a mandatory self-isolation for a minimum of 14 days (Olarn, 2020). In the United States, the army temporarily banned any travel for soldiers and their families to or from South Korea and Italy (Starr and LeBlanc, 2020; Wallace, 2020).

REFERENCES

ADB. (2020a) ADB Approves Another $2 Million to Help Asia and the Pacific Tackle Coronavirus. Available at: https://www.adb.org/news/adb-approves-another-2-million-help-asia-and-pacific-tackle-coronavirus.

ADB. (2020b) ADB Initiates Coronavirus Response. Available at: https://www.adb.org/news/adb-initiates-coronavirus-response.

Africanews. (2020) Egypt Records Africa's First Coronavirus-Related Death. Available at: https://www.reuters.com/article/us-health-coronavirus-egypt-idUSKBN20U0TK.

Al Arabiya. (2020) Coronavirus Death Toll in Iran Rises to 34, 388 People Infected: Health Ministry. Available at: https://english.alarabiya.net/en/News/middle-east/2020/02/28/Coronavirus-death-toll-rises-to-34-388-people-infected-Health-Ministry.html.

Alfaisal L. (2020) Iranian MP Mahmoud Sadeghi Says He Tested Positive for Coronavirus. Available at: https://english.alarabiya.net/en/News/middle-east/2020/02/25/Iranian-MP-Mahmoud-Sadeghi-says-he-tested-positive-for-coronavirus.

Aljazeera. (2020a) China Coronavirus Outbreak: AL the Latest Updates. Available at: https://www.aljazeera.com/news/2020/02/cloneofcloneofcloneofcloneofcloneof2002152244372-200220231446112.html.

Aljazeera. (2020b) Egypt Confirms Coronavirus Cases, the First in Africa. Available at: https://www.aljazeera.com/news/2020/02/egypt-confirms-coronavirus-case-africa-200214190840134.html.

Aljazeera. (2020c) Iran's Deputy Health Minister Tests Positive for Coronavirus. Available at: https://www.aljazeera.com/news/2020/02/iran-deputy-health-minister-tests-positive-coronavirus-200225131520852.html.

Aljazeera. (2020d) Iran Shuts Schools, Cultural Centres as Coronavirus Kills Six. Available at: https://www.aljazeera.com/news/2020/02/iran-shuts-schools-cultural-centres-coronavirus-kills-200223000740899.html.

Aljazeera. (2020e) UAE Confirms First Cases of New Coronavirus. Available at: https://www.aljazeera.com/news/2020/01/uae-confirms-cases-coronavirus-200129063305587.html.

Aljazeera. (2020f) UK Confirms First Two Coronavirus Cases. Available at: https://www.aljazeera.com/news/2020/01/uk-confirms-coronavirus-cases-200131100102626.html.

ANSA R. (2020) Coronavirus: 229 Infected in Italy. Available at: https://www.ansa.it/english/news/general_news/2020/02/24/coronavirus-229-infected-in-italy_4b864afb-11d1-4d42-884f-f51211b4af35.html.

AP. (2020) Germany in Warning Over a Virus Epidemic. Available at: https://apnews.com/230fa2d2e2891ab2ccb6d9c8a5f479bf.

Apple. (2020) Investor Update on Quarterly Guidance. Available at: https://www.apple.com/newsroom/2020/02/investor-update-on-quarterly-guidance/.

Associated Press. (2020) China Scientists Want to Patent Gilead Drug to Treat Coronavirus Patients. Available at: https://www.marketwatch.com/story/china-scientists-want-to-patent-gilead-drug-to-treat-coronavirus-patients-2020-02-06.

AU. (2020) African Union Mobilizes Continent-Wide Response to COVID-19 Outbreak. Available at: https://au.int/en/pressreleases/20200224/african-union-mobilizes-continent-wide-response-covid-19-outbreak.

Axelrod T. (2020) San Francisco Declares State of Emergency Over Coronavirus. Available at: https://thehill.com/policy/healthcare/484602-san-francisco-declares-state-of-emergency-over-coronavirus.

Backer JA, Klinkenberg D and Wallinga J. (2020) Incubation Period of 2019 Novel Coronavirus (2019-nCoV) Infections Among Travellers From Wuhan, China, 20–28 January 2020. Euro Surveillance: bulletin Europeen sur les maladies transmissibles = European Communicable Disease Bulletin 25: 2000062.

Bangkok Post. (2020) Thailand Report 1 New Cases of Coronavirus, Bring Total to 33. Available at: https://www.bangkokpost.com/thailand/general/1855184/thailand-reports-1-new-case-of-coronavirus-brings-total-to-33.

Bangkok Post and Reuters. (2020) Fifth Coronavirus Case in Thailand. Available at: https://www.bangkokpost.com/thailand/general/1842939/fifth-coronavirus-case-in-thailand.

Barrett E. (2020) Billionaires Are Donating Millions to Fight China's Coronavirus. But Where Is the Money Going? Available at: https://fortune.com/2020/02/20/coronavirus-donations-china/.

Baseel C. (2020) Osaka Cancels One of Japan's Biggest Anime Cosplay Events Over Coronavirus Fears. Available at: https://soranews24.com/2020/02/20/osaka-cancels-one-of-japans-biggest-anime-cosplay-events-over-coronavirus-fears/.

BBC. (2020a) Coronavirus: China to Pump Billions into Economy Amid Growth fears. Available at: https://www.bbc.com/news/business-51347497.

BBC. (2020b) Coronavirus: Five Britons in French Ski Chalet Catch Virus. Available at: https://www.bbc.com/news/uk-51425702.

BBC. (2020c) Coronavirus: Four New UK Cases Among Ship Evacuees. Available at: https://www.bbc.com/news/uk-51606368.

BBC. (2020d) Coronavirus: Iran Temporarily Frees 54,000 Prisoners to Combat Spread. Available at: https://www.bbc.com/news/world-middle-east-51723398.

BBC. (2020e) Coronavirus: Northern Italy quarantines 16 million people. Available at: https://www.devex.com/news/dfid-goes-quiet-on-covid-19-response-96851.

BBC. (2020f) Coronavirus: Passengers Leave Diamond Princess Amid Criticism of Japan. Available at: https://www.bbc.com/news/world-asia-51555420.

BBC. (2020g) Coronavirus: South Korea declares highest alert as infections surge. Available at: https://www.bbc.com/news/world-asia-51603251.

BBC. (2020h) Coronavirus: UK Cases Double as Four More People Diagnosed. Available at: https://www.bbc.com/news/uk-51442314.

BBC. (2020i) Coronavirus: Woman in 70s Becomes First Virus Fatality in UK. Available at: https://www.bbc.com/news/uk-51759602.

BBC News. (2020a) China Coronavirus: Lockdown Measures Rise Across Hubei Province. Available at: https://www.bbc.com/news/world-asia-china-51217455.

BBC News. (2020b) Coronavirus: Ivory Coast Tests Woman for China Virus. Available at: https://www.bbc.com/news/world-africa-51258014.

BBC Sport. (2020) Formula E: China Race Called off Amid Coronavirus Outbreak. Available at: https://www.bbc.com/sport/motorsport/51344513.

Beijing Municipal Health Commission. (2020) Four New Cases of Imported New Coronary Pneumonia in Beijing. Available at: http://wjw.beijing.gov.cn/xwzx_20031/wnxw/202003/t20200306_1681226.html.

Bill & Melinda Gates Foundation. (2020) Press Release and Statement: Bill & Melinda Gates Foundation Dedicates Additional Funding to the Novel Coronavirus Response. Available at: https://www.gatesfoundation.org/Media-Center/Press-Releases/2020/02/Bill-and-Melinda-Gates-Foundation-Dedicates-Additional-Funding-to-the-Novel-Coronavirus-Response.

BJnews. (2020) 1.3 Million Civilian Masks in Hubei Invested 1 Yuan in the Market and 2 Yuan in Retail. Available at: http://www.bjnews.com.cn/news/2020/02/13/688878.html.

Bocci M. (2020) Coronavirus, 325 Cases in Italy. *Three More Died in Lombardy and One in Veneto, the Victims Become 11*. Available at: https://www.repubblica.it/cronaca/2020/02/25/news/coronavirus_toscana-249520102/?ref=RHPPTP-BH-I249554472-C12-P1-S1.12-T1.

Branswell H. (2020) WHO Says Coronavirus Is Not Yet a Pandemic But Urges Countries to Prepare. Available at:

https://www.scientificamerican.com/article/who-says-coronavirus-is-not-yet-a-pandemic-but-urges-countries-to-prepare/.

CDC. (2020a) Global COVID -19 Pandemic Notice. Available at: https://www.cdc.gov/.

CDC. (2020b) HHS and CDC Receive Additional Flights Carrying Passengers From China. Available at: https://www.cdc.gov/media/releases/2020/s0205-china-passengers.html.

CDC. (2020c) Update on the Diamond Princess Cruise Ship in Japan. Available at: https://www.cdc.gov/media/releases/2020/s0218-update-diamond-princess.html.

Chalmers V. (2020) Fashion Retailer Burberry Closes a THIRD of its Chinese Stores Because of the Killer Coronavirus Outbreak Cutting Demand for Luxury Coats and Scarves. Available at: https://www.dailymail.co.uk/health/article-7978129/Burberry-closes-one-three-Chinese-stores-coronavirus-outbreak.html.

Chan M. (2020) Coronavirus: Chinese Military Takes Control of Medical Supplies in Wuhan. Available at: https://www.scmp.com/news/china/society/article/3048778/coronavirus-chinese-military-takes-control-medical-supplies.

Chang JY. (2020) Full Border Shutdown With Mainland China is Discriminatory, Carrie Lam Says. Available at: https://www.scmp.com/video/hong-kong/3048508/full-border-shutdown-mainland-china-discriminatory-carrie-lam-says.

Chappell B. (2020) 65 More Coronavirus Cases on Diamond Princess Cruise Ship Stuck in Japan. Available at: https://www.scpr.org/news/2020/02/10/90843/65-more-coronavirus-cases-on-diamond-princess-crui/.

Chee K. (2020) Coronavirus: Singapore Confirms 4 New Cases, Including 6-Month-Old Child of Infected Couple. Available at: https://www.straitstimes.com/singapore/health/coronavirus-4-more-confirmed-cases-in-singapore-28-cases-so-far.

Cheung E and Lum A. (2020) Coronavirus: Confirmed Hong Kong Cases Now 65 as Mother-in-Law of Infected Engineer Becomes One of Three More Struck Down in Virus Outbreak. Available at: https://www.scmp.com/news/hong-kong/health-environment/article/3051312/second-hongkonger-dies-after-becoming-infected.

Choi D. (2020) Face Mask and Hand Sanitizer Hoarders Face $42,108 Fine and Up to 2 Years in Prison Under New South Korean Law Amid Coronavirus Spread. Available at: https://markets.businessinsider.com/news/stocks/face-mask-hand-sanitizer-hoarders-south-korea-2020-2-1028874053.

Chung K, Lok-kei S, Ho-him C, et al. (2020) China Coronavirus: Hong Kong Will Ban Anyone Who Has Been to Hubei Province From Entering City in Response to Mounting Calls to Tighten Border Checks. Available at: https://www.scmp.com/news/hong-kong/health-environment/article/3047689/china-coronavirus-hong-kong-has-its-sixth-patient.

Chung L. (2020) Taiwan Slaps Coronavirus Entry Ban on Foreigners Travelling From Mainland China. Available at: https://www.scmp.com/news/china/society/article/3048798/coronavirus-taiwan-deadly-virus-h1n1-flu.

Churchill O, Wu W, Zhen L, et al. (2020) Coronavirus: Infant Tests Positive Just 30 Hours After Birth. Available at: https://www.scmp.com/news/china/society/article/3049011/coronavirus-death-toll-jumps-65-479-chinas-hubei-province.

CNA. (2020a) Coronavirus Outbreak: Hong Knog to Quarantine all Arrivals From Mainland China. Available at: https://www.channelnewsasia.com/news/asia/wuhan-coronavirus-hong-kong-quarantine-mainland-china-visitors-12396568.

CNA. (2020b) Coronavirus: South Korea, Israel Advise Citizens to Defer Travel to Singapore. Available at: https://www.japantimes.co.jp/news/2020/02/09/world/coronavirus-sars-diamond-princess#.XkACJXlGT3A.

CNA. (2020c) Cruise Ship Stranded by COVID-19 Fears to Dock in Cambodia. Available at: https://www.channelnewsasia.com/news/asia/wuhan-coronavirus-covid-19-westerdam-ship-dock-cambodia-12427660.

CNA. (2020d) Fourth Passenger From Cruise Ship Dies in Japan: Reports. Available at: https://www.channelnewsasia.com/news/asia/covid-19-coronavirus-japan-diamond-princess-cruise-death-12467980.

CNA. (2020e) Honda to Keep Vehicle Plants in Wuhan Suspended Through Feb 13. Available at: https://www.channelnewsasia.com/news/business/honda-to-keep-vehicle-plants-in-wuhan-suspended-through-feb-13-12404200.

CNA. (2020f) Japan Confirms its First COVID-19 Death: Health Minister. Available at: https://www.channelnewsasia.com/news/asia/japan-confirms-first-covid-19-coronavirus-death-12432316.

CNA. (2020g) Lockheed Martin Pulls Out of Singapore Airshow Over Coronavirus Concerns. Available at: https://www.channelnewsasia.com/news/singapore/wuhan-virus-coronavirus-singapore-airshow-lockheed-martin-12407710.

CNA. (2020h) Novel Coronavirus: Hong Kong Leader Carrie Lam Announces Suspension of 10 Border Crossings With Mainland China. Available at: https://www.channelnewsasia.com/news/asia/wuhan-virus-hong-kong-carrie-lam-suspension-border-crossings-12386054.

CNA. (2020i) South Korea Reports 52 New COVID-19 Cases, Bring Total to 156. Available at: https://www.channelnewsasia.com/news/asia/covid19-south-korea-52-new-coronavirus-cases-total-156-12456158.

CNA. (2020j) Taiwan Records its First COVID-19 Death as Global Toll Passes 1,600. Available at: https://www.channelnewsasia.com/news/asia/coronavirus-covid19-taiwan-first-death-12439978.

CNA. (2020k) Thailand Reports 7 Confirmed Cases of Wuhan Virus, Airport Continues to Limit Temperature Scans. Available at: https://www.channelnewsasia.com/news/asia/thai-airport-virus-scans-patient-confirm-case-12338150.

CNA. (2020l) Wuhan Virus: 3 New Cases Confirmed in Singapore, Bringing Tally to 13. Available at: https://www.channelnewsasia.com/news/singapore/wuhan-virus-singapore-new-confirmed-cases-13-12369838.

CNBC. (2020) France Confirms First Three Casess of Coronavirus in Europe. Available at: https://www.cnbc.com/2020/01/24/france-confirms-2-cases-of-virus-from-china-1st-in-europe.html.

Cockrane E, Weiland N and Sanger-Katz M. (2020) U.S. Health Workers Responding to Coronavirus Lacked Training and Protective Gear, Whistle-Blower Says. Available at:

nytimes.com/2020/02/27/us/politics/coronavirus-us-whistleblower.html.
Cohen A. (2020) Oil Markets Brace for WHO's Global Health Emergency Declaration. Available at: https://www.forbes.com/sites/arielcohen/2020/01/30/oil-markets-brace-for-whos-global-health-emergency-declaration/#4edef1357058.
Commission E. (2020) The EU's Response to COVID-19. Available at: https://ec.europa.eu/commission/presscorner/detail/en/qanda_20_307.
Culbertson A. (2020) Coronavirus: South Korea New COVID-19 Front as 100 Fresh Cases Confirmed. Available at: https://news.sky.com/story/coronavirus-south-korea-new-covid-19-front-as-100-fresh-cases-confirmed-11939479.
Daily Mirror Online. (2020) Two Suspected Cases of Coronavirus Invetigated at IDH. Available at: http://www.dailymirror.lk/top_story/Two-suspected-cases-of-Coronavirus-investigated-at-IDH/155-181921.
Daly T, Zhang M and Fullick N. (2020) China's Wuhan Opens Another Makeshift Hospital to Fight Virus. Available at: https://www.reuters.com/article/us-china-health-hospital/chinas-wuhan-opens-another-makeshift-hospital-to-fight-virus-idUSKBN20209Z.
Daoud E. (2020) Monash Medical Centre Treating First Australia Case of Coronavirus. Available at: https://7news.com.au/news/health/first-australian-coronavirus-case-confirmed-in-victoria-c-664530.
Development Aid. (2020a) USAID Commits $37m to Respond to Novel Coronavirus COVID-19. Available at: https://www.developmentaid.org/#!/news-stream/post/60191/usaid-commits-37m-to-respond-to-novel-coronavirus-covid-19.
Development Aid. (2020b) Who and Find Formalize Strategic Collaboration to Drive Universal Access to Essential Diagnostics. Available at: https://www.developmentaid.org/#!/news-stream/post/58879/who-and-find-formalize-strategic-collaboration-to-drive-universal-access-to-essential-diagnostics.
Doherty B. (2020) Coronavirus: Three Cases in NSW and on in Victoria as Infection Reaches Australia. Available at: https://www.theguardian.com/science/2020/jan/25/coronavirus-five-people-in-nsw-being-tested-for-deadly-disease.
Dongwang. (2020) Two Cases of Pneumonia in Wuhan and in Hong Kong. Available at: https://hk.news.yahoo.com.
DW. (2020a) Coronavirus: Austria Briefly Halts Trains From Italy Over COVID-19 Concerns. Available at: https://www.dw.com/en/coronavirus-austria-briefly-halts-trains-from-italy-over-covid-19-concerns/a-52493063.
DW. (2020b) EU Health Ministers Hold Coronavirus Meeting — As it Happened. Available at: https://www.dw.com/en/eu-health-ministers-hold-coronavirus-meeting-as-it-happened/a-52362168.
Edwards E. (2020a) Americans Should Prepare for Coronavirus Crisis in U.S., CDC Says. Available at: https://www.nbcnews.com/health/health-news/americans-should-prepare-coronavirus-spread-u-s-cdc-says-n1142556.
Edwards E. (2020b) Coronavirus Case Confirmed in California is 13th in the U.S. Available at: https://www.nbcnews.com/health/health-news/coronavirus-case-confirmed-san-diego-13th-u-s-n1134561.
Ellis-Petersen H. (2020) China Promises Tougher Crackdown to Stop Spread of Disease. Available at: https://www.theguardian.com/science/live/2020/jan/26/coronavirus-outbreak-death-toll-rises-to-54-as-canada-confirms-first-case.
Ellyatt H. (2020) Russia Closes Border With China to Prevent Spread of the Coronavirus. Available at: https://www.cnbc.com/2020/01/30/coronavirus-russia-closes-border-with-china-to-prevent-spread.html.
Emma C and Scholtes J. (2020) House Swiftly Passes Bipartisan $8.3B Coronavirus Package. Available at: https://www.politico.com/news/2020/03/04/house-coronavirus-funding-121065.
Farrer M. (2020) Chinese Shares Drop Nearly 9% Amid Fears of Coronavirus Impact. Available at: https://www.theguardian.com/business/2020/feb/03/asia-pacific-shares-plunge-stock-markets-ftse-wall-street-uk-economy-fears-coronavirus-impact-on-global-economy.
Faucon B and Said S. (2020) Russia Blocks OPEC Response to Coronavirus. Available at: https://www.wsj.com/articles/russia-blocks-opec-response-to-coronavirus-11580992799.
Fazeli Y. (2020) 23 Iran MPs Have Coronavirus: Deputy Speaker. Available at: https://english.alarabiya.net/en/News/middle-east/2020/03/03/23-Iran-MPs-have-coronavirus-Deputy-Speaker.html.
FDA. (2020) FDA Takes Significant Steps in Coronavirus Response Efforts, Issues Emergence Use Authorisation for the First 2019 Novel Coronavirus Diagnostic. Available at: https://www.fda.gov/news-events/press-announcements/fda-takes-significant-step-coronavirus-response-efforts-issues-emergency-use-authorization-first.
Feiner L. (2020) Apple Extends its Store Closure in China Due to the Coronavirus. Available at: https://www.cnbc.com/2020/02/07/apple-extends-its-store-closures-in-china-due-to-the-coronavirus.html.
Follley A. (2020) Florida Governor Declares Public Health Emergency After State Records First Coronavirus Cases. Available at: https://thehill.com/policy/healthcare/485421-florida-governor-declares-public-health-emergency-after-state-gets-its.
FQ. (2020) Coronavirus, the Direct — 2502 Infections in Italy, 79 Died, 55 Only in Lombardy. A Few Weeks Old Baby in Bergamo. Available at: https://www.ilfattoquotidiano.it/2020/03/03/coronavirus-la-diretta-sono-2502-i-contagi-in-italia-79-i-morti-55-solo-in-lombardia-a-bergamo-positivo-un-bambino-di-poche-settimane/5723602/.
France-Presse A. (2020a) Chinese Banks Disinfect Banknotes to Stop Spread of Coronavirus. Available at: https://www.theguardian.com/world/2020/feb/15/chinese-banks-disinfect-banknotes-to-stop-spread-of-coronavirus.
France-Presse A. (2020b) Coronavirus: Woman on Diamond Princess Cruise Ship Tested Positive After Disembarking. Available at: https://www.theguardian.com/world/2020/feb/23/coronavirus-woman-on-diamond-princess-cruise-ship-tested-positive-after-disembarking.
France-Presse A. (2020c) Iranian MP Dies as Coronavirus Cases Hit 100, 000. Available at: https://www.newagebd.net/article/101522/iranian-mp-dies-as-coronavirus-cases-hit-100000.
France 24. (2020) First European Coronavirus Deaths in Italy Send Towns into Lockdown. Available at: https://www.

france24.com/en/20200222-first-coronavirus-death-in-europe-sends-italian-towns-into-lockdown.

Frew C. (2020) Armed Robbers Steal 600 Rolls of Toilet-Paper From Hong Kong Supermarket. Available at: https://www.unilad.co.uk/news/armed-robbers-steal-600-rolls-of-toilet-paper-from-hong-kong-supermarket/.

Gajanan M and Mansoor S. (2020) Cruise Ship Docks in Mexico, Passengers Allowed to Disembark After Being Denied Entry in Jamaica, Cayman Islands Amied Coronavirus Fears. Available at: https://time.com/5790955/cruise-ship-coronavirus-jamaica-cayman-islands/.

Garda. (2020a) Singapore: First Case of 2019-nCoV Confirmed January 23/Update 2. Available at: https://www.garda.com/crisis24/news-alerts/307966/singapore-first-case-of-2019-ncov-confirmed-january-23-update-2.

Garda. (2020b) Vietnam: Two Cases of 2019-nCoV Confirmed January 23. Available at: https://www.garda.com/crisis24/news-alerts/307976/vietnam-two-cases-of-2019-ncov-confirmed-january-23.

Giuffrida A and Cochrane L. (2020) Italy Imposes Draconian Rules to Stop Spread of Coronavirus. Available at: https://www.theguardian.com/world/2020/feb/23/italy-draconian-measures-effort-halt-coronavirus-outbreak-spread.

Giuffrida A and Willsher K. (2020) Outbreaks of Xenophobia in West as Coronavirus Spreads. Available at: https://www.theguardian.com/world/2020/jan/31/spate-of-anti-chinese-incidents-in-italy-amid-coronavirus-panic.

Global News. (2020) U.S. Woman Previously on Westerdam Cruise Ship Tests Positive for New Coronavirus. Available at: https://globalnews.ca/news/6555892/westerdam-cambodia-coronavirus-passenger/.

Gopal P. (2020) U.S. 30-Year Mortgage Rates Tumble to a Record Low of 3.29. Available at: https://www.bloomberg.com/news/articles/2020-03-05/u-s-mortgage-rates-sink-to-a-record-low-on-coronavirus-fears.

Government of Philippines. (2020) DOH Reveals More Negative 2019-nCoV Cases; Confirms First nCoV Ard Death in PH. Available at: https://www.doh.gov.ph/press-release/DOH-reveals-more-negative-2019-nCoV-cases-confirms-first-nCoV-ARD-death-in-PH?fbclid=IwAR19gEIAXIhpEfyjOFOEfblGXW_2yqu1nNchzcgSfrNbkz4EIWK7yJPlR5c.

Grady D. (2020) Coronavirus Tests Kits Sent to States are Flawed, C.D.C. Says. Available at: https://www.nytimes.com/2020/02/12/health/coronavirus-test-kits-cdc.html.

Gregorio X. (2020) Philippines Confirms First Case of Novel Coronavirus. Available at: https://www.indiatoday.in/india/story/kerala-reports-first-confirmed-novel-coronavirus-case-in-india-1641593-2020-01-30.

Griffiths J. (2020) Hospital Director Dies in Wuhan as China Designates Dead Nurses and Doctors as 'Martyrs'. Available at: https://edition.cnn.com/2020/02/17/asia/coronavirus-covid-19-update-intl-hnk/index.html.

Guidelli M. (2020) Coronavirus in Italy: Isolation of Outbreaks Started, 43 Gates and 500 Men. Available at: https://www.ansa.it/canale_saluteebenessere/notizie/sanita/2020/02/23/coronavirus-in-italia-aumentano-i-contagi.-scuole-chiuse-in-lombardia-e-veneto.-stop-al-carnevale-di-venezia_40e888b6-8418-406a-9771-7a6c3c0b45fd.html.

Gulf Insider. (2020) Kuwait Urges Citizens to Delay Travel Plans to Singpare. Available at: https://www.japantimes.co.jp/news/2020/02/09/world/coronavirus-sars-diamond-princess#.XkACJXlGT3A.

Hai H. (2020) The 15th case of corona virus infection is a 3-month-old girl in Vinh Phuc. Available at: https://www.reuters.com/article/us-china-health-germany-cases/germany-confirms-two-more-cases-of-coronavirus-raising-overall-number-to-16-idUSKBN2052GT.

Hansler J. (2020) Trump Proposes Cuts to Global Health Programs During Coronavirus. Available at: https://edition.cnn.com/asia/live-news/coronavirus-outbreak-02-10-20-intl-hnk/h_3e6957b38dd51cbb62b0d55c07b8a42a.

Harkov L. (2020) South Korean Gov't Summons Israeli Diplomat Following Israel Travel Ban. Available at: https://www.jpost.com/Israel-News/South-Koreans-refused-entry-to-Israel-over-coronavirus-fears-618419.

Harun HN. (2020) Another Chinese National Tests Positive for 2019-nCoV. Available at: https://www.nst.com.my/news/nation/2020/01/560955/another-chinese-national-tests-positive-2019-ncov.

Hopkins CD. (2020) American With Coronavirus Dies at Hospital Near Centre of Epidemic. Available at: https://www.npr.org/2020/02/08/804048544/american-with-coronavirus-dies-at-hospital-near-center-of-epidemic.

HSS. (2020) Secretary Azar Declares Public Health Emergency for United State for 2019 Novel Coronavirus. Available at: https://www.hhs.gov/about/news/2020/01/31/secretary-azar-declares-public-health-emergency-us-2019-novel-coronavirus.html.

Huang C, Wang Y, Li X, et al. (2020) Clinical Features of Patients Infected With 2019 Novel Coronavirus in Wuhan, China. The Lancet 395: 497-506.

IMF. (2020) IMF Makes Available $50 Billion to Help Address Coronavirus. Available at: https://www.imf.org/en/News/Articles/2020/03/04/sp030420-imf-makes-available-50-billion-to-help-address-coronavirus.

Impelli M. (2020) What U.S. States Have Declared a State of Emergency Amid Coronavirus Outbreak. Available at: https://www.newsweek.com/what-us-states-have-declared-state-emergency-amid-coronavirus-outbreak-1491299.

Japan Time. (2020) Japan Confirms Six More Cases From Quarantined Cruise Ship as Coronavirus Deaths Surpass SARS Toll. Available at: https://www.japantimes.co.jp/news/2020/02/09/world/coronavirus-sars-diamond-princess#.XkACJXlGT3A.

Japan Times. (2020) Countries Rush to Build Diagnostic Capacity as Coronavirus Spreads But Live Samples Elude. Available at: https://www.japantimes.co.jp/news/2020/02/11/asia-pacific/science-health-asia-pacific/countries-rush-build-diagnostic-capacity-coronavirus-spreads-live-samples-elude/.

Jeong-ho L, Zheng W and Zhou L. (2020) Chinese Scientists Race to Develop Vaccine as Coronavirus Death Toll Jumps. Available at: https://www.scmp.com/news/china/society/article/3047676/number-coronavirus-cases-china-doubles-spread-rate-accelerates.

Jiao Z. (2020) Risk Aversion Releases RMB to USD Exchange Rate Breaking "7". Available at: http://www.cs.com.cn/xwzx/hg/202002/t20200204_6021968.html.

Jiemian. (2020a) China News. Available at: https://www.jiemian.com/article/3970636.html.

Jiemian. (2020b) Li Keqiang: Introduce Measures to Encourage the Employment of College Graduates and Migrant Workers. Available at: https://www.jiemian.com/article/4028846.html.

Jiemian. (2020c) State Council: Exemption of VAT for Small-Scale Taxpayers in Hubei for 3 Months. Available at: https://www.jiemian.com/article/4028874.html.

Johnson CK. US Virus Cases Climb to 35 With Return of Cruise Passengers. Available at: https://abcnews.go.com/Health/wireStory/us-virus-cases-climb-35-return-cruise-passengers-69133172.

Johnson M. (2020) Hyundai Suspending Productin in South Korea Due to Coronovirus. Available at: https://thehill.com/policy/transportation/automobiles/481397-hyundai-suspending-production-in-south-korea-due-to.

Joseph A. (2020) Study Reports First Case of Coronavirus Spread by Asymptomatic Person. Available at: https://www.scientificamerican.com/article/study-reports-first-case-of-coronavirus-spread-by-asymptomatic-person/.

Julie. (2020) Updated Statement Regarding Westerdam. Available at: https://www.hollandamerica.com/blog/ships/ms-westerdam/statement-regarding-westerdam-in-japan/.

Junga S. (2020) South Korea Places More Than 7,000 Soldiers in Quarantine. Available at: https://www.ft.com/content/13fc82b8-56c2-11ea-a528-dd0f971febbc.

Khalik S and Goh T. (2020) Singapore Confirms 2 More Wuhan Virus Cases, Bringing Total to 3 Infected. Available at: https://www.straitstimes.com/singapore/health/singapore-confirms-2-more-wuhan-virus-cases-bringing-total-to-three-infected.

Kindred A and Hawken A. (2020) Contagion Coranavirus – 41 Million Quarantined in 14 Cities as China Closes Great Wall, Forbidden City and Disneyland. Available at: https://www.thesun.co.uk/news/10803076/coronavirus-china-lockdown-huanggang-ezhou-wuhan/.

Law V. (2020) Hong Kong Medical Workers Strike to Demand Total Border Closure. Available at: https://www.aljazeera.com/news/2020/02/hong-kong-medical-workers-strike-demand-total-border-closure-200203165501416.html.

Lee YN. (2020) Singapore Downgrades 2020 Economic Forecast Amid Coronavirus Outbreak. Available at: https://www.cnbc.com/2020/02/17/singapore-releases-fourth-quarter-full-year-2019-gdp-data.html.

Leng S and Huifeng H. (2020) Coronavirus: Atleast Three Cases Among 4,000 Passengers on China-Vietnam Cruise, Doctor Says. Available at: https://www.scmp.com/economy/china-economy/article/3048784/coronavirus-least-three-cases-among-4000-passengers-china.

Linnane C. (2020) Vans Parent VF Corp. Says 60% of China Stores Are Closed Over Coronavirus, to Update Guidance in May. Available at: https://www.marketwatch.com/story/vans-parent-vf-corp-says-60-of-china-stores-are-closed-over-coronavirus-to-update-guidance-in-may-2020-02-07.

Lok-kei S, Ho-him C and Chung K. (2020) Coronavirus: Seven More Cases Confirmed in Hong Kong, Taking City's Total Number to 49. Available at: https://www.reuters.com/article/us-china-health-germany-cases/germany-confirms-two-more-cases-of-coronavirus-raising-overall-number-to-16-idUSKBN2052GT.

Loo E. (2020) Japan's Biggest Cosplay Event Canceled Due to COVID-19 Coronavirus. Available at: https://www.animenewsnetwork.com/news/2020-02-19/japan-biggest-cosplay-event-canceled-due-to-covid-19-coronavirus/.156609.

Lovelace B and Feuer W. (2020) Pace of New Coronavirus Cases in Hubei on the Rise Again; Cruise Lines Ban Chinese Nationals. Available at: https://www.cnbc.com/2020/02/07/coronavirus-latest-updates.html.

Lum A and Chung K. (2020) Wuhan Coronavirus: Macau Confirms First Case as New Disease Looms Over Hong Kong. Available at: https://www.scmp.com/news/hong-kong/health-environment/article/3047140/china-coronavirus-macau-reports-first-case-new.

Luna F. (2020) First Confirmed nCoV Death Outside China is in Philippines. Available at: https://www.philstar.com/headlines/2020/02/02/1989762/doh-confirms-second-case-novel-coronavirus-philippines.

Macau News. (2020) Government Confirms 5 Cases of Coronavirus so far in Macau. Available at: https://macaunews.mo/government-confirms-5-cases-of-coronavirus-so-far-in-macau/.

Maresca T. (2020) South Korea Coronavirus Cases Near 1,000; 11 Dead. Available at: https://www.upi.com/Top_News/World-News/2020/02/25/South-Korea-coronavirus-cases-near-1000-11-dead/4761582619827/.

McCurry J and Ratcliffe R. (2020) Diamond Princess Cruise Ship in Japan Confirms 99 New Coronavirus Cases. Available at: https://www.theguardian.com/world/2020/feb/17/coronavirus-japan-braces-for-hundreds-more-cases-as-another-china-city-locked-down.

Mclean R, He L and Tappe A. (2020) Dow Plunges 1,000 Points, Positing its Worst Day in Two Years as Coronavirus Fears Spike. Available at: https://edition.cnn.com/2020/02/23/business/stock-futures-coronavirus/index.html.

Medical Express. (2020) South Korea Confirms Second Coronavirus Cases. Available at: https://medicalxpress.com.

Middle East Monitor. (2020) 8th Case of Coronavirus Confirmed in UAE. Available at: middleeastmonitor.com.

Ministry of Health Italy. (2020a) Covid-19 -Situation in Italy. Available at: http://www.salute.gov.it/portale/nuovocoronavirus/dettaglioContenutiNuovoCoronavirus.jsp?lingua=italiano&id=5351&area=nuovoCoronavirus&menu=vuoto/.

Ministry of Health Italy. (2020b) Covid-19: the Cases in Italy at 6 pm on March 5th. Available at: http://www.salute.gov.it/portale/nuovocoronavirus/dettaglioNotizieNuovoCoronavirus.jsp?lingua=italiano&menu=notizie&p=dalministero&id=4157.

Ministry of Health Singapore. (2020) Fourth Confirmed Imported Case of Wuhan Coronavirus Infection in Singapore. Available at: https://web.archive.org/web/20200220163229/https://www.moh.gov.sg/news-highlights/details/fourth-confirmed-imported-case-of-wuhan-coronavirus-infection-in-singapore.

Mizumoto K, Kagaya K, Zarebski A, et al. (2020) Estimating the Asymptomatic Proportion of Coronavirus Disease 2019

(COVID-19) Cases on Board the Diamond Princess Cruise Ship, Yokohama, Japan. 25: 2000180.

MSN. (2020) Who Is Jean-Luc Reitzer, the Deputy Contaminated by the Coronavirus? Available at: https://www.msn.com/fr-fr/actualite/france/qui-est-jean-luc-reitzer-le-d%c3%a9put%c3%a9-contamin%c3%a9-par-le-coronavirus/ar-BB10PrRW.

Murphy B. (2020) Chief Medical Officer's Update on Novel Coronavirus. Available at: https://www.health.gov.au/news/chief-medical-officers-update-on-novel-coronavirus-2.

NBC Los Angeles. (2020) California, Arizona Cases Push US Tally of New Virus to 5. Available at: https://www.nbclosangeles.com/news/los-angeles-countys-first-case-of-deadly-novel-coronavirus-confirmed/2298402/.

Nebehay S. (2020) WHO Advance Team on Coronavirus on Way to China: Tedros Tweet. Available at: https://www.reuters.com/article/us-china-health-who-team/who-advance-team-on-coronavirus-on-way-to-china-tedros-tweet-idUSKBN2030QX.

New Straits Times. (2020) [Breaking] 3 Coronavirus Cases Confirmed in Johor Baru. Available at: https://www.nst.com.my/news/nation/2020/01/559563/breaking-3-coronavirus-cases-confirmed-johor-baru.

Newey S. (2020) China Allocates $10bn to Contain Coronavirus as Death Toll Outstrips 2003 Sars Outbreak. Available at: https://www.telegraph.co.uk/news/2020/02/09/china-allocates-10bn-contain-coronavirus-death-toll-outstrips/.

News B. (2020) China Coronavirus: Death Toll Rises as More Cities Restrict Travel. Available at: https://www.bbc.com/news/world-asia-china-51230011.

Nguyen P. (2020) Vietnam Quarantines Rural Community of 10,000 Because of Coronavirus. Available at: https://www.usnews.com/news/world/articles/2020-02-13/vietnam-quarantines-rural-community-of-10-000-over-coronavirus-fears-officials.

NHK. (2020) 6 New Infection Confirmed Fukui Prefecture Interview. Available at: https://web.archive.org/web/20200201165246/https://www3.nhk.or.jp/news/html/20200130/k10012266331000.html?utm_int=news-new_contents_list-items_091.

Nienaber M and Reese C. (2020) Germany Confirms Two More Cases of Coronavirus, Raising Overall Number to 16. Available at: https://www.reuters.com/article/us-china-health-germany-cases/germany-confirms-two-more-cases-of-coronavirus-raising-overall-number-to-16-idUSKBN2052GT.

Nikkei. (2020) Mongolia President Under Quarantine After China Trip. Available at: https://asia.nikkei.com/Spotlight/Coronavirus/Mongolian-president-under-quarantine-after-China-trip.

Office of the Governor. (2020a) Governor Larry Hogan Declares State of Emergency, Expands Statewide Response to Novel Coronavirus. Available at: https://governor.maryland.gov/2020/03/05/governor-larry-hogan-declares-state-of-emergency-expands-statewide-response-to-novel-coronavirus/.

Office of the Governor. (2020b) No. 202: Declaring a Disaster Emergence in the State of New York. Available at: https://www.governor.ny.gov/news/no-202-declaring-disaster-emergency-state-new-york.

Office of the President. (2020) Request. Available at: https://www.whitehouse.gov/wp-content/uploads/2020/02/Coronavirus-Supplemental-Request-Letter-Final.pdf.

Olarn K. (2020) Thailand Requires Travelers From South Korea, China, Iran and Italy to Self-isolate for 14 Days. Available at: https://edition.cnn.com/asia/live-news/coronavirus-outbreak-03-08-20-intl-hnk/h_79fe9ec1c9f62239cf3b4e8385160171.

Parsey M. (2020) Gilead Partnering with China on Trial of Remdesivir as Coronavirus Treatment. Available at: https://www.genengnews.com/topics/drug-discovery/gilead-partnering-with-china-on-trial-of-remdesivir-as-coronavirus-treatment/.

Peace Corps. (2020) Peace Corps China Volunteers Evacuated Safely. Available at: https://www.peacecorps.gov/news/library/peace-corps-china-volunteers-evacuated-safely/.

Peltier E. (2020) France Confirms First Death in Europe From Coronavirus. Available at: https://www.nytimes.com/2020/02/15/world/europe/france-coronarivus-death.html.

Penh P. (2020) Cambonia Confirms First Case of Coronavirus. Available at: https://www.bangkokpost.com/world/1844884/cambodia-confirms-first-case-of-coronavirus.

Perma.cc record. (2020) Public Health, England: The Health Protection (Coronavirus) Regulation 2020. England, UK: Secretary of State, UK. Government, 1-11.

Pham S. (2020) Airlines Around the World Are Suspending Flights to China as the Coronavirus Spreads. Available at: https://edition.cnn.com/2020/01/29/business/british-airways-coronavirus/index.html.

Pompeo MR. (2020) The United States Announces Assistance to Combat the Novel Coronavirus. Available at: https://www.state.gov/the-united-states-announces-assistance-to-combat-the-novel-coronavirus/.

PPTV Online. (2020) Ministry of Health Confirmed That the Patient of the "Corona Virus" is the 8 Case. Available at: https://www.pptvhd36.com/news/%E0%B8%9B%E0%B8%A3%E0%B8%B0%E0%B9%80%E0%B8%94%E0%B9%87%E0%B8%99%E0%B8%A3%E0%B9%89%E0%B8%AD%E0%B8%99/118387.

Promchertchoo P. (2020) Wuhan Virus: 2 More Cases Confirmed in Thailand. Available at: https://www.channelnewsasia.com/news/asia/wuhan-virus-china-two-more-cases-found-thailand-12301606.

Qin A, Myeers SL and Yu E. (2020) China Tightens Wuhan Lockdown in "Wartime" Battle with Coronavirus. Available at: https://www.nytimes.com/2020/02/06/world/asia/coronavirus-china-wuhan-quarantine.html.

Quito A. (2020) How China Cna Build a Hospital for Coronavirus Patients in a Week. Available at: https://qz.com/1792705/coronavirus-the-engineering-behind-wuhans-rapidly-built-hospitals/.

Rabin RC. (2020) First Patient With Wuhan Coronavirus Is Identified in the U.S. Available at: https://www.nytimes.com/2020/01/21/health/cdc-coronavirus.html.

Ravelo JL and Jerving S. (2020) COVID-19 — A Timeline of the Coronavirus Outbreak. Available at: https://www.devex.com/news/covid-19-a-timeline-of-the-coronavirus-outbreak-96396.

Reed S. (2020) Saudi-Russian Alliance is Strained as Coronavirus Saps Demand for Oil. Available at: https://www.nytimes.com/2020/02/07/business/opec-russia-saudi-arabia.html.

Reuters. (2020a) Coronavirus: Lockheed, Raytheon Among 70 to Pull Out of Singapore Airshow. Available at: https://www.business-standard.com/article/international/coronavirus-lockheed-raytheon-among-70-to-pull-out-of-singapore-airshow-120020900104_1.html.

Reuters. (2020b) Coronavirus: Russia to Ban Chinese Citizens From Entry Amid Outbreak Fears. Available at: https://www.scmp.com/news/world/russia-central-asia/article/3051240/coronavirus-russia-ban-chinese-citizens-entry.

Reuters. (2020c) Egypt Confirms 33 New Cases of Coronavirus on Nile Cruise Ship. Available at: https://www.reuters.com/article/us-health-coronavirus-egypt-idUSKBN20U0TK.

Reuters. (2020d) Iran Says Coronavirus Death Toll Reaches 16, 95 Infected. Available at: https://nationalpost.com/pmn/health-pmn/iran-says-coronavirus-death-toll-reaches-16-95-infected.

Reuters. (2020e) Japan Confirms Second Case of Wuhan Virus: Health Ministry. Available at: https://www.reuters.com/article/us-china-health-japan-idUSKBN1ZM35W.

Reuters. (2020f) Japan Confirms Third Case of Wuhan Virus. Available at: https://www.reuters.com/article/us-china-health-japan-idUSKBN1ZO08O.

Reuters. (2020g) Nepal Confirms First Case of New Coronavirus. Available at: https://www.reuters.com/article/us-china-health-nepal/nepal-confirms-first-case-of-new-coronavirus-idUSKBN1ZN1S2.

Reuters. (2020h) Qatar Bans Arrivals From 14 Countries Over Coronavirus Fears. Available at: https://www.reuters.com/article/us-health-coronavirus-qatar/qatar-bans-arrivals-from-14-countries-over-coronavirus-fears-idUSKBN20V116.

Reuters. (2020i) Russia Reports First Coronavirus Cases. Available at: https://www.themoscowtimes.com/2020/01/31/russia-reports-first-coronavirus-cases-a69123.

Reuters. (2020j) Saudi Arabia Suspends Travel to and From Nine Countries Including UAE, Bahrain and Egypt. Available at: https://www.reuters.com/article/us-health-coronavirus-saudi-travel/saudi-arabia-suspends-travel-to-and-from-nine-countries-including-uae-bahrain-and-egypt-idUSKBN20V14D.

Reuters. (2020k) Sri Lanka Confirms First Case of Coronavirus: Health Official. Available at: https://www.reuters.com/article/us-health-china-sri-lanka/sri-lanka-confirms-first-case-of-coronavirus-health-official-idUSKBN1ZQ1WF.

Reuters. (2020l) Third Person Dies in Coronavirus Outbreak in Northern Italy: Official. Available at: https://www.reuters.com/article/us-china-health-italy-death/third-person-dies-in-coronavirus-outbreak-in-northern-italy-official-idUSKCN20H0N1.

Reuters AFP. (2020) Iranian Mayor Tests Positive for Coronavirus With New Cases Reported. Available at: https://www.arabnews.com/node/1631516/middle-east.

Rothe C, Schunk M, Sothmann P, et al. (2020) Transmission of 2019-nCoV Infection from an Asymptomatic Contact in Germany. New England Journal of Medicine 382: 970-971.

Saey TH. (2020) The First Case of Coronavirus Being Spread by a Person With no Symptoms Has Been Found. Available at: https://www.sciencenews.org/article/first-case-coronavirus-spread-person-no-symptoms-found-germany.

Safi M, Jones S and Willsher K. (2020) China Braces for Return to Work as Coronavirus Deaths Exceed SARS. Available at: https://www.theguardian.com/world/2020/feb/09/coronavirus-global-death-toll-overtakes-sars-epidemic.

Salo J. (2020) US Confirms 53 Coronavirus Cases, Including Evacuated Cruise Passengers. Available at: https://nypost.com/2020/02/24/us-confirms-53-coronavirus-cases-including-evacuated-cruise-passengers/.

Samuels B and Hellmann J. (2020) CDC Has Tested 1,583 People for Coronavirus. Available at: https://thehill.com/homenews/administration/486452-cdc-has-tested-1583-people-for-coronavirus.

Sang-Hun C. (2020) North Korea Bans Foreign Tourists Over Coronavirus, Tour Operator Says. Available at: https://www.nytimes.com/2020/01/21/world/asia/coronavirus-china-north-korea-tourism-ban.html.

Schnirring L. (2020) WHO Sees no Sign of nCoV Peak in China as Cases Rise Overseas. Available at: https://www.cidrap.umn.edu/news-perspective/2020/02/who-sees-no-sign-ncov-peak-china-cases-rise-overseas.

Selsky A. (2020) Wash. State Sees 1st Virus Death in US, Declares Emergency. Available at: https://apnews.com/f175d89567a26d59cab27725c9e8a0d7.

Sgueglia K. (2020) US National Security Adviser: "There Is no Reason for Americans to Panic". Available at: https://edition.cnn.com/asia/live-news/coronavirus-outbreak-02-02-20-intl-hnk/index.html.

Shear MD, Weiland N and Rogers K. (2020) Trump Names Mike Pence to Lead Coronavirus Response. Available at: https://www.nytimes.com/2020/02/26/us/politics/trump-coronavirus-cdc.html.

Shenzen China. (2020) Shenzhen Special Economic Zone Prohibits the Consumption of Wild Animals. Available at: http://www.sz.gov.cn/cn/xxgk/zfxxgj/zwdt/content/post_6740871.html.

Shin H and Yi HY. (2020) Secretive Church at Centre of South Korea's Explosive Coronavirus Outbreak. Available at: https://www.reuters.com/article/us-china-health-southkorea-church/secretive-church-at-center-of-south-koreas-explosive-coronavirus-outbreak-idUSKCN20L0Q8.

Sim W. (2020) Coronavirus: Japan Reports 41 More Positive Cases on Cruise Ship, Total Cases on Diamond Princess Now 61. Available at: https://www.straitstimes.com/asia/east-asia/coronavirus-another-41-on-japan-cruise-tested-positive-nhk.

Sipalan J. (2020) Malaysis Confirms Fourth Case of Coronavirus Infection. Available at: https://www.cnbc.com/2020/01/24/france-confirms-2-cases-of-virus-from-china-1st-in-europe.html.

Smith R. (2020) Iran Rejects Offer for U.S. Humanitarian Aid. Available at: https://www.bloomberg.com/news/articles/2020-04-24/reckitt-warns-against-using-disinfectants-to-treat-coronavirus.

Standaert M. (2020) Coronavirus Outbreak: Doctor in Wuhan Hospital Dies as Army Medics Flown in Available at: https://www.theguardian.com/science/2020/jan/25/

coronavirus-outbreak-doctor-in-wuhan-hospital-dies-as-army-medics-flown-in.

Starr B and LeBlanc P. (2020) US Army Suspends Soldier Travel to and From South Korea and Italy Amid Mounting Coronavirus Concern. Available at: https://edition.cnn.com/2020/03/08/politics/us-army-coronavirus-south-korea-italy/index.html.

Sun LH. (2020) CDC Sends Test Kits to More Than 100 U.S. labs. Available at: https://www.washingtonpost.com/world/asia_pacific/coronavirus-china-live-updates/2020/02/05/114ced8a-479c-11ea-bc78-8a18f7afcee7_story.html.

Sunnybrook. (2020) Patient Admitted With Novel Coronavirus. Available at: https://sunnybrook.ca/media/item.asp?c=1&i=2043&f=novel-coronavirus-2020.

Surging News. (2020) 6 Angle Masks Sold 1 Yuan Was Fined 40,000? Honghu Hubei Has Started a New Investigation of the Penalty. Available at: https://www.sohu.com/a/372724100_260616.

Tan H. (2020) Coronavirus Whistleblower Doctor Dies, Sparking Outpouring — and Censorship — on Social Media. Available at: https://www.cnbc.com/2020/02/07/hashtag-censored-after-coronavirus-whistleblower-doctors-death.html.

Taylor A. (2020) White House Unveils $2.5B Emergency Coronavirus Plan. Available at: https://apnews.com/39d9c237bfc75c93016870b00ac6dab8.

The Brussels Times. (2020) First Case of Coronavirus Confirmed in Belgium. Available at: https://www.brusselstimes.com/all-news/belgium-all-news/93361/first-case-of-coronavirus-confirmed-in-belgium/.

The Canadian Press. (2020) B.C. Confirms Seventh Case of COVID-19, Bringing Total Number of Canadian Cases to 11. Available at: https://nationalpost.com/news/canada/canadian-press-newsalert-seventh-case-of-covid-19-diagnosed-in-b-c.

The Government of the Hong Kong Specia Administrative Region. (2020) CHP Investigates Three Additional Imported Cases of Novel Coronavirus Infection. Available at: https://www.info.gov.hk/gia/general/202001/25/P2020012500012.htm.

The Local. (2020) Italy Suspends all China Flights as Coronavirus Cases Confirmed in Rome. Available at: https://www.thelocal.it/20200131/italy-suspends-all-china-flights-after-coronavirus-cases-confirmed-in-rome.

The Moscow Times. (2020) Russia Quarantines Chinese Diplomat as Coronavirus Precaution. Available at: https://www.themoscowtimes.com/2020/02/10/russia-quarantines-chinese-diplomat-as-coronavirus-precaution-interfax-a69224.

The Straits Times. (2020a) Coronavirus Silences Hyundai's Car Plant in South Korea – The World's Biggest Capacity Vehicle Factory. Available at: https://www.straitstimes.com/business/economy/coronavirus-claims-worlds-biggest-capacity-car-plant.

The Straits Times. (2020b) Coronavirus Vaccine Could be Ready in 18 Months: WHO Chief. Available at: https://www.straitstimes.com/asia/east-asia/coronavirus-vaccine-could-be-ready-in-18-months-who-chief.

The Straits Times. (2020c) Coronavirus: China Warns Against Travel to US, Citing Unfair Treatment in Virus Control. Available at: https://edition.cnn.com/2020/02/23/business/stock-futures-coronavirus/index.html.

The Straits Times. (2020d) Coronavirus: Qatar, Kuwait advices Citizens to Avoid Unnecessary Travel to Singapore. Available at: https://www.japantimes.co.jp/news/2020/02/09/world/coronavirus-sars-diamond-princess#.XkACJXlGT3A.

The Straits Times. (2020e) Coronavirus: South Korea Confirms 70 More Coronavirus Cases, Total 833; 7th Death Reported. Available at: https://www.straitstimes.com/asia/east-asia/coronavirus-south-korea-reports-161-new-cases-bringing-total-to-763.

The Straits Times. (2020f) Coronavirus: South Korea Raises Alert to Highest Level as Number of Cases Jumps to 602, With 5 Deaths. Available at: https://www.straitstimes.com/asia/east-asia/south-korea-reports-123-more-coronavirus-cases-2-deaths.

The Straits Times. (2020g) South Korea Coronavirus Cases Surge to 2,337, BTS Cancel Gigs. Available at: https://www.straitstimes.com/asia/east-asia/south-korea-reports-256-new-coronavirus-cases-total-tally-now-2022.

The Wall Street Journal. (2020) China Expels Three Wall Street Journal Reporters. Available at: https://www.wsj.com/articles/china-expels-three-wall-street-journal-reporters-11582100355.

The World Bank. (2020a) Statement on the Novel Coronavirus in China Available at: https://www.worldbank.org/en/news/statement/2020/02/03/statement-on-the-novel-coronavirus-in-china-february-3-2020.

The World Bank. (2020b) World Bank Group Announces Up to $12 Billion Immediate Support for COVID-19 Country Response. Available at: https://www.worldbank.org/en/news/press-release/2020/03/03/world-bank-group-announces-up-to-12-billion-immediate-support-for-covid-19-country-response.

Thomson Reuters. (2020) Only Three U.S. States Can Test for Coronavirus – Public Lab group. Available at: https://news.trust.org/item/20200221170633-5papx/.

Timiraos N. (2020) Federal Reserve Cuts Rates by Half Percentage Point to Combat Virus Fear. Available at: https://www.wsj.com/articles/federal-reserve-cuts-interest-rates-by-half-percentage-point-11583247606?mod=livecoverage_web.

U.S. Embassy in Georgia. (2020) Coronavirus Aid From U.S. Groups Arrives in China. Available at: https://ge.usembassy.gov/coronavirus-aid-from-u-s-groups-arrives-in-china-february-6/.

U.S. Department of State. (2020a) China Travel Advisory. Available at: https://travel.state.gov/content/travel/en/traveladvisories/traveladvisories/china-travel-advisory.html.

U.S. Department of State. (2020b) Joint Statement by U.S. Department of State and U.S. Department of Health and Human Services on Repatriation of American Passengers From the Diamond Princess Cruise Ship. Available at: https://www.state.gov/joint-statement-by-u-s-department-of-state-and-u-s-department-of-health-and-human-services-on-repatriation-of-american-passengers-from-the-diamond-princess-cruise-ship/.

UN. (2020) Coronavirus Update: 290 Million Students Now Stuck at Home. Available at: https://news.un.org/en/story/2020/03/1058791.

UNICEF. (2020) UN Releases $15 Million to Help Vulnerable Countries Battle the Spread of the Coronavirus. Available at: https://www.unicef.org/press-releases/un-releases-15-million-help-vulnerable-countries-battle-spread-coronavirus.

University S. (2020) Shenzhen University Develops the World's First Single-Agent Chemiluminescence COVID-19 Antibody Detection Kit. Available at: https://en.szu.edu.cn/info/1010/1192.htm.

Unnithan PSG. (2020) Kerela Reports First Confirmed Coronavirus Case in India. Available at: https://www.indiatoday.in/india/story/kerala-reports-first-confirmed-novel-corona virus-case-in-india-1641593-2020-01-30.

USCDC. (2020a) CDC Confirms Person-to-Person Spread of New Coronavirus in the United States. Available at: https://www.cdc.gov/media/releases/2020/p0130-coronavirus-spre ad.html.

USCDC. (2020b) Second Travel-related Case of 2019 Novel Coronavirus Detected in United States. Available at: https://www.cdc.gov/media/releases/2020/p0124-second-travel-coronavirus.html.

Waldrop T. (2020) The 1st Group of American Evacuated From Wuhan and Quarantined Over Coronavirus Just Got Released. Available at: https://edition.cnn.com/2020/02/10/us/coronavirus-american-evacuees-release/index.html.

Wallace D. (2020) Army Suspends Travel for Soldiers, Families to and From South Korea Amid Coronavirus Outbreak. Available at: https://www.foxnews.com/health/coronavirus-us-army-south-korea-suspends-travel-soldiers.

Wang V and Wee S-L. (2020) China to Ease Coronavirus Lockdown on Hubei 2 Months After Imposing it. Available at: https://www.nytimes.com/2020/03/24/world/asia/china-coronavirus-lockdown-hubei.html.

Westcott B and Deng S. (2020) China Has Made Eating Wild Animals Illegal After the Coronavirus Outbreak. But Ending the Trade Won't be Easy. Available at: https://edition.cnn.com/2020/03/05/asia/china-coronavirus-wildlife-consum ption-ban-intl-hnk/index.html.

White House. (2020) Remarks by Vice President Pence at the White House Initiative on Asian Americans and Pacific Islanders Lunar New Year Celebration. Available at: https://www.whitehouse.gov/briefings-statements/remarks-vice-pr esident-pence-white-house-initiative-asian-americans-paci fic-islanders-lunar-new-year-celebration/.

WHO. (2020a) Coronavirus Disease 2019 (COVID-19): Situation Report- 31. Available at: https://www.who.int/docs/default-source/coronaviruse/situation-reports/20200220-sitrep-31-covid-19.pdf?sfvrsn=dfd11d24_2.

WHO. (2020b) Coronavirus Disease 2019 (COVID-19): Situation Report- 40. Available at: https://www.who.int/docs/default-source/coronaviruse/situation-reports/20200229-sitrep-40-covid-19.pdf?sfvrsn=7203e653_2.

WHO. (2020c) Coronavirus Disease 2019 (COVID-19): Situation Report- 49. Available at: https://www.who.int/docs/default-source/coronaviruse/situation-reports/20200309-sitrep-49-covid-19.pdf?sfvrsn=70dabe61_4.

WHO. (2020d) Coronavirus Disease 2019 (COVID-19): Situation Report -30. Available at: https://www.who.int/docs/default-source/coronaviruse/situation-reports/20200219-sitrep-30-covid-19.pdf?sfvrsn=6e50645_2.

WHO. (2020e) Coronavirus Disease 2019 (COVID-19): Situation Report -36. Available at: https://www.who.int/docs/default-source/coronaviruse/situation-reports/20200225-sitrep-36-covid-19.pdf?sfvrsn=2791b4e0_2.

WHO. (2020f) Coronavirus Disease 2019 (COVID-19): Situation Report -41. Available at: https://www.who.int/docs/default-source/coronaviruse/situation-reports/20200301-sitrep-41-covid-19.pdf?sfvrsn=6768306d_2.

WHO. (2020g) Coronavirus Disease 2019 (COVID-19): Situation Report -42. Available at: https://www.who.int/docs/default-source/coronaviruse/situation-reports/20200302-sitrep-42-covid-19.pdf?sfvrsn=224c1add_2.

WHO. (2020h) Coronavirus Disease 2019 (COVID-19): Situation Report -43. Available at: https://www.who.int/docs/default-source/coronaviruse/situation-reports/20200303-sitrep-43-covid-19.pdf?sfvrsn=2c21c09c_2.

WHO. (2020i) Coronavirus Disease 2019 (COVID-19): Situation Report -44. Available at: https://www.who.int/docs/default-source/coronaviruse/situation-reports/20200304-sitrep-44-covid-19.pdf?sfvrsn=783b4c9d_2.

WHO. (2020j) Coronavirus Disease 2019 (COVID-19): Situation Report -46. Available at: https://www.who.int/docs/default-source/coronaviruse/situation-reports/20200306-sitrep-46-covid-19.pdf?sfvrsn=96b04adf_2.

WHO. (2020k) Coronavirus Disease 2019 (COVID-19): Situation Report - 23. Available at: https://www.who.int/docs/default-source/coronaviruse/situation-reports/20200212-sitrep-23-ncov.pdf?sfvrsn=41e9fb78_2.

WHO. (2020l) Coronavirus Disease 2019 (COVID-19): Situation Report - 24. Available at: https://www.who.int/docs/default-source/coronaviruse/situation-reports/20200213-sitrep-24-covid-19.pdf?sfvrsn=9a7406a4_4.

WHO. (2020m) Coronavirus Disease 2019 (COVID-19): Situation Report - 28. Available at: https://www.who.int/docs/default-source/coronaviruse/situation-reports/20200217-sitrep-28-covid-19.pdf?sfvrsn=a19cf2ad_2.

WHO. (2020n) Coronavirus Disease 2019 (COVID-19): Situation Report - 35. Available at: https://www.who.int/docs/default-source/coronaviruse/situation-reports/20200224-sitrep-35-covid-19.pdf?sfvrsn=1ac4218d_2.

WHO. (2020o) Global Research and Innovation Forum to Mobilize Internaitonal Action in Response to the Novel Coronavirus (2019-nCoV) Emergency. Available at: https://www.who.int/news-room/events/detail/2020/02/11/defau lt-calendar/global-research-and-innovation-forum-to-mobil ize-international-action-in-response-to-the-novel-coronavirus-(2019-ncov)-emergency.

WHO. (2020p) Munich Security Conference. Available at: https://www.who.int/dg/speeches/detail/munich-security-conference.

WHO. (2020q) Novel Coronavirus (2019-nCoV): Situation Report -22. Available at: https://www.who.int/docs/default-source/coronaviruse/situation-reports/20200211-sitrep-22-ncov.pdf.

WHO. (2020r) Novel Coronavirus (2019-nCoV) Situation Report-3. Available at: https://www.who.int/docs/default-source/coronaviruse/situation-reports/20200123-sitrep-3-2019-ncov.pdf.

WHO. (2020s) Novel Coronavirus (2019-nCoV) Situation Report-5. Available at: https://www.who.int/docs/default-source/coronaviruse/situation-reports/20200125-sitrep-5-2019-ncov.pdf?sfvrsn=429b143d_8.

WHO. (2020t) Novel Coronavirus (2019-nCoV) Situation Report-6. Available at: https://www.who.int/docs/default-source/coronaviruse/situation-reports/20200126-sitrep-6-2019–ncov.pdf?sfvrsn=beaeee0c_4.

WHO. (2020u) Novel Coronavirus (2019-nCoV) Situation Report-9. Available at: https://www.who.int/docs/default-source/coronaviruse/situation-reports/20200129-sitrep-9-ncov-v2.pdf?sfvrsn=e2c8915_2.

WHO. (2020v) Novel Coronavirus (2019-nCoV) Situation Report-15. Available at: https://www.who.int/docs/default-source/coronaviruse/situation-reports/20200204-sitrep-15-ncov.pdf?sfvrsn=88fe8ad6_2.

WHO. (2020w) Novel Coronavirus (2019-nCoV) Situation Report- 1. Available at: https://www.who.int/docs/default-source/coronaviruse/situation-reports/20200121-sitrep-1-2019-ncov.pdf?sfvrsn=20a99c10_4.

WHO. (2020x) Novel Coronavirus (2019-nCoV) Situation Report - 7. Available at: https://www.who.int/docs/default-source/coronaviruse/situation-reports/20200127-sitrep-7-2019–ncov.pdf?sfvrsn=98ef79f5_2.

WHO. (2020y) Novel Coronavirus (2019-nCoV): Situation Report- 2. Available at: https://www.who.int/docs/default-source/coronaviruse/situation-reports/20200122-sitrep-2-2019-ncov.pdf?sfvrsn=4d5bcbca_2.

WHO. (2020z) Novel Coronavirus (2019-nCoV): Situation Report -10. Available at: https://www.who.int/docs/default-source/coronaviruse/situation-reports/20200130-sitrep-10-ncov.pdf?sfvrsn=d0b2e480_2.

WHO. (2020aa) Novel Coronavirus (2019-nCoV): Situation Report -11. Available at: https://www.who.int/docs/default-source/coronaviruse/situation-reports/20200131-sitrep-11-ncov.pdf?sfvrsn=de7c0f7_4.

WHO. (2020ab) Novel Coronavirus (2019-nCoV): Situation Report -12. Available at: https://www.who.int/docs/default-source/coronaviruse/situation-reports/20200201-sitrep-12-ncov.pdf?sfvrsn=273c5d35_2.

WHO. (2020ac) Novel Coronavirus (2019-nCoV): Situation Report -13. World Health Organisation, 1-7.

WHO. (2020ad) Novel Coronavirus (2019-nCoV): Situation Report -17. Available at: https://www.who.int/docs/default-source/coronaviruse/situation-reports/20200206-sitrep-17-ncov.pdf?sfvrsn=17f0dca_4.

WHO. (2020ae) Novel Coronavirus (2019-nCoV): Situation Report -18. Available at: https://www.who.int/docs/default-source/coronaviruse/situation-reports/20200207-sitrep-18-ncov.pdf?sfvrsn=fa644293_2.

WHO. (2020af) Novel Coronavirus (2019-nCoV): Situation Report -19. Available at: https://www.who.int/docs/default-source/coronaviruse/situation-reports/20200208-sitrep-19-ncov.pdf?sfvrsn=6e091ce6_2.

WHO. (2020ag) Novel Coronavirus (2019-nCoV): Situation Report -20. Available at: https://www.who.int/docs/default-source/coronaviruse/situation-reports/20200208-sitrep-19-ncov.pdf?sfvrsn=6e091ce6_2.

WHO. (2020ah) Novel Coronavirus (2019-nCoV): Situation Report -21. Available at: https://www.who.int/docs/default-source/coronaviruse/situation-reports/20200210-sitrep-21-ncov.pdf?sfvrsn=947679ef_2.

WHO. (2020ai) Novel Coronavirus (2019-nCoV): Situation Report - 8. Available at: https://www.who.int/docs/default-source/coronaviruse/situation-reports/20200128-sitrep-8-ncov-cleared.pdf?sfvrsn=8b671ce5_2.

WHO. (2020aj) Novel Coronavirus (2019-nCoV): Situation Report - 14. Available at: https://www.who.int/docs/default-source/coronaviruse/situation-reports/20200203-sitrep-14-ncov.pdf?sfvrsn=f7347413_4.

WHO. (2020ak) Novel Coronavirus (2019-nCoV): Situation Report - 16 - ERRATUM. Available at: https://www.who.int/docs/default-source/coronaviruse/situation-reports/20200205-sitrep-16-ncov.pdf?sfvrsn=88fe8ad6_2.

WHO. (2020al) Press Conference of WHO-China Joint Mission on COVID-19. Beijing, China: WHO, 1-26.

WHO. (2020am) Shortage of Personal Protective Equipment Endangering Health Workers Worldwide. Available at: https://www.who.int/news-room/detail/03-03-2020-shortage-of-personal-protective-equipment-endangering-health-workers-worldwide.

WHO. (2020an) Statement on the Meeting of the International Health Regulations (2005) Emergency Committee Regarding the Outbreak of Novel Coronavirus (2019-nCoV). Available at: https://www.who.int/news-room/detail/23-01-2020-statement-on-the-meeting-of-the-international-health-regulations-(2005)-emergency-committee-regarding-the-outbreak-of-novel-coronavirus-(2019-ncov).

WHO. (2020ao) Statement on the Second Meeting of the International Health Regulation (2005) Emergency Committe Regarding the Outbreak of Novel Coronavirus (2019-nCoV). Geneva, Switzerland: WHO.

WHO. (2020ap) Updated WHO Recommendations for International Traffic in Relation to COVID-19 Outbreak. Available at: https://www.who.int/news-room/articles-detail/updated-who-recommendations-for-international-traffic-in-relation-to-covid-19-outbreak/.

WHO. (2020aq) US$675 Million Needed for New Coronavirus Preparedness and Response Global Plan. Available at: https://www.who.int/news-room/detail/05-02-2020-us-675-million-needed-for-new-coronavirus-preparedness-and-response-global-plan.

WHO. (2020ar) Virtual Press Conference 6 March, 2020 on COVID-19. Available at: https://www.who.int/docs/default-source/coronaviruse/transcripts/who-audio-emergencies-coronavirus-press-conference-full-06mar2020.pdf?sfvrsn=6e557eb1_4.

WHO. (2020as) WHO Director-General's Opening Remarks at the Media Briefing on COVID-19 — 28 February 2020. Available at: https://www.who.int/dg/speeches/detail/who-director-general-s-opening-remarks-at-the-media-briefing-on-covid-19—28-february-2020.

WHO. (2020at) WHO Director-General's Remarks at the Media Briefing on COVID-2019 Outbreak on 17th February

2020. Available at: https://www.who.int/dg/speeches/detail/who-director-general-s-remarks-at-the-media-briefing-on-covid-2019-outbreak-on-17-february-2020.

WHO. (2020au) WHO Pledges to Support African Countries on Joint Coronavirus Disease Preparedness and Response Strategy. Available at: https://www.afro.who.int/news/who-pledges-support-african-countries-joint-coronavirus-disease-preparedness-and-response.

WHO. (2020av) WHO to Accelerate Research and Innovation for New Coronavirus. Available at: https://www.who.int/news-room/detail/06-02-2020-who-to-accelerate-research-and-innovation-for-new-coronavirus.

William Wan, Katie Mettler, Berger M, et al. (2020) First Coronavirus Death in U.S. and New Cases Detected as Testing Expands. Available at: https://www.washingtonpost.com/health/first-us-coronavirus-death-prompts-new-travel-restrictions-from-trump/2020/02/29/4d492a7c-5b2b-11ea-9b35-def5a027d470_story.html.

Winsor M and Schumaker E. (2020) Northern Italy Closes Schools and Suspends Gatherings as Coronavirus Case Mount. Available at: https://abcnews.go.com/International/hundreds-chinese-inmates-infected-coronavirus-outbreak-spreads-prisons/story?id=69120484.

Worley W. (2020) DFID Goes Quiet on COVID-19 Response. Available at: https://www.devex.com/news/dfid-goes-quiet-on-covid-19-response-96851.

Wu Z and McGoogan JM. (2020) Characteristics of and Important Lessons From the Coronavirus Disease 2019 (COVID-19) Outbreak in China: Summary of a Report of 72 314 Cases From the Chinese Center for Disease Control and Prevention. Journal of the American Medical Association 323: 1239-1242.

Xinghui K. (2020) Singapore Closes Borders to all Foreign Travellers From China to Stem Spread of Coronavirus. Available at: https://www.themoscowtimes.com/2020/01/31/russia-reports-first-coronavirus-cases-a69123.

Xinhua. (2020a) China's Top Legislature Postpones Annual Session. Available at: http://www.xinhuanet.com/english/2020-02/24/c_138814164.htm.

Xinhua. (2020b) S. Korea Confirms 851 More Cases of COVID-19, 5,186 in Total. Available at: http://www.xinhuanet.com/english/2020-03/03/c_138839677.htm.

Xinhua. (2020c) Xi Inspects Novel Coronavirus Prevention, Control Work in Beijing. Available at: http://www.xinhuanet.com/english/2020-02/10/c_138771195.htm.

Xinhua News Agency. (2020) The National Development and Reform Commission Urgently Issued 200 Million Yuan to Support Hubei to Improve the Treatment Capacity of Severely Infected Patients. Available at: https://www.jiemian.com/article/3958370.html.

Xiong Y, Alam HA and Gan N. (2020) Wuhun Hospital Announces Death of Whilstleblower Doctor Li Wenliang. Available at: https://edition.cnn.com/2020/02/06/asia/li-wenliang-coronavirus-whistleblower-doctor-dies-intl/index.html.

Xu Y. (2020) Public Transport in Wuhan Suspended Due to Coronavirus Concerns. Available at: https://www.npr.org/sections/goatsandsoda/2020/01/22/798602296/public-transport-in-wuhan-suspended-due-to-coronavirus-concerns.

Yan S. (2020) Wuhan Mayor Offers to Resign After Admitting Slow Respose to Coronavirus Outbreak. Available at: https://www.telegraph.co.uk/news/2020/01/27/chinese-premier-li-keqiang-wuhan-lead-emergency-efforts-coronavirus/.

Yeping Y. (2020) Stacks of Cash Wait Destruction Due to Coronavirus. Available at: https://www.globaltimes.cn/content/1179654.shtml.

Yle. (2020) Finland's First Coronavirus Case Confirmed in Lapland. Available at: https://yle.fi/uutiset/osasto/news/finlands_first_coronavirus_case_confirmed_in_lapland/11182855.

Yonhap. (2020a) (LEAD) S. Korea Reports 3 More Deaths From Coronavirus, Death Toll Rises to 16. Available at: https://en.yna.co.kr/view/AEN20200228009851325.

Yonhap. (2020b) S. Korea Reports 2 More New Coronavirus Cases, Total Now at 6. Available at: http://www.koreaherald.com/view.php?ud=20200130000905.

Yuan S. (2020) Local Red Cross Under Fire Over China Coronavirus Donation Mess. Available at: https://www.aljazeera.com/news/2020/02/local-red-cross-fire-china-coronavirus-donation-mess-200202055418491.html.

Yusof A. (2020) Malaysia Confirms Sixth Citizen Case of Coronavirus, Man Worked in Macau Before Coming Home Unwell. Available at: https://www.channelnewsasia.com/news/asia/coronavirus-malaysia-confirms-sixth-citizen-case-macau-12415998.

Zere AT. (2020) Trump's Travel Ban: Thousands of Lives in Limbo. Available at: https://www.aljazeera.com/indepth/opinion/trump-travel-ban-thousands-lives-limbo-200213123339756.html.

Zhong R and Mozur P. (2020) To Tame Coronavirus, Mao-Style Social Control. Available at: https://www.nytimes.com/2020/02/15/business/china-coronavirus-lockdown.html.

Zhou C, Wu W, Pinghui Z, et al. (2020) Coronavirus: WHO Enlists Internet Giants in War on Rumours as Mainland China Death Toll Hits 361. Available at: https://www.scmp.com/news/china/society/article/3048643/coronavirus-57-more-deaths-and-2829-new-cases-china-authorities.

CHAPTER 3

The Third 50 Days: A Detailed Chronological Timeline and Extensive Review of Literature Documenting the COVID-19 Pandemic From Day 100 to Day 150

INTRODUCTION

The past 100 days of the COVID-19 pandemic had been eventful, as the reality of the disease was clear globally, where no single continent had been spared. The next 50 days (day 100 to day 150) were marked with major milestones, challenging and most trying in different spheres of life as is demonstrated in succeeding sections. To start with, during this period, the number of confirmed cases increased from slightly above 100,000 to a high of 3 million and counting (Spotlight, 2020), with the number of casualties increasing from 3809 deaths to over 215,000 deaths across the globe by the end of the 150 days. In addition, the number of affected countries increased from 105 countries to 210 countries and territories (Worldometer, 2020). Another change that was witnessed within the third 50 days is the shifting of the COVID-19 pandemic epicenter from Europe to the United States, where the numbers of confirmed cases in the country, being—by that time—more than a quarter of the confirmed cases in the rest of the world (Kirby and Stewart, 2020).

As the impacts of the coronavirus continued to be felt, there was evidence of an economic downturn in different countries, including in developed economies, where the number of people filing for unemployment claims increased. Due to the economic hardships, it became apparent that many countries were trying to ease the lockdown restrictions to allow for reopening of economies, but in a gradual and cautious manner to avoid the reemergence of cases. It is within these 50 days that governments were seen to propose economic stimulus packages to bail out their citizens and economies, including companies that were already struggling due to reduced activities. At the same time, due to the economic and social strives, there was evidence of political tension between countries as they trade blame on responsibilities toward containing the coronavirus before it spread, and become global pandemic (Business Today, 2020a; Davidson, 2020a; Smith, 2020).

During these 50 days, it also became clear that the world was a long way before a vaccine could be developed and thus, the demand for personal protective equipment (PPEs) would continue, and we see countries and regions formulating policies to control the exportation of PPEs and medical supplies to other countries. With the increasing scarcity of PPEs and other basic, medical essentials, these were seen to rely on the World Health Organization (WHO) and well-wishers for the supplies.

Within these 50 days, there is also evidence of there was no safe-haven against coronavirus, as even those in cruise ships and aircraft carriers were infected and with cases in such places spreading faster (CNA, 2020c; Gajanan and Mansoor, 2020; Kaneko and Kim, 2020; Willsher and Sabbagh, 2020). It also dawned that even those in positions of power and authority are not immune to the virus, where some even succumbed to their injuries. Within these 50 days, it also became apparent that every single sector is highly dependent on the health sector, as those like sports and entertainment, religious sectors and others remained "grounded" with some high profile events such as professional football leagues, Olympics, and Wrestling being canceled, postponed, or suspended indefinitely (BBC Sport, 2020; Cacciola and Deb, 2020; Schad, 2020).

During this period also, it becomes apparent that it is possible for technology companies to set aside their

Surveying the Covid-19 Pandemic and Its Implications. https://doi.org/10.1016/B978-0-12-824313-8.00003-6

competition and come together for the common goal of humanity (Apple, 2020). Therefore, even as events of these third 50 days had been devastating and heartbreaking, there is much that humanity can learn, and have learned, and going forward, even after the COVID-19 is finally phased out, as people, governments, regions, and economies embark on rebuilding, some of the positives that have been learned will need to be kept alive. The following sections document the unfolding of the pandemic.

DAY 102—MARCH 11, 2020

During this month, every effort counted in the fight against the spread of COVID-19, and this was emphasized by the events of March 11. On this day, finally, the WHO conceded that without a doubt, coronavirus amounted to a global pandemic (WHO, 2020ad). The build-up to this global pandemic announcement saw a national wide lockdown declared in Italy on 9th following an uncontrollable and astronomic increase in the number of new cases and deaths in the country (BBC, 2020c). Following this, the country was beginning to experience unprecedented abandonment by its neighbors and country members of the EU who had continued to issue a travel advisory to their citizens against traveling into or from Italy (Gov.UK, 2020a). Unsurprisingly, by 10th, all 26 EU member states had experienced the outbreak of the COVID-19 disease, and most of the first cases were related to travelers fleeing Italy after the situation therein started to worsen (WHO, 2020ad).

In North America, the situation in the United States was also getting out of hand, with over 24 states including Arizona, Washington D.C., Michigan, Colorado, Vermont and Rhode Island, and others declaring states of emergency (Razek, 2020). Here, on March 10, the United Nations Headquarters in New York closed its doors to the public for fear of spreading the virus (Krisel, 2020). As the situation escalated, with over 1000 confirmed cases in the country, and over 31 deaths from the virus, the National Basketball Association (NBA), one of the most popular and fancied sporting activity in North America abruptly suspended its season, as of March 11, when a player of the Utah Jazz tested positive for coronavirus, just before their game with Oklahoma City began (Cacciola and Deb, 2020). These unfolding attracted a host of intervention measures in the country to ensure people would observe the health guidelines, especially by staying at home and keeping social distancing. First, on March 10, Vice President Pence announced that medical insurance companies had agreed to waive all copayments on COVID-19 testing and also extended their coverage for the treatment of the disease (Office of the President, 2020b). Similarly, the country, through Homeland Security, announced a level 3 travel advisory and subsequently temporarily restricting entry to all foreign travelers from China, Iran, and certain countries of Europe. The restrictions also demanded that all American citizens and legal permanent residents and their immediate families returning from countries already affected by the virus must undergo a self-quarantine for a minimum of 14 days upon arrival (Homeland Security, 2020). This announcement was affirmed by the Oval Office address by President Trump stating that travel advisory applied to all the 26 countries in the Schengen Area (Collinson, 2020). The decision by Trump was disapproved by the EU leaders (Gaouette et al., 2020).

Elsewhere, to control and reduce the spread of the virus, the schooling system in different countries was seen to be disrupted. As of March 11, a UN report indicated that about 20% of students across the globe were out of school and this included countries like Italy, Czech Republic, part of Spain (Madrid region), Greece, and Austria among many others that took the decision of closing the school to protect students and their families, as a mean to comply with WHO's health guidelines (WHO, 2020p). Surprisingly, as countries hastened to close down schools—highlighting the worsening of this situation, reports from China indicated that normalcy was returning to a point that some schools were reopening especially in Qinghai Province (CGTN, 2020).

In regard to financing efforts against this disease and supporting technological advancement in the development of test kits and vaccine development, on March 10, the *Bill & Melinda Gates Foundation*, *Mastercard*, and *Wellcome* together committed approximately $125 million (Bill and Melinda Gates Foundation, 2020). On the same date, The *Coalition for Epidemic Preparedness Innovations* on its part committed an extra $4.4 million to render the organization's total investment in vaccine development to $23.7 million, with the funds expected to help both the company Novavax and the University of Oxford to research and develop a vaccine for this disease (KFF, 2020). Furthermore, on March 11, the United Kingdom announced more funding ($192.4 million), this time from its national budget to aid vulnerable countries in their efforts against COVID-19 (Gov.UK, 2020b).

DAY 104—MARCH 13, 2020

Two days after declaring the coronavirus a global pandemic, circumstances in the western part of the globe have led the WHO to make another declaration; this time, the *new epicenter* of the outbreak of coronavirus was Europe (WHO, 2020ae). This announcement was not surprising as of then, Italy was already overwhelmed (17,660 cases and 1266 deaths already) (Snuggs, 2020), and Spain had in the day declared a state of emergency (CNBC, 2020). Things in other member countries of the union were also worsening, with the region recording over 300 deaths in a span of 24 h from the disease, and over 6000 new cases in the same period (WHO, 2020c). And surprisingly, from the situation report by the WHO (WHO, 2020c), all the cases in each of these countries were of local transmission; thus, warranting the decision different countries were making to restrict movements, and where possible, instituting total lockdowns like the case of Italy.

On the western side of the globe, more states in the United States were declaring a state of emergencies, restricting the number of people in gatherings, closing all learning institutions, and restricting movements among other things. These happenings were more pronounced on March 13, and when the worse came to worst, Present Donald Trump, under the Robert T. Stafford Disaster Relief and Emergency Assistance Act (Stanford Act), declared a state of National Emergency (Office of the President, 2020a). By then, the number of cases in the United States had increased to 1678 and those who died from the disease reached 41 deaths, with transmission happening locally (WHO, 2020j).

In total, the global number of confirmed cases had reached a high of 142,534 cases, with 9764 of those reported in the past 24 h. Of the sum, 61,513 had been confirmed from 134 countries, of which 12 were reporting their first cases. The remaining cases were reported in China, where situations were coming back to normal, with only 18 new cases reported in the populous country, and 14 deaths were reported in the 24-h period. Wuhan, the former epicenter only recorded five confirmed cases (Reuters, 2020c). Outside China, the deaths increased by 423, raising the total tally to 2198 cases (WHO, 2020c).

Following these unprecedented unfolding globally, economies were facing numerous challenges, as most economic activities had stalled or were nonexistent. For instance, in the United States, the stock exchange recorded the lowest point, only reminiscence with situations of 1987 (McCabe and Ostroff, 2020). For this reason, different agencies introduced financial packages to offer some support. For instance, the ADB announced a $200 million package that could be accessed by companies to supply critical essentials for combating COVID-19 (ADB, 2020). In Europe, The European Bank for Reconstruction and Development is reported to have approved a $1.1 billion financial package to help companies in the region to remain afloat during this period the region was experiencing the most trying moment in the recent history (Williams, 2020).

Amid the challenges of COVID-19 and its impacts, some countries like Taiwan found some solace in the use of technology to track and instill the mandatory quarantine, especially for those coming from certain areas. With technology, enforcement officers were able to know those who were flaunting rules and their whereabouts, and this helped reduce the spread of the virus, despite it being just kilometers from China where things were worse some days ago (Yun, 2020). In Europe, there was some use of technology, especially mobile Apps, that helped in mapping and tracking cases, and to bolster this even further, the European Commission (EC) was offering funding to a tune of €164m ($177.46) for start-ups or Small Medium Enterprises (SMEs) developing technologies with capacities to treat, test, monitor, or offer other aspects that could help in the fight against COVID-19 (Euroean Commission, 2020a).

DAY 105—MARCH 15, 2020

In the past 1 month since the first case was confirmed in Africa, the number of countries affected in the continent increased to 26 by March 15, with seven reporting their first case in a span of 24 h. Also, a week prior, the number of cases in the continent was only 27, but they increased to 273 with six deaths reported to have been imported, except for South Africa, Algeria, Senegal, and Cameroon (WHO, 2020k).

In Europe, most countries were receiving unprecedented numbers of new cases, especially in Italy, Spain, France, and Germany, which recorded 3497, 1,522, 828, and 733 new cases, respectively, and almost all cases in most of these EU countries were locally transmitted (WHO, 2020k). The number of deaths in the region was also rising with Italy losing 173 people in a single day (Snuggs, 2020), while Spain lost 16, France 12, and the United Kingdom lost 11 lives. In Germany, which was reported to have embarked on mass testing as early as the situation warranted so, the number of deaths was relatively low (only two reported by 15th) (WHO, 2020k). Following the dire state in the region, the European Commission published guidelines (European Commission, 2020b) on the exportation of PPEs out of the region. Among such guidelines were the restriction of exportation of the said equipment unless with express green light from the EU member states.

However, the EU was categorical that the measures taken were only within a specified period, especially during that period when those PPEs were greatly needed locally; and thus, it was not a total ban on export, which would contravene the region's international obligations in matters of trade (Euroean Commission, 2020b).

In the Middle East, the severity of the disease was still present in Iran, which until 15th had a total of 14,991 confirmed cases and 854 deaths, with a high of 245 deaths having been reported in a period of 24 h. The situation in other countries within the region was controlled with only 13 deaths reported (9 in Iraq, 3 in Lebanon, and 1 in Bahrain). In the American region, only a few confirmed cases were reported, and only 2 deaths were reported in Ecuador. However, the government there continued to institute proactive response measures to ensure the spread would be contained. For instance, the CDC announced that no gathering would be allowed in the United States that have more than 50 people, thus putting into disarray functions such as weddings, concerts, and sporting events among others that are known to attract a large crowd (The New York Times, 2020a). More states declared a state of emergencies, while more schools in different states (more than 30 states), including New York City with over 1.1 students (Shapiro, 2020) calling for the closure of schools. One major news in the United States on that day was the negative test results for the country's President, who a few days ago had some contact with a Brazilian official who turns positive after the test—prompting President Trump to undergo testing (Education Week, 2020).

In other places, country borders were being closed. For instance, after confirming their first COVID-19 cases, Kazakhstan and Uzbekistan closed their borders (Reuters, 2020j). Colombia also closed its border with Venezuela, while Turkey, with one of the leading airline services globally, suspended flights to nine European countries (Liptak, 2020). Lebanon reported to have called for a 14-day lockdown in the entire country to curb the spread of the virus, which for the past week had claimed the lives of three people (France 24, 2020b).

The other goods news of the day came from South Korea, which had shown a great resolve in bringing down the number of new cases, and this was bearing fruits after it implemented a number of strategies that involved the use of advanced technologies. First, it adopted the use of drive-thru clinics where people could be tested within 10 min and receive their results the following day. This allowed them to test over 300 people per hour, as there were 50 such clinics countrywide, where six people were being tested in an hour per clinic (Choon, 2020). The strategy also reduced local transmissions as contacts were greatly reduced. The country also implemented the use of mobile Apps to enforce quarantines and track the spread of the virus (Park, 2020). The success of the drive-thru clinics and Apps were later adopted by the United States and Germany (Yamey, 2020).

DAY 108—MARCH 17, 2020

By March 16, the situation globally had worsened such that the number of deaths outside China was increasing at alarming rates (3388) to a point of exceeding those who died in China (3218). In only a period of 24 h, China reported 14 new deaths, while the rest of the world reported 848 new deaths, with a majority of these coming from Europe. The global number of confirmed cases had increased to 167,515, with 13,903 reported in a period of past 24 h (only 29 new cases in China) (WHO, 2020l).

On 17th, the health landscape in different regions changed even further, with the Western Pacific Region having the highest number of confirmed cases, mostly because of China. The European Region was on its knees, health-wise, with 64,188 confirmed cases, with 8506 of these being reported in a single day. The number of deaths in this region had also increased by 428 to take the region's tally to 3108 deaths. Both North and South American regions had 4910 cases, and a total of 68 deaths (18 deaths reported in a day). The African and the South-East Asia regions were relatively saved until then, with only 228 and 508 confirmed cases, respectively, and total deaths for both regions being 13 (WHO, 2020l).

Following the dire need in the European region, the EU closed its borders except for essential travels. Russia also closed its borders, only allowing its citizens and legal permanent residents to travel back. Spain was also reported to have instituted border restrictions for all noncitizens and residents. In France, besides instituting border restrictions like a majority of its EU counterparts, it also announced a countrywide lockdown, which meant that no gathering of any size would be allowed, with people expected to remain at home with some exceptions (Onishi and Méheut, 2020). Similar events of widespread lockdowns and border restrictions were also observed in Latin America, with countries such as Venezuela and Peru leading the cue in countrywide lockdowns. Colombia and Costa Rica also instituted border restrictions and control. However, Brazil, which by then (March 16) had the most confirmed cases in the region, overlooked all the measures that the rest of the world were implementing, and had a section of its population (supporters of their president; Jair Bolsonaro) demonstrate against his opponents (Harris and Schipani, 2020). In Iran, the government was forced to release over 85,000 prisoners as a way of curbing the spread of the virus in the country, which was already at alarming levels (Hawkins, 2020).

As the global social fabric was being dismantled by the disease, its impacts were being felt in the economic sphere. For instance, on 16th, the airline industry in the United States was seeking government financial assistance of up to $50 billion to help them remain afloat (Sider and Mann, 2020). The Dow Jones Industry also recorded its historical low after dropping 2997.10 points; the worst day crash since the 1987 "Black Monday" crash (Millhiser, 2020).

Following those uncertainties and the threat COVID-19 posed to the global fabric, a number of well-wishers and philanthropists were seen to be in the frontline of helping countries win this war. On 16th, the Jack Ma Foundation donated assorted PPEs and testing kits to the United States (Ward, 2020), which greatly needed these following the increasing demand, and the disruption of supply chain following the slow activities in China. On 17th, the World Bank Group committed another $2 billion to help in the fight against the diseases (The World Bank, 2020b), while on the same day, Bloomberg Philanthropies gave a financial package of $40 million, especially to help low-x and middle-income economies (Bloomberg Philanthropies, 2020).

DAY 110—MARCH 19, 2020

As the dark crowd of coronavirus continued to spread in Italy, its impacts were becoming evident, as in a month, the number of deaths (3405) in the country surpassed those in China (3242) since the onset of the outbreak to March 19 (Quinn, 2020b). Its health sector was completely overwhelmed with images of dejected nurses trending on social media, and while that was happening, China reported no new confirmed cases attributable to local infection, as the 34 new cases that it confirmed were suspected to have been imported from other countries (Siobhán O'Grady et al., 2020b), as it had started to ease its border restrictions. The number of new cases in Italy also increased by 5322 cases, bringing their country total to 41,035, becoming the second most affected country after China.

As for the European regions, Italy recorded a total of over 10,000 cases on both 18th 19. The number of deaths for both days totaled 1195, far much more than the rest of the regions combined. In the Americas, new cases on 19th were 4166: almost double of what was recorded the previous day (2243 new cases on 18th). The Eastern Mediterranean region recorded 1430 new cases to push their region total to 19,518, and the number of deaths in the region reached 1161 after (150 died on 19th), with most of these coming from Iran. In total, the global confirmed cases had increased to 209,839 cases on 19th after 16,556 more cases were reported. The number of total deaths globally increased by a total of 828 to reach a global tally of 8778 cases (WHO, 2020m).

On local scenes, the disease affected some prominent people, celebrities, and sports personalities. For instance, in the US NBA teams, Denver Nuggets (Wimbish, 2020), Los Angele Lakers (Whitcomb, 2020b), Philadelphia 76ers (Zagoria, 2020), and Boston Celtics (Ward-Henninger, 2020) reported that each had some of their players confirmed positive, but they decline to give the names of those players. On the same land, Congress Representatives, Ben McAdams (D-Utah) and Mario Diaz Balart of Florida, confirmed that they had also contracted the disease (Helsel, 2020). In Washington, two employees of the World Bank Group tested positive on the 18th with fears that more could have been affected. On the 19th, there were reports that Prince Albert of Monaco also tested positive for COVID-19 (Romo, 2020). Another person is the Executive Director of the World Food Program, David Beasley, who also tested positive after returning from Canada (World Food Program, 2020).

To respond to the numerous cases and scenarios prompted by the COVID-19 case, different regions, individual countries, and agencies adopted different and diverse measures. For instance, in India, the government was reported to have banned any export of PPEs, ventilators, and certain medications and supplements as such were not enough locally (Suneja, 2020). In addition to this, to reduce further spread, especially from imported cases, it closed its borders for incoming flights (Business Today, 2020b). In the United States, the number of interventions was observed, for instance, the two June scheduled party primaries in Connecticut were postponed (Pramuk and Dzhanova, 2020). President Trump also signed into law the Family First Coronavirus Response Act that would see most Americans receive a family relief of $2000. The act also gave $300 billion to be accessed by SMEs (Erica Werner et al., 2020). The University of Hong Kong received $620,000 from the Coalition for Epidemic Preparedness Innovations to continue with vaccine testing for COVID-19 (Galford, 2020). On the 19th, the Rockefeller Foundation committed a $20 million to assist in response to COVID-19, especially in cities such as Nairobi, New York, Washington, Bangkok, and Bellagio (Rockefeller Foundation, 2020).

DAY 111—MARCH 20, 2020

Since the onset of the coronavirus, there had been a theory that it was mostly affecting older people, but the WHO debunked this, by indicating that data on those affected in different countries and regions have shown that a significant proportion of those in hospitals are aged below 50 years; hence, calling the younger generation to be also extra cautious. The organization also launched a health alert messaging services through WhatsApp and Facebook, demystifying the importance of technology in the fight against COVID-19, especially in sharing data and information (WHO, 2020d). The organization also reported that it had reached an agreement with different producers in China who were ready to supply the organization with PPEs, so that it could continue supporting countries in need of such across the world (Schnirring, 2020). While that was going on, they delivered an extra 1.5 million laboratory test kits for COVID-19 to different parts of the world (Watts and Simon, 2020). There was also news that first vaccine trials had begun, and the WHO together with its partners was to organize an international study dubbed *Solidarity Trial* in different countries aimed at trying different treatments that could be adopted to win over COVID-19 (WHO, 2020d).

Regarding the reports on the spread and impacts of the coronavirus on this day (March 20), the situation reported by World Health Organization indicated that the world was still in great danger of recording even more cases. For instance, Italy reported the single largest number of deaths, where 627 people died, and those confirmed increasing to 47,021 cases. In the United States, the CDC indicated that it had confirmed a total of 18,487 cases (CDC, 2020). As that was happening, President Trump invoked the Defense Production Act, to force General Motors (GM) to produce ventilators to fill the gap after the situation in the hospital become dire (Haynes, 2020). On this, earlier on the day, GM rejected the move, prompting the President to apply his executive authority on them, and the New York governor equated the ventilators to missiles during World War II (Klein and Raju, 2020). The controversies in the United States were not over as it was reported that Canada, through its Prime Minister, Justin Trudeau, would return all asylum seekers to the United States (Austen, 2020). Elsewhere, Cuba invoked border restrictions for all noncitizens and nonresidents. It had delayed this decision to "keep its key tourism industry alive," but the threat of the coronavirus forced the President to take that crucial and bold decision (France 24, 2020a).

DAY 114—MARCH 23, 2020

As time passes, the spread of the coronavirus virus took hold across the globe. On March 11, the WHO declared the virus outbreak as a global pandemic, and 12 days later (on 13th), the Director-General declared that the "pandemic is accelerating" (Chappell, 2020). And true to his word, in the past 3 days, the number of new confirmed cases each day were averaging 30,000 new cases, to push the global total to 332,930 confirmed cases. The number of new deaths in those 3 days was also increasing at an average of almost 1500 each day, and by 23rd, the total number of deaths had reached 14,500 globally (WHO, 2020n). Of great concern on those numbers is that most of them were coming from the European region, which by 23rd had reached a high of 171,424 confirmed cases and 8742 total deaths. The only regions that had shown a lot of resilience were the African region with only 990 total confirmed cases and 23 total reported deaths. The South-East Asia Region was also relatively spared having confirmed only 1776 cases and 58 total deaths. The Region of Americas was showing worrisome trends, having reported a high of 17,331 new cases in a single day (March 23) to push its total tally of confirmed cases to 37,016 cases and a total tally of 465 deaths (213 deaths) reported in a single day (WHO, 2020n).

While a majority of countries, especially in Europe writhed in desperation from the impacts of COVID-19, China reported a third consecutive day with no local new case of coronavirus (The straits Times, 2020c). This meant that they could slowly transition back to their previous economic routine, and it also gave hope to those whose situation was worsening. In the other regions, including Africa where confirmed cases were low, they were responding to the spread by escalating lockdowns and border restrictions (Aljazeera, 2020b). Other countries followed this trend. For instance, on March 21–23, Bolivia (Reuters, 2020b), Greece (Stamouli, 2020), Cuba (Oppmann, 2020), and the United Kingdom (Sparrow et al., 2020) imposed total lockdown in their countries (Aljazeera, 2020b). Egypt on the other hand called off all religious activities in mosques and churches for 14 days (Mourad, 2020). During this period still, other countries including Pakistan (Reuters, 2020n), Vietnam, Singapore (Benner, 2020),

UAE, Panama (Aljazeera, 2020b), India, Nigeria (Reuters, 2020m), and Zimbabwe (The Citizen, 2020) closed their borders to all foreign travels and nonresidents and banned international flights to or from their soils for a minimum of 14 days. Germany, on the other hand, banned gatherings of more than two persons, as cases in the country started to soar, while on the same day, Spain extended the state of emergency for 15 more days, as the situation internally was getting out of hand, with thousands hospitalized, and cases soaring each day (Picheta, 2020).

The decision taken by each individual country was meant for the good of the citizens, but such also had a far-reaching impact on the economy. For instance, the banning of the international flights in these 3 days, and others that had been instituted earlier mean that sectors such as tourism, hospitality industry, and others are grounded, with millions of workers employed in those sectors uncertain of what the future holds. In such circumstances, governments were forced to rely on external organizations—like the Jack Ma Foundation, which on 22nd delivered a consignment of assorted PPEs, and test kits to African countries to fight the COVID-19 (Meseret and Meldrum, 2020). On 23rd, the World Bank Group's President was also pleading with bilateral creditors to extend debt relief to low-income economies to help them build some capacity that could allow them to fight the disease (Bank, 2020). While this was going on, African finance ministers were pleading for a $100 billion economic stimulus in addition to the suspension of external debt to allow their individual countries to fight the coronavirus pandemic (UNECA, 2020).

DAY 115—MARCH 24, 2020

China's progression toward containing the virus received a boost after the province of Hubei was freed from the lockdown after almost 2 months since the lockdown was instituted (Associated Press, 2020). It was a relief to the residents who, for such a long period, lived in fear and uncertainty of when they would return to their previous routines. The good news was that Wuhan, the first epicenter of coronavirus was to open a month later, as the number of new cases had reduced significantly. In the last 24 h, the entire country of China reported on 78 new cases, of which, 74 cases were reported to have been imported (CNA, 2020a). The number of deaths had also increased, with seven reported in the city of Wuhan (The Star, 2020).

The other good news came from Germany where the Chancellor's, Angela Merkel, the first test came back negative for coronavirus, but would undergo the same process a few days later to confidently confirm this result (Mischke, 2020). The fear that she would have contracted the disease came after a doctor who had attended her turned positive, forcing the Chancellor into a safety procedure of self-isolation (Mischke, 2020).

The day however did not present the good news to everyone, especially to governments, health workers, and security forces implementing lockdowns and other measures in different countries and to the general global population. On this, in the past 24 h alone, the number of newly laboratory-confirmed cases neared 40,000 and the deaths on a single day accumulated to 1722 globally (CNA, 2020a). The most unfortunate report on this is that half of the new cases and deaths reported came from European countries (24,085 cases and 1447 deaths), with the American regions also experiencing a high of 12,428 new cases and 100 deaths (WHO, 2020e). Regarding the accumulation of confirmed cases, it took at least 3 months for cases to climb to 100,000 confirmed, and only 12 days to reach 200,000 cases. From here, it only took 3 days for the global total to surpass 300,000 confirmed cases, and even more startling, only 2 days for the total to reach almost 400,000 confirmed cases.

Such trends prompted the International Olympics Committee and Japan's Olympic authority, led by Prime Minister Shinzo Abe, to postpone the Olympics scheduled for summer 2020 to 2021 as more countries had expressed their fears of the virus (Ramsay, 2020), while others cited lack of preparation and other technicalities (Aarons, 2020). They also prompted the Prime Minister of India, Narendra Modi, to lock down the country for 21 days, only a day after the later declared an immediate grounding of all flights in or out of India (Shroff, 2020). New Zealand also went into lockdown (BBC, 2020e), as Australia announced a ban on all overseas travel (Whiteman and Sharma, 2020). While in the United States, a troop of 11,400 US National Guards was mobilized in 50 states to help in response to the disease (Gresik and Altman, 2020), as it had already infected more than 50,000 people countrywide. While those were being mobilized, three of their colleagues in the navy (sailors) contracted the virus, when an aircraft carrier they were boarding—together with approximately 4000 other people—set sail from Vietnam.

DAY 117—MARCH 26, 2020

By now, the situation of COVID-19 globally reached fever-pitch where the U.N. Secretary-General António Guterres argued that the disease was ravaging the whole of humanity, with approximately one-third of the population experiencing one or more COVID-19-related restriction (UNICEF, 2020). Following this, there was shortages in all sectors, with the WHO warning that already, the world was facing a "significant shortage" of assorted medical supplies. On the social sphere, there was a shortage in the health sector prompting the UN to launch a $2 billion financial package on March 25 targeting global humanitarian responses, especially to be advanced to vulnerable countries (UN Secretary-General, 2020). With the funds, those countries would manage to bolster their laboratory equipment, build and increase available sanitation (handwashing) stations, and increase medical supplies among other things. Besides the financial package, the WHO was calling on developed economies to assist African countries with health machines such as ventilators and respirators as the continent cannot satisfy the demand for such, especially if cases of COVID-19 were to increase (Ighobor, 2020).

Those calls and interventions come at a time when most countries, especially in Europe and America, were experiencing one of the darkest moments of their history. For instance, in Spain, as of 26th, the number of reported deaths (3434 deaths) surpassed those reported in China (3293). But still, Italy was leading in the number of people who had died with a total of 7505, with 685 having died in a span of only 24 h. France had also started to lose a significant number of people as a result of the COVID-19, with 231 already having succumbed in the past 24 h. The Islamic State of Iran and the United States were also affected with 143 (total deaths 2077) and 211 (total deaths 884) deaths having died in the past 24 h. In regard to the number of confirmed cases, which were averaging 40,000 cases per day in the past 4 days, the global total had increased to 462,684 by 26th according to the WHO data. Africa was still showing some resilience despite reports of weak health system, with only 31 deaths reported coming from 1937 confirmed cases across the globe (WHO, 2020o).

The economic situation globally was worsening, but even more in the United States where it was reported that by March 26, over 3.3 million American had filed for their employment benefit (Casselman et al., 2020); a figure that is thought to be the highest in the history of the country. This could be attributed to the increasing number of people who were contracting the coronavirus especially in New York, which had become the epicenter of the outbreak in the Northern American region, with the United States having more cases than any other country (Kirby and Stewart, 2020; The New York Times, 2020b). But, fortunately, the Trump Administration's stimulus plan—worth $2 trillion—was unanimously passed the Senate (Carney, 2020), thus allowing the government to offer some financial support, especially to those who continued to lose their livelihoods. Elsewhere, more countries were responding to the pandemic by instituting lockdowns or other strict measures that would somehow suppress the local transmission. On this, on March 26, Panama was reported to have suspended any form of domestic flights (Moreno et al., 2020), 4 days after, it had suspended international flights (Aljazeera, 2020b). In Thailand, the government declared a state of emergency forcing more areas within the country to shut down (Techakitteranun, 2020), while Iraq and Lebanon extended their curfews by 14 days in each country. In Russia, Moscow shut down all forms of businesses and activities for a week (March 28 to April 5), except for essential businesses such as pharmacies and grocery stores (Astapkovich, 2020).

DAY 118—MARCH 27, 2020

The highlight of the day was the testing positive for coronavirus of UK Prime Minister Boris Johnson, which he announced to the world via a video on Twitter (BBC, 2020g). He reported that, henceforth, he would be in self-isolation and will continue working from. But, while this was breaking news, the greatest and most unfortunate news came from Italy and Spain. In Spain, it had earlier been reported that it had recorded the highest number of deaths in a single day (769) (RTVE, 2020), but later only Italy released its official report of the day where it indicated that approximately 919 (WHO later reported 971 (WHO, 2020f)) people had died within a span of only 24 h. Italy had also confirmed 5959 new cases while Spain reported 7871 new cases bringing the total confirmed cases to 86,498 and 64,059 cases, respectively. However, the United States reported the highest number of new confirmed cases (16,894), taking its total tally to 85,228 according to the data by WHO (WHO, 2020f) but according to the US CDC data (CDC, 2020), the total number of cases reported in the country by 27th had reached 103,321, thus leading globally. In the Middle East, Iran was reporting the highest numbers of new cases, with 2926 cases reported within 24 h and 144 new deaths during the same period (WHO, 2020f). Other countries in the region were relatively calm with no other reporting more than a 100 cases a day. In Africa, Algeria reported the highest number of deaths (4) (WHO, 2020f) while South Africa reported the first death from the virus. This death and the increasing number of confirmed cases in the country prompted the government to announce a 3-week nationwide lockdown (Neuman, 2020b). Elsewhere, China reported 117 new cases and 5 new deaths, in what seemed like a signal to a second wave of infection. Following this, the government announced a ban on all foreigners, suspecting that they were the cause of this new trend in rise of cases, as out of those new cases, none were from local transmission (BBC, 2020a; Mai, 2020).

On the same date, the African Development Bank (AFDB) provided aid to the continent with a $3 billion social bond targeted to economic and social sectors facing stiff challenges from the impacts of COVID-19 (AFDB, 2020). At the same time, the WHO announced that the vaccine trial dubbed Solidarity Trial—that it had announced about on March 20—was to begin shortly, with the first trials administered to patients drawn from Norway and Spain, but overall, the trials would be extended to more than 45 countries that had agreed to be part of the program (WHO, 2020af). In the United States, the Food and Drug Administration authorized the use of a 15-min diagnostic kit for coronavirus intended to speed-up the testing process, but a shortage of necessary equipment for collecting specimens was feared to derail the use of this kit (Azad, 2020). On the same land, Donald Trump, President of America, signed the $2 trillion stimulus that was passed the previous day by the Senate (Foran et al., 2020).

DAY 121—MARCH 30, 2020

Even as the month of March came to an end, the incidences related to COVID-19 continued almost unthwarted. For instance, the number of new confirmed cases for the past 3 days has been increasing at an average of above 61,000 each day, and the number of deaths occurring each day likewise increased at an average of 3250 deaths. Within the 3 days, the total number of confirmed cases globally increased from 571,659—as captured by the WHO on March 28 (WHO, 2020f)—to 693,224 by March 30. Another astonishing occurrence—especially on March 28—was the number of people that died in a single day in both Spain and Italy, which recorded 832 and 889 new deaths, respectively (WHO, 2020p). This happened while the number of patients being admitted to different hospitals in both countries exceeded their bed capacity and human resources allocation (Cheng, 2020). The United States was also going through thick and thin, as the number of new cases in the country continued to soar at alarming rates. Even in Africa—which had shown some levels of resilience against the spread of this pandemic—the numbers for the past 3 days seemed to increase at an average of almost 300 daily, with Egypt, Algeria, and South Africa being the most affected (WHO, 2020q). In fact, the WHO's Director-General highlighted the plight of the global health system and argued that there was a chronic global shortage of medical supplies such as PPEs, ventilators, and other basic amenities required to saving lives (WHO, 2020af).

These unfolding events were happening amidst numerous responses and interventions both at local, regional, and international levels by government, international organizations like the WHO, the World Bank, and others. Among the new interventions that countries were implementing include the extension of the social distancing guidelines in the United States by President Donald Trump until the end of the following month (April 30), and perhaps with a possible extension to June (Shear, 2020). The country had also accelerated the testing of individuals, and by 30th, the President announced that over one million people had been tested despite earlier hiccups in regard to faulty testing kits (Tirrell et al., 2020). In Africa, on 29th, Nigeria was reported to have directed the cessation of movement in two of its most populous cities, Lagos and Abuja, to reduce the chances of importation of the coronavirus to rural areas (Akwagyiram, 2020a). In Mexico, in a bid to reduce the soaring confirmed cases and growing number of deaths as a result of COVID-19, the government declared a health emergency (Reuters, 2020l). In Portugal, the government had resulted in treating everyone including foreigners with pending applications as permanent residents of the country so they could access public health facilities without encountering hitches (Reuters, 2020o).

But despite all those negatives, there was good news from the city of Wuhan, which after undergoing a "dark moment" in the past 2 months, saw authorities relaxing some quarantine measures, including rail services in and out of the city, meaning that people could eventually access the rest of the country (Beaumont, 2020). Authorities in the province of Hubei also announced that they would allow domestic flights to resume in all airports, except Tianhe International Airport in Wuhan (Xinhua, 2020c). The other goods news is that on 29, the Bill & Melinda Gates Foundation, Wellcome, and Mastercard together granted three institutions (the University of Washington, University of Oxford, and La Jolla Institute for Immunology) financial support worth $20 million to facilitate clinical trials for immunotherapies they were developing (Mastercard, 2020).

DAY 124—APRIL 2, 2020

In the wake of the new months, the reality of devastation of the COVID-19 in different countries, regions, and globally was becoming clear. For instance, in Spain, by April 1, the number of those affected reached 102,136. But, by then, Italy had more than these cases with 110,574 confirmed cases, while the United States, which had become the new epicenter, had 213,144 confirmed cases, as per the CDC data (CDC, 2020), while the WHO reported 187,302 (WHO, 2020r). Regionally, cases in Europe reached more than half a million people (503,006), where 33,604 of those had succumbed to the virus. The region of the Americas was the second most affected with a total of 216,912 confirmed cases and 4565 deaths. The Western Pacific region was the third hardest hit, with 107,626 infected and 3723 deaths. The Eastern Mediterranean regions had 58,168 confirmed cases and 3279 recorded deaths, while the African region had 4702 confirmed cases and 127 reported deaths from the virus. Overall, the global total number of confirmed cases had reached 896,450, and an addition of 72,839 from the previous reported numbers. The number of deaths had also reached 45,525, with a high of 4923 dying in the past 24 h (WHO, 2020r). By April 2, the global total exceeded the 1,000,000 mark as per the John Hopkins data, nCoV2019.Live, and other websites, but WHO reported the total numbers at 972,303 confirmed cases (WHO, 2020g).

The reality was reflected in the economic sector with the World Bank reporting that the impacts of COVID-19 pandemic would force more than 11 million people into poverty (The world Bank, 2020a). The reality of this statement was affirmed in the happenings in the United States, where it was reported that in a period of just 1 week, 6.6 million more people filed for unemployment benefits, taking the number of those who had filed for the benefits to over 10 million people (Long and Dam, 2020a). The same trends of unemployment were also being experienced in Austria where the unemployment levels jumped to 66% in the country within the 3 months since the onset of the pandemic (Reuters, 2020a).

The said reality prompted several unprecedented actions in different countries and organizations. For instance, on April 1, the UN announced the postponement of the climate conference (COP26) scheduled for November due to COVID-19 (UN, 2020). In the sporting world, the All England Club announced that the Wimbledon Tennis Tournament was canceled due to COVID-19, and this was the first time since World War II that the championship was called off. On the same day, the Health Minister in Italy announced that the countrywide lockdown would continue to be in force until the 13th of the month as the number of confirmed cases, and deaths continued to increase (Reuters, 2020i). The announcement was also confirmed by the country's Prime Minister Giuseppe Conte said that the situation in the country forced him to sign the decree to extend the measures (Orihuela et al., 2020). The same measures were taken by Germany. On April 2, more actions continued, with Saudi Arabia extended its curfew to 24 h on its most visited and the holiest cities in Islam: Mecca and Medina (Aljazeera, 2020c). A similar action was taken in Thailand involving the entire country, with exception of medical personnel, and those transporting essential products, and for people moving to quarantine or health facilities (The Nation, 2020). Peru and Panama establish a different strategy for reducing the number of people outside by imposing a gender divide, where certain days were set aside for only men and the others for men. This way, it would be impossible for those living together leaving their homes together (Aquino and Moreno, 2020). In the United States, the white house was encouraging people going out to wear masks (Sun and Dawsey, 2020), and this came while most of the citizens were trying to come to terms with stay-at-home orders that had been declared in almost 12 states in the country (Nottingham, 2020).

DAY 128—APRIL 6, 2020

The highlight of the day is the worsening health status of the UK Prime Minister Boris Johnson, prompting him to be moved into intensive care. He was taken to hospital in London the previous day (April 5), after the COVID-19 symptoms persisted, 9 days after he tested positive (BBC, 2020g). On the same day, in the same country, 439 new deaths were reported, taking the country's total death toll to 5373 while the total number of confirmed cases increased to 51,612 after 3802 new cases were reported in a period of 24 h. Within the European region, the total number of confirmed cases had increased to 686,338 after 30,999 more cases were reported in a span of 24 h. The number of deaths also had increased by a total of 3330 deaths to take the total tally for the region to 52,809, and these were far much more than the total deaths of all other regions combined. On the same day, the United States reported 26,493 new cases to take their country's total to 333,811 (WHO, 2020s) and also reported a high of 1201 deaths increasing the total deaths recorded in the country to 9559, while other data showed that deaths had reached 10,530 (Siobhán O'Grady et al., 2020a). In the previous day (April 5), it had reported 1300 cases and 33,510 new cases; the highest reported data in the region since the onset of the pandemic (WHO, 2020a). As these occurred, President Trump reported that hydroxychloroquine, an antimalaria drug, could be used against COVID-19 (Crowley et al., 2020). In the Middle East, the total number of confirmed cases in Iran increased to 60,500 after 2274 more people tested positive. Globally, the total confirmed cases stood at 1,279,722 and the total deaths reported were 72,614 (WHO, 2020s).

In Africa, where cases had started to increase significantly—reaching 7092 and 294 deaths, it was reported that the former Libya Prime Minister Mahmoud Jibril died of coronavirus the previous day after fighting the COVID-19 disease for approximately 2 weeks (Aljazeera, 2020d). In China, which reported 75 new cases and only 2 deaths, fears were that the country would be experiencing asymptomatic transmissions of the virus; hence, the increase in newly reported cases. These were experienced though the country had already introduced border restrictions with other countries, and following the fear of asymptomatic cases, the government vowed to tighten border control measures even further (Zhang and Munroe, 2020). The most astonishing news reported on April 5 was that of the positive testing for coronavirus of four tigers and three lions in the Bronx Zoo, bringing the total number of cats reported to have contracted the virus to 9 (Daly, 2020). This raised alarms as no known research had shown that the virus could be passed from humans to animals.

This far, a report by the WHO indicated that more than 90% (approximately 1.5 billion) of students globally have had to remain at home following the closure of school. To offer some intervention on this, the organization, together with UNICEF and the International Publishers Association, launched the "Read the World" initiative to allow student access learning materials even during the difficult times (WHO, 2020a). In the sporting sector, to safeguard the lives of participants and to comply with the health guidelines of social distancing and others, the Open Golf Championship was called off; being the second time, it was canceled since 1945 during the WW2 (The Open, 2020).

DAY 130—APRIL 8, 2020

After 76 days of uncertainties, the Chinese authorities finally lifted the lockdown on Wuhan as promised, after the city successfully saw a reduction in the number of new confirmed cases for the coronavirus (Aljazeera, 2020a). In fact, the report from the entire country was that the new cases that were being reported were all imported ones, and the government had vowed to take extra measures to control its borders (Zhang and Munroe, 2020). The good news on the country is that on the previous day (April 7), despite reporting 66 new confirmed cases—which were all imported, the country reported zero death for the first time since it started publishing figures of the death related to COVID-19 (WHO, 2020b). Even on 8th, the number of new cases was only 86: all imported and only two deaths. The situation was, however, totally different in other regions, especially in Europe where France, on a single day, reported 1417 new deaths to push its total death toll to 10,313, while those whose tests turned positive in the past 24 h increased by 3738 to take the country's total to 77,226 (WHO, 2020t). This total was however smaller compared to Germany, Italy, and Spain whose totals had increased to 103,228, 135,586, and 140,510 cases, respectively. Belgium and the Netherlands also witnessed an increase in the number of deaths with 403 and 234 new recorded deaths, respectively (WHO, 2020b). On this, despite Germany having more confirmed cases, it had managed to keep the death toll relatively low, with reports showing that it is due to the mass testing initiative it had embarked on; thus, cases were getting identified before becoming critical (Perrigo, 2020). Until eighth, it had only lost 1861 people, while its European counterparts were worse off (WHO, 2020t).

The other nation that saw the number of casualty increase was the U.S, which, since a few days ago had started to witness numerous deaths, and confirmed cases. On this day, the country lost 1286 lives to the disease, and 29,510 were the newly confirmed cases taking the country's total to 363,321, according to WHO data (WHO, 2020t), but the USCDC reported the total number as 427,460 cases (CDC, 2020), where the difference could be due to difference in reporting time between WHO on Central European Time (CET) and US EDT time zones. While this was happening, the country's President, Donald Trump who had frequently attacked the WHO for failing in its mandate in detecting the virus earlier threatened to withdraw funding to the agency (Sevastopulo and Manson, 2020). He categorically said that the organization had withheld information about the virus and was wrong about the outbreak in China (Davidson, 2020a). But, in a quick rejoinder, the WHO's Director-General warned that it would be disastrous to politicize the fight against the pandemic (Wise, 2020).

Following the health situation in France, authorities announced that they were imposing a ban on daytime outdoor exercise in Paris, which had allowed its citizens to enjoy despite the country being on lockdown (BBC, 2020f). On the same day (April 7), the Egyptian authorities announced that the ban on mosques and churches would still continue even during the Ramadan period as the country was still facing the challenge of coronavirus, with new cases increasing and more deaths being witnessed (Egypt Independent, 2020). In the Asian region, Japan joined the list of many other countries who had declared a state of emergency as the number of cases in the country had started to rise in the month (Rich et al., 2020). In Singapore, to contain the spread of the COVID-19, the Health Minister Gan Kim Yong announced that the government was banning any form of social gathering whether at home or in public (Zhang, 2020). The ban came just a day after a motion to outlaw social gathering in the country was rushed and passed to the law in Parliament the previous day.

Elsewhere, as the impacts of the virus continued to be felt, the Wellness Trust, on April 7, started an initiative aimed to raise a minimum of $8 billion from the private sector by the end of April to fill the financial gap being experienced in search vaccines, drugs, and tests for COVID-19 (Wellcome, 2020). A similar initiative dubbed "AfroChampions Initiative" was launched by African Union and Africa Centres for Disease Control and Prevention to raise over $400 million for medical responses, with $150 million required urgently for the same purpose (Africanews, 2020).

DAY 132—APRIL 10, 2020

After spending three nights in the intensive care unit, the UK Prime Minister Boris Johnson was finally discharged from the unit and transferred to a normal ward where he recovered. In fact, it was reported that he could manage short walks, though he needed some time to feel better (The Sun, 2020). While the report of his improvement was encouraging, it was not the case for over 980 families in the country, from England who had lost their loved ones as a result of the disease on that particular day. In Italy, a total of 570 people lost their lives on 10th (WHO, 2020h), while 612 had died the previous day (WHO, 2020u). In total, the number of deaths in Italy had reached a high of 18,851 by 10th with 100 of these being doctors who had contracted the virus while in line of duty (Aljazeera, 2020g). In Spain, hopes of flattening the curve were high after the country saw a decline in the number of deaths for the third consecutive day (Landauro and Keeley, 2020). However, the number of new cases in the country was increasing and had climbed to 157,022 cases after 4576 more cases were confirmed on 10th. The renewed hope was also being experienced in China after it continued to witness a reduced number of deaths in the country, as well as more recoveries, which had reached 77,000 (Regencia et al., 2020).

While that was happening, the spread of the virus has gone as far as in deep rural areas where a 13-year-old boy from the indigenous tribe of Yanomami found in Brazil, Amazon forest was confirmed with the coronavirus on t9th, and on 10th, unfortunately, he passed away (Phillips, 2020). Another rare place where the virus was reported was in the Cook County Jail in Chicago where 450 new cases involving inmates and staff were reported (Whitcomb, 2020a). In America still, the number of death from COVID-19 were increasing at an alarming rate, where 1931 new deaths were reported on 10th (WHO, 2020h) and 1895 more had died the previous day (WHO, 2020u). Following these increases, with most of them coming from New York cities, the state had resulted in burials in mass graves as the numbers kept on increasing (Anderson, 2020), with its confirmed cases being more than any other country globally (BBC, 2020d). The situation in the United States prompted the German Foreign Minister to criticize the US handling of the virus (Connor, 2020). Another rare place that was affected by coronavirus is a French navy airplane carrier, where 50 servicemen tested positive to COVID-19 (Aljazeera, 2020e).

As the cases globally increased to over 1.6 million people, the economic impact of the virus continued to bite. For instance, in the United States, another 6.6 million people filed for unemployment claims bringing the total number of those in the same predicaments into almost 17 million in only 3 weeks (Long and Dam, 2020b). In Vietnam, it was reported that the country was in dire need of almost $1 billion to caution its economy against the budget deficit that continued to widen (Reuters, 2020r). Albania was also trending on a tight economic path, prompting it to seek financial support from the IMF, which extended a loan of $190.5 million (IMF, 2020). In Zimbabwe, following the ban on all international flights in or out of the country, Air Zimbabwe sent its employees on leave, which was, unfortunately, unpaid (The Herald, 2020). On the same continent, Senegal adopted a directly opposite approach of protecting its workers against being laid off by companies in excuse of the COVID-19 crisis (France-Presse, 2020).

On other news, there were reports that Google and Apple would cooperate to develop a mobile app that would help in tracking coronavirus spread (Apple, 2020). Although that was good news especially coming from the tech world, in Singapore, the use of technology faced concerns when online learning platforms that the government had initiated were suspended after the video conferencing ZOOM platform was hacked during a learning session, and the hackers displayed explicit images to the students (Lee, 2020).

DAY 136—APRIL 14, 2020

Although the death tolls in at least four countries crossed the 15,000 mark, others have witnessed significant declines in the number of new cases being reported daily, and thus planning to ease lockdown stances and other strict measures that had been put in place. Until April 14, countries like the United States (23,476 deaths), Spain (18,056 deaths), Italy (21,069 deaths), and France (15,708 deaths) were most affected, with the situation in the United Kingdom worsening (12,107) (WHO, 2020w). Indeed, a report by the Office for National Statistics highlighted that UK numbers were underreported by 52%, the number in the country would be reading over 20,000 cases (Bruce, 2020). On this, it was highlighted that the number of deaths reported did not reflect the actual number represented in over 232 care homes, where most of the elderly population were (McIntyre and Duncan). Although those numbers are many, there was hope in Spain and Italy as the number of deaths kept on decreasing each day, and from the report, these were optimistic that they would ease their stand on lockdown—Spain by end of June (BBC, 2020h). On this, other more countries including Greece (by May 4) (Tugwell, 2020), Portugal (by May 3), Australia (had already started by then), Pakistan, and Austria (with already thousands of shops reopened (Niesner and Murphy, 2020)) were considering this move (DW, 2020).

Although those countries were eager to lift lockdown measures, Germany was considering reintroducing it after community infection cases over the past few days started to rise after the country had cautiously tried to ease the lockdown (Mayberry et al., 2020). In Moscow, President Putin strengthened the lockdown measures until May 11 to counter the rising cases of infections (Davidson, 2020b). Similar measures were also being taken in China, in the Heilongjiang province bordering Russia, where 79 cases were reported on April 14, where Chinese nationals who had fled to Russia tried to return home (Wu, 2020). Following this, the cases in the province increased to 409, and Chinese authorities in the province promised to reward locals who would report the "illegal migrants" (The straits Times, 2020b). Georgia, on its part, was planning to lock down four of its largest cities, including its capital Tbilisi for 10 days (Today, 2020a) as local transmission started to increase with the county's total cases reaching 306 (WHO, 2020w), an addition of 10 more confirmed cases (WHO, 2020v).

On the economic front, the IMF warned that the global economy would shrink by approximately 3% following unprecedented measures like lockdowns, and ban on transportations, and closing down of manufacturing and other industries (Rapperport and Smialek, 2020). In a way to ease the economic pressure, President Donald Trump started issuing stimulus checks to Americans, amid some delays after he realized that his name did not appear on the checks (Rein, 2020). The situation of the economy is also pointed by activities in Heathrow Airports where passenger demands were expected to reduce by almost 90% this month (April), after having plummeted by 52% last month and cargo volume reduced by 32.5% (Rojas, 2020). The economy was worsening also for the WHO after President Trump retaliated that he was halting funds to the agency following its mismanagement of the coronavirus (Mayberry et al., 2020).

On the societal fronts, the racial discrimination of blacks in China continued, with the McDonald outlets in China forced to apologize after the store displayed posters banning black people from accessing the China store (Folley, 2020). Elsewhere, Turkey was planning to temporarily release over 45,000 inmates, after getting approval from Parliament to ease overcrowding; thus, void the risk of coronavirus infection in the facilities (Wilks, 2020).

DAY 138—APRIL 16, 2020

As of 16th, COVID-19 had spread to 210 countries and territories across the globe with over 2,074,529 confirmed cases and 139,378 deaths reported. Of those cases and deaths, 50% were reported in Europe, while more than 80% of the remaining cases (743,607 confirmed cases and 33,028 deaths) reported in regions of the Americas. The Eastern Mediterranean region had 115,824 confirmed cases and 5662 deaths while the South-East Asia region had a count of 23,560 confirmed cases and 1051 deaths. Africa, which had started to experience some significant increase in infections, had 12,360 confirmed cases with 517 of those newly reported and 586 deaths of which 36 of those occurred in a span of 24 h (WHO, 2020aa). Still in Africa, it was noted that 11 out of the 17 countries that had reported cases of COVID-19 were drawn from the Western and Central part of the continent, and WHO officials reported that they had teams on the ground to establish the real reason why this was happening

(WHO, 2020ac). Of the total reported deaths, the highest number occurred in the United States with a high of 2350 deaths, while the United Kingdom had the second tally of the day with 861 cases. France had 753 cases while Italy and Spain, two countries that had for past days shown remarkable improvement, had 551 and 525 cases, respectively (WHO, 2020aa). On 10th, the French navy reported that an airplane carrier had 50 soldiers affected, and in less than a week, on 16th, the number of those had increased to a total of 668 (Willsher and Sabbagh, 2020).

Although reports in the health sector showed that the world was still unsafe, as had also been warned by the WHO, other issues were coming up in other sectors. For instance, in Japan, whose total confirmed cases tallied to 9167—which included three cabinet officials—and the number of deaths increasing to 148, the Prime Minister Shinzo Abe declared a nationwide state of emergency (McCurry, 2020). He also advanced a handout worth ¥100,000 to every resident of the country regardless of their economic status to caution them during the period of this emergency (The Japan Times, 2020a). In the United States, on the same day, 5.6 million people filed unemployment claims bringing the total number of those in this situation to more than 22 million people in a period of only 4 weeks (Long, 2020). Following this, President Donald Trump unveiled guidelines aimed to help some economic activities in the country to resume, but he left the final decision of opening the economy, by easing the restrictions on each individual state, to the individual State Governors (White House, 2020). In Germany, after experiencing prior issues after easing lockdown measures resulted to increased number of confirmed cases, the government was planning to reopen the economy as from April 20 by allowing some nonessential stores to open and also allowing schools to resume as from May (Morris and Beck, 2020). In Brazil, President Jair Bolsonaro fired the Minister for Health after the minister insisted on strict social isolation guidelines, a move that the president was against. Unfortunately, the president had been seen to have regularly downplayed the outbreak of the virus in his country despite the country having 28,320 confirmed cases and 1048 deaths by April 16 (Quinn, 2020a).

In sports, following the situation in France, the Tour de France scheduled for June and July was postponed to a tentative date between 29th August and 20th September, as the government banned public gatherings to reduce the spread of the coronavirus (Tour de France, 2020). For World Wrestling Entertainment, the company was planning to lay off some employees including wrestlers and producers such as Kurt Angle (Russell, 2020). The move was to caution the company against the financial decline it was facing following the impacts of the pandemic.

DAY 141—APRIL 19, 2020

After months of extreme pressure, anxiety, and uncertainties, Wuhan settled and revised its official data relating to the coronavirus. After the review, the death toll from the COVID-19 pandemics increased by 50% meaning that its number increased from 1290 deaths to 3869 deaths, pushing the country total by April 17 to 4642 deaths. The errors in reporting were attributed to delays, omissions, and incorrect reporting that are understandable following all the many things that are happening during that period (Neuman, 2020a). The number of reported deaths also increased in the African continent after 55 more deaths were reported, taking the total tally to 1080, while new confirmed cases increased by 1047, pushing the continent's total to 21,317, according to Africa Centres for Disease Control and Prevention (Africa CDC) (Xinhua, 2020a), but data by the WHO for the same period show a total of 13,892 cases and 628 deaths (WHO, 2020x). Death tolls were rising by higher margins in the European regions and had exceeded 100,000 deaths, from 1,122,189 cases reported in the region. This increase, observed throughout Spain and Italy, however, continued to experience improvements with death rates reducing each day. The United Kingdom, France, and Belgium still reported increasing numbers of deaths (888, 635, and 290, respectively). However, the United States still leads in the number of confirmed cases (695,535 on April 19) and death tolls (2043 on the same day) per day for more than two consecutive weeks (WHO, 2020x). Globally, the total number of cases had increased to a high of over 2.3 million, with the number of deaths exceeding 157,000 by April 19 (WHO, 2020x).

Despite the risk of the disease being live, the Orthodox churches in Georgia were observed to flaunt the state of emergency declaration to hold Easter masses, where hundreds of congregants attended (Antidze, 2020). In the United States, a day after the President had outlined a set of rules for reopening the economy, but left the final say on the hands of the Governor, some protesters were observed in States of Michigan, Minnesota, and Ohio and others, calling their Governors to lift the restrictions in their states (Gabbatt, 2020). At the same time, Texas Governor is said to have signed an executive order to allow a reopening as from May (Office of the Texas Governor, 2020). This was happening, even as the US Secretary of Defense extended the travel ban for one more month to void the earlier expiry scheduled for May 2; thus, showing that the country was still not ready to ease the restrictions it had set. Further South, in Chile, the government started issuing "immunity cards" for all those who had infected and recovered from the virus. With the card, these could comfortably return to their work stations (Thomson, 2020). As this was happening, the number of cases in the country rose to 10,888, taking the country as the third most affected in Latin America (WHO, 2020x). However, the WHO, through Dr. Michael Ryan, one of the executive directors, warned that there was no evidence that those who were recovering from COVID-19 were developing any immunity that could prevent them from being reinfected (WHO, 2020ab). During the same press conference, the Director-General emphasized that as Chinese authorities allowed the wet market to reopen, they would ensure conformity to food safety and highest levels of hygiene and that the law banning any trade in wildlife for food was to be implemented strictly to save the world from future pandemics like the coronavirus (WHO, 2020ab).

Elsewhere, more countries were slowly and cautious easing restrictions, with France allowing visitors to care homes, albeit some conditions (DodMan, 2020). Croatia also eased some restrictions allowing people to travel within their districts. In other countries such as the United Kingdom and Zimbabwe, the lockdown measures were to remain intact until when the government is confident the situations are controlled (Today, 2020b). In Saudi Arabia, despite the start of Ramadan, the top religious authorities of the country were recommending people to pray at home to reduce the spread of the virus among the faithful (Reuters, 2020p). This was necessary, as already, deaths were not sparing countries' leadership. For instance, in Nigeria, President Buhari's Chief of Staff, Abba Kyari became the latest top-ranking official to die from COVID-19 (Akwagyiram, 2020b). A similar case was reported in Guinea where a top official and ally of the President Alpha Condé also died (AFP, 2020a).

DAY 143—APRIL 21, 2020

Within a period of 48 h (April 19—21), the number of infections globally increased from 2.3 million cases to over 2.5 million, while the number of deaths increased to above 170,000 globally (Reuters, 2020g). In Europe, the number of those infected increased over this period to over 1.2 million, with a daily average increase of approximately 35,000 new cases, while the number of new deaths in the areas also increased by an average of above 3200 each day—taking the total deaths in the region to 109,952 according to data by the WHO (WHO, 2020y). In the American regions, cases increased by an average of 33,000 confirmations pushing the total confirmed cases to 925,291 cases (WHO, 2020y). The number of deaths increased to approximately 44,775 by April 21, with a majority of these reported in the United States, which was the new epicenter for the coronavirus. The Eastern Mediterranean region had its total confirmed cases increase to 139,349 cases with 6326 people dying from COVID-19. The Western Pacific region had a total of 136, 271 cases after 1765 new cases were confirmed while the number of deaths increased to 5793. The South-East Asia region and African regions, though have had their cases increase, have shown remarkable levels of resilience despite having some of the weakest health systems. Their total confirmed cases increased to 33,912 and 16,115 cases, respectively, while the number of people who succumbed to the COVID-19 in the regions increased to 1427 and 720 deaths, respectively, (WHO, 2020y).

Following the unprecedented increase of infections in the United States, President Donald Trump had reported on April 20 that he would be signing an executive order to suspend immigration to the United States for the next 60 days. And, true to his word, on 21st, he signed the order meaning that Green card recipients would be blocked from moving into the country, with only workers holding nonimmigrant visas allowed (Nick Miroff et al., 2020). He supported his decision by arguing that the unprecedented effects on COVID-19 had pushed many Americans out of jobs, and he would wish to see them access the available job opportunities without having to compete with migrants (Nick Miroff et al., 2020). And to ensure that job opportunities would be available, on the same day, his office and Congressional leaders agreed on a $484 billion small business and hospitals stimulus package, that now only awaited approval from the House of Representatives (Roberts, 2020). In Africa, South Africa took a similar approach of bailing out the economy by unveiling a $26 billion relief plan that would also aid the most vulnerable in the society during the period that the country was struggling with increasing cases of coronavirus and the lockdown measures (Channelstv, 2020). The economic struggles saw Iran start to reopen its economy with major shopping centers in the capital Tehran being the first (Press, 2020). Similar actions were observed in Israel, which eased lockdown restrictions to allow small shops and stores to open and allow people to move around, but on condition mask-wearing in public (Haaretz, 2020). This came as the number of recoveries in those countries started to increase, while the death toll contained (Efrati and Rabinowitz, 2020). In the poorest countries in the world, the World Bank supported the pandemic bond, launched in 2017, with an amount of $195.84 million to assist 64 nations from the impacts of COVID-19 (Baker, 2020). This came as the UN World Food Programme warned that the impacts of COVID-19 would result in the doubling of world hunger, representing a total of 265 million people (Anthem, 2020).

The economy was however not worsening for individuals only, but on this day, it was seen to have particularly worsened for US oil-producing economies and companies, with the prices per barrel going down to $0, a historical event that has never happened (Suleymanova, 2020). The only sector that was seen to be doing well, especially in the United States is the gaming industry, probably due to the "stay-at-home" orders and also due to the closure of schools. But, while the market increased, there were fewer games produced due to the impacts sparked by the coronavirus (Schreier, 2020). The other sector that was seen to benefit from the impacts of COVID-19 was the environment, where it was reported that following the reduced activities in the manufacturing and transport sector, less emissions (6% drop) are expected during the year (Marchand and Faigle, 2020).

DAY 146—APRIL 24, 2020

As over 210 countries continued to fight the spread, and the impacts of COVID-19 in their countries, the United States was the most hit with over 895,766 cases and over 50,000 reported deaths as up to April 24. The new cases in the country had increased at an average number of approximately 28,000 (CDC, 2020). As the number of cases continued to increase, and other more "staying-at-home" measures following the lockdowns in different states, the number of those filing for unemployment claims continued to increase with over 4.4 million additional claims reported over the past week, which was the fifth consecutive week since this trend started (Lambert, 2020). These new numbers raised the total of those who had filed for their employment benefits to over 26 million people (Chaney and Guilford, 2020).

Outside the United States, there were mixed responses to the virus. Some were seen to ease and lift the lockdown and subsequent measures they had implemented, while others were seen to be in haste to institute those measures. For instance, in the Netherlands, after experiencing some "relative calm" over the past weeks in respect to infections in the country, its number had started to rise with new deaths averaging over 120 each day and reaching a high of 4177 deaths and 35,729 confirmed cases by April 24 (WHO, 2020z). To minimize further infection, a stern decision was taken to ban any form of public gather until September 1 (3 months extension) the first of such a ban globally. That means that events such as sports, music festivals, and religious grouping would not be resuming anytime soon (Reuters, 2020e). But, it was not the only one extending such measure as in Pakistan, the lockdown was extended by two more weeks until May 9, as the country was still experiencing increasing numbers of local transmission of the virus, and the lockdown extension would somehow reverse these trends (Cherian, 2020). Indonesia also joined the list of those that were strengthening their measures after the government announced that it would be temporarily suspending nonessential domestic and international air and sea travel until the end of May to curtail the spread of the coronavirus in the country (Bangkok Post, 2020). Others that extended their lockdown include Liberia (Garda, 2020), Lebanon (Reuters, 2020k), and Czech, which sought parliamentary intervention to allow the extension of the state of emergency until May 25 (Xinhua, 2020b).

On the same breath, some countries and states in the United States started easing restrictions to allow the reopening of their economy. These include states such as Georgia, Oklahoma, and others in the United States, which took these decisions despite the disapproval of President Trump (Smith, 2020). Belgium was ready to start reopening some businesses and schools as from May, but gradually and cautiously (Martens, 2020).

Although countries were reacting to COVID-19 situations in different ways, some unfortunate news besides new cases and deaths were also reported. For instance, in the United Kingdom, which had seen the confirmed cases increase significantly and the number of deaths rising to beyond 20 000, there were reports that among the dead were 69 National Health Service personnel who had paid the ultimate price in a bid to save their country from the pandemic (Express and Star, 2020). In Bangladesh, it was reported that 251 frontline doctors had tested positive for the coronavirus due to strains that the COVID-I9 had put on the healthcare system, with most of those in the frontline experiencing a shortage of PPEs, test kits, and hospital beds, among other basic essentials (Mahmud, 2020).

Elsewhere in Japan, after a dreadful experience with the Diamond Princess Cruise ship, on 21st, another fateful incidence involving an Italian cruise ship (*Costa Atlantica)* happened in Nagasaki shipyard (The Japan Times, 2020b). It started when one of the crew members tested positive for coronavirus, while 20 of his colleagues were also showing signs, especially high fever. The following day, after contact tracing from the first confirmed cases, another 33 cases tested positive (The Straits Times, 2020a). 24 h later, another 14 people tested positive (Kaneko and Kim, 2020) and by 24th, a total of 96 people; all crew members were confirmed as testing positive (CNA, 2020b). Following this, the Japanese government stated that it would test 260 people, out of the 630 who were on board the cruise ship and those who turned negative would be repatriated back to their home countries.

DAY 148—APRIL 26, 2020

As the fifth month, since the onset of the coronavirus, is almost over, the number of those confirmed to have contracted the virus increased to over 3 million people globally, and at least 209,000 were reported to have succumbed to the disease. Over the same period, of the 3 million, over 884,000 patients had recovered (Spotlight, 2020). One country where success against COVID-19 have, and continued to be celebrated, was in Wuhan, Hubei Province, China, where healthy officials reported that they had treated all cases and those who recovered were discharged from hospital (O'Donnell, 2020). In fact, as previously reported, the restrictions and lockdown in the provinces were lifted including in Wuhan, on April 8 (Aljazeera, 2020a). Following this, on 23rd, China pledged additional funding, amounting to $30 million, to the WHO (Shih, 2020), as already, it could manage the few cases emerging, and the funds could help other areas that were experiencing high pressure from the pandemic. In the new cases, between 24th and 26th, China was reported to have only recorded a total of 33 new cases and 29 asymptomatic cases, but no death was reported in the 2 days (WHO, 2020i). As cases in China reduced, those in the European region seemed to have continued increasing reaching a high of 1,341,851 cases after the addition of 27,185 new cases on 26th, and the number of deaths increased to 122,218. In the American region, the number of cases was 1,094, 846 and 56,063 deaths reported, according to data by the WHO (WHO, 2020i). The Eastern Mediterranean, Western Pacific, and South-East Asia regions had 160,586, 142,639, and 43,846 confirmed cases, respectively. The African region continued to show high levels of resilience with only 20,316 confirmed cases and 839 deaths reported (WHO, 2020i).

But as the number of cases continued to increase, reports of more countries planning to ease up the lockdown also increased. As of 26th, Italy and Spain, two of the most affected countries by the COVID-19 pandemic, with cases of death in each exceeding 20,000 (Italy 26,384 deaths, Spain 22,524) unveiled plans of how they would open up their country as from May 4. In Italy, according to Prime Minister Giuseppe Conte, the manufacturing industry would gradually open as from May 4, but schools would remain closed for three more months until September (Kayali, 2020). In Spain, people would be allowed to walk out for physical activities, but social distancing will have to be observed, as infections in the country were still real (Reuters, 2020q). Saudi Arabia is another country that considered lifting the nationwide curfew, except for Mecca, which remained under 24-h curfew (Aljazeera, 2020h).

In Germany, after easing the restrictions a few days ago, it is reported that Volkswagen was gearing to resume production in their Wolfsburg factory on April 27 (Allan, 2020), the same decision was also taken by BMW company and other companies such as Mercedes, Jaguar Land Rover, and others reopening in a few days (Reuters, 2020f). This came as some protests were witnessed in Berlin as people demanded the easing of lockdown measures to allow them to return to work (Reuters, 2020d). In the United States, as some states started reopening businesses, the airline industry, which was yet to resume, received support funds amounting to $9.5 billion -taking their bailout total from the US Treasury to $12.4 billion, with the first disbursement received on April 20 (Landay and Shephardson, 2020).

Although those countries were gearing to resume business, others insisted on strict measures as cases continued to rise. For instance, the United Kingdom maintained the lockdown as it was still not safe from the virus infections (BBC, 2020i). Sri Lanka also extended the lockdown in the country to counter the increasing number of cases (AFP, 2020b). Honduras was even considering extending the lockdown by at least one more week until May 3 (Reuters, 2020h). In India, Prime Minister Modi urged his citizens to piously adhere to the nationwide lockdown to contain the rising cases that came amid the month-long curfew (The Straits Times, 2020d).

DAY 150—APRIL 28, 2020

By April 28, it became official that the number of COVID-19 infection cases had exceeded the 3 million (the WHO reported 2.95 million cases and 202,597 deaths) people and caused the death of over 211,000 people globally. Of the confirmed cases, over 1 million were reported in the United States while a quarter of reported deaths from the virus coming from the United States. The number of deaths in the country (59,266) even surpassed the total of those who died during the Vietnam War between 1955 and 1975, where nearly 58,200 people died (Woodward, 2020). In New York, it was reported that for every four people, one of them had contracted the coronavirus. This is after almost 300,000 cases had been confirmed, and more than 17,500 deaths were reported in the city alone. These numbers in the United States eclipse those of other reported regions. For instance, as of 28th, the total number of reported cases in Africa (35,676) was far much less than the total number of deaths (59,266) reported in the United States on the same day. In addition, they were more than the total number of deaths (52,661) in Italy and the United Kingdom, which were leading in terms of reported deaths in Europe (Worldometer, 2020). To reduce these unprecedented trends, some states in the United States started testing for asymptomatic residents such as delivery drivers, rideshare drivers, and others. This came as most of the states were planning to reopen by easing the lockdown restrictions, amidst opposition from President Trump, and the latest, Judge Clay Jenkins of Dallas County, who mentioned the solution, for now, was to follow science and people to stay at home (Holcombe, 2020).

Besides the United States, other countries that are yet to experience some reductions in a number of cases include Russia, where President Vladimir Putin stated that the country was bracing for a new and grueling phase of the pandemic (Llyushina, 2020). His statement came at a time when the number of confirmed cases had continued to stabilize, and the country performed significantly well to reduce casualties. Italy, though determined to ease its lockdown restrictions, was experiencing some new cases, with its numbers reaching beyond the 200,000 mark. According to the WHO, Africa, Eastern Europe, Latin America, and parts of Asia were still not yet out of risk; hence, caution was required even as some actions such as easing the restriction were being taken.

This came as EU experts warned that the world would have to wait longer for the vaccine, which would not be ready until the end of 2021, especially considering the cost implications, and other processes that have to be accomplished (Cullen, 2020). In relation to this, in New York City, it was reported that medical personnel had started testing *Famotidine*; an over-the-counter heartburn medication could cure COVID-19 (Lentile, 2020). This came as human trials had also started in Germany where BioNTech, a pharmaceutical company was testing its vaccine on volunteers, with 12 participants already having received the dose as from April 23 (Aljazeera, 2020f). As solutions for the COVID-19 continued to be sought, some diplomatic disharmony was witnessed when India canceled orders for 500,000 rapid test kits from China after claiming that they were "faulty," and also went forth to withdraw some of the kits that were already in use in several states (BBC, 2020b). China responded harshly and claimed that it was unfair and irresponsible for India to label Chinese products as "faulty" (Business Today, 2020a).

In sports, following the unseen end for the pandemic, French authorities stated that there was no hope for "big sporting affairs" to come back until September in the years, thus, throwing the French Football season in disarray, thus, causing them to be canceled (Aarons and Lowe, 2020). The cancellation came as other countries like Germany had already announced that the football season (Bundesliga) would return in a date to be confirmed albeit under closed doors (Bassell, 2020). Regarding the Olympics, the Olympics International Committee stated that it would cancel the event coming in the next year if the pandemic would not have ended (Schad, 2020).

REFERENCES

Aarons E. (2020) Olympics Must be Delayed to Ensure "Equal" Competition. Available at: https://www.theguardian.com/sport/2020/mar/18/ioc-counting-on-solidarity-of-athletes-as-dissent-grows-over-2020-olympics.

Aarons E and Lowe S. (2020) French Football Season Will Not Resume But La Liga Has New Hope of Restart. Available at: https://www.theguardian.com/football/2020/apr/28/french-football-season-cancelled-with-no-games-until-at-least-august-prime-minister-coronavirus.

ADB. (2020) ADB to Provide $200 Million to Support Strained Supply Chains in Fight Against COVID-19. Available at: https://www.adb.org/news/adb-provide-200-million-support-strained-supply-chains-fight-against-covid-19.

AFDB. (2020) African Development Bank launches record breaking $3 billion "Fight COVID-19" Social Bond. Available at: https://www.afdb.org/en/news-and-events/press-releases/african-development-bank-launches-record-breaking-3-billion-fight-covid-19-social-bond-34982.

AFP. (2020a) Leading Member of Guinea Government Dies From Coronavirus. Available at: https://guardian.ng/news/leading-member-of-guinea-government-dies-from-coronavirus/.

AFP. (2020b) Sri Lanka Extends Virus Lockdown. Available at: https://www.france24.com/en/20200426-sri-lanka-extends-virus-lockdown.

Africanews. (2020) Coronavirus – Africa: African Union and African Private Sector Launch COVID-19 Response Fund. Available at: https://www.africanews.com/2020/04/07/coronavirus-africa-african-union-and-african-private-sector-launch-covid-19-response-fund//.

Akwagyiram A. (2020a) Nigeria Orders 14-Day Cessation of Movement in Lagos, Abuja to Fight Coronavirus. Available at: https://www.reuters.com/article/us-health-coronavirus-nigeria-buhari/nigeria-orders-14-day-cessation-of-moveme nt-in-lagos-abuja-to-fight-coronavirus-idUSKBN21G0UA.

Akwagyiram A. (2020b) Nigerian President's Chief of Staff Dies From Coronavirus. Available at: https://www.reuters.com/article/us-health-coronavirus-nigeria/nigerian-presidents-chi ef-of-staff-dies-from-coronavirus-presidency-spokesman-idU SKBN220001.

Aljazeera. (2020a) China's Wuhan Ends Coronavirus Lockdown But Concerns Remain. Available at: https://www.aljazeera.com/news/2020/04/china-wuhan-ends-coronavirus-lockdo wn-concerns-remain-200408021319019.html.

Aljazeera. (2020b) Coronavirus: Travel Restrictions, Border Shutdowns by Country. Available at: https://www.aljazeera.com/news/2020/03/coronavirus-travel-restrictions-border-shutdo wns-country-200318091505922.html.

Aljazeera. (2020c) Curfew in Mecca, Medina Extended to 24 Hours Over Coronavirus. Available at: https://www.aljazeera.com/news/2020/04/curfew-mecca-medina-extend ed-24-hours-coronavirus-200402140517634.html.

Aljazeera. (2020d) Former Libya Prime Minister Mahmoud Jibril Dies From Coronavirus. Available at: https://www.aljazeera.com/news/2020/04/libya-prime-minister-mahm oud-jibril-dies-coronavirus-200405162834328.html.

Aljazeera. (2020e) France Reports 50 COVID-19 Cases on Board Aircraft Carrier. Available at: https://www.aljazeera.com/news/2020/04/france-reports-50-covid-19-cases-aboa rd-aircraft-carrier-200410115829402.html.

Aljazeera. (2020f) Germany Company Begins Human Trials of Coronavirus Vaccine. Available at: https://www.independent.co.uk/news/world/americas/us-coronavirus-death-toll-vietna m-war-american-fatalities-a9489241.html.

Aljazeera. (2020g) One Hundered Italian Doctors Have Died of Coronavirus. Available at: https://www.aljazeera.com/news/2020/04/italian-doctors-died-coronavirus-20040921 1435347.html.

Aljazeera. (2020h) Saudi Arabia Partially Lifts Curfew Except in Mecca. Available at: https://www.aljazeera.com/news/2020/04/saudi-arabia-partially-lifts-curfew-mecca-200426 063100986.html.

Allan M. (2020) Volkswagen Restart Production as European Car Factories Reopen. Available at: https://www.thescarboroughnews.co.uk/lifestyle/cars/volkswagen-restarts-production-european-car-fa ctories-reopen-2550910.

Anderson M. (2020) Burials on New York Island Are Not New, But Are Increasing During Pandemic. Available at: https://www.npr.org/sections/coronavirus-live-updates/2020/04/10 /831875297/burials-on-new-york-island-are-not-new-but-ar e-increasing-during-pandemic.

Anthem P. (2020) Risk of Hunger Pandemic as COVID-19 Set to Almost Double Acute Hunger by End of 2020. Available at: https://insight.wfp.org/covid-19-will-almost-double-people-in-acute-hunger-by-end-of-2020-59df0c4a8072.

Antidze M. (2020) Hundreds of Parishioners attend Orthodox Easter Vigil in Georgia. Available at: https://www.reuters.com/article/us-health-coronavirus-georgia-easter/hundreds-of-parishioners-attend-orthodox-easter-vigil-in-georgia-idUS KBN2200Y3.

Apple. (2020) Apple and Google Partner on COVID-19 Contact Tracing Technology. Available at: https://www.apple.com/ke/newsroom/2020/04/apple-and-google-partner-on -covid-19-contact-tracing-technology/.

Aquino M and Moreno E. (2020) Gender Divide: Peru, Panama Limit Men and Women to Alternate Days Out to Stall Virus. Available at: https://www.reuters.com/article/us-health-coronavirus-peru/gender-divide-peru-panama-limit-men-and -women-to-alternate-days-out-to-stall-virus-idUSKBN21K39N.

Associated Press. (2020) China to End Lockdown of Coronavirus-Hit Hubei province; Wuhan to Open Next Month. Available at: https://www.foxnews.com/world/china-end-lockdown-coronavirus-hubei-wuhan.

Astapkovich V. (2020) Moscow Shuts Down All Non-Essential Shops & Restaurants to Stop Spread of Covid-19. Available at: https://www.rt.com/russia/484133-moscow-shops-restaurants-coronavirus/.

Austen I. (2020) In Shift, Trudeau Says Canada Will Return Asylum Seekers to U.S. Available at: https://www.nytimes.com/2020/03/20/world/canada/trudeau-asylum-seekers-coronavirus.html.

Azad A. (2020) FDA Authorizes 15-Minute Coronavirus Test. Available at: https://edition.cnn.com/world/live-news/coronavirus-outbreak-03-27-20-intl-hnk/index.html.

Baker M. (2020) Poorest Countries Finally Set to Get World Bank Pandemic Bond Funds. Available at: https://www.euromoney.com/article/b1ld7jd2y7w2rd/poorest-countri es-finally-set-to-get-world-bank-pandemic-bond-funds.

Bangkok Post. (2020) Indonesia Bans Air, Sea Travel Until June Over Virus Fears. Available at: https://www.bangkokpost.com/world/1906755/indonesia-bans-air-sea-travel-until-ju ne-over-virus-fears.

Bank TW. (2020) World Bank Group President Malpass: Remarks to the Development Committee. Available at: https://www.worldbank.org/en/news/statement/2020/04/17/world-bank-group-president-malpass-remarks-to-the-development-committee.

Bassell A. (2020) Bundesliga Return in May Now Looks Inveitable But Fans Far From Happy. Available at: https://www.theguardian.com/football/2020/apr/23/bundesliga-retur n-in-may-now-looks-inevitable-but-fans-are-far-from-hap py.

BBC. (2020a) Coronavirus Travel: China Bars Foreign Visitors as Imported Cases Rise. Available at: https://www.bbc.com/news/world-asia-china-52059085.

BBC. (2020b) Coronavirus: India Cancels Order for "Faulty" China Rapid Test Kits. Available at: https://www.bbc.com/news/amp/world-asia-india-52451455.

BBC. (2020c) Coronavirus: Italy Extends Emergency Measures Nationwide. Available at: https://www.bbc.com/news/world-europe-51810673.

BBC. (2020d) Coronavirus: New York Has More Cases Than Any Country. Available at: https://www.bbc.com/news/world-us-canada-52239261.

BBC. (2020e) Coronavirus: New Zealand Announces Lockdown. Available at: https://www.bbc.com/news/av/world-52001578/coronavirus-new-zealand-announces-lockdown.

BBC. (2020f) Coronavirus: Paris Bans Daytime Outdoor Exercise. Available at: https://www.bbc.com/news/world-europe-52202700.

BBC. (2020g) Coronavirus: Prime Minister Boris Johnson Tests Positive. Available at: https://www.bbc.com/news/uk-52060791.

BBC. (2020h) Coronavirus: Spain Plans Return to 'New Normal' by End of June. Available at: https://www.bbc.com/news/world-europe-52459034.

BBC. (2020i) Coronavirus: UK Must Find 'New Normal' to Ease Lockdown – Raab. Available at: https://www.bbc.com/news/uk-52431501.

BBC Sport. (2020) Formula E: China Race Called Off Amid Coronavirus Outbreak. Available at: https://www.bbc.com/sport/motorsport/51344513.

Beaumont P. (2020) Wuhan Eases Quarantine as Coronavirus Cases in US Pass 100,000. Available at: https://www.theguardian.com/world/2020/mar/28/quarantine-eased-in-wuhan-as-coronavirus-cases-in-us-pass-100000.

Benner T. (2020) Singapore Closes Borders to Keep Virus at Bay, But No Shutdown. Available at: https://www.aljazeera.com/news/2020/03/singapore-closes-borders-virus-bay-shutdown-200322061359901.html.

Bill & Melinda Gates Foundation. (2020) Bill & Melinda Gates Foundation, Wellcome, and Mastercard Launch Initiative to Speed Development and Access to Therapies for COVID-19. Available at: https://www.gatesfoundation.org/Media-Center/Press-Releases/2020/03/COVID-19-Therapeutics-Accelerator.

Bloomberg Philanthropies. (2020) Michael R. Bloomberg Accelerates Fight Against Global Coronavirus Pandemic. Available at: https://www.bloomberg.org/press/releases/michael-r-bloomberg-accelerates-fight-against-global-coronavirus-pandemic/.

Bruce A. (2020) UK Coronavirus Death Toll Could be Far Higher Than Previously Shown. Available at: https://www.reuters.com/article/us-health-coronavirus-england-casualties/uk-coronavirus-death-toll-could-be-far-higher-than-previously-shown-idUSKCN21W0YA.

Business Today. (2020a) Coronavirus Crisis: China Fumes Over ICMR Clampdown on 'Faulty' Rapid Testing Kits, Calls it 'Unfair'. Available at: https://www.businesstoday.in/current/economy-politics/coronavirus-crisis-china-fumes-over-icmr-clampdown-faulty-rapid-testing-kits-calls-it-unfair/story/402221.html.

Business Today. (2020b) Coronavirus Outbreak: India Bans International Flights Till March 28. Available at: https://www.businesstoday.in/sectors/aviation/coronavirus-outbreak-india-bans-international-flights-for-a-week-from-march-22/story/398709.html.

Cacciola S and Deb S. (2020) N.B.A. Suspends Season After Player Tests Positive for Coronavirus. Available at: https://www.nytimes.com/2020/03/11/sports/basketball/nba-season-suspended-coronavirus.html.

Carney J. (2020) Senate Unanimously Passes $2T Coronavirus Stimulus Package. Available at: https://thehill.com/homenews/senate/489590-senate-passes-2-trillion-coronavirus-stimulus-package.

Casselman B, Chen P and Hsu T. (2020) 'It's a Wreck': 3.3 Million File Unemployment Claims as Economy Comes Apart. Available at: https://www.nytimes.com/2020/03/26/business/economy/coronavirus-unemployment-claims.html.

CDC. (2020) Coronavirus Disease 2019: Cases in the US. Available at: https://www.cdc.gov/coronavirus/2019-ncov/cases-updates/cases-in-us.html.

CGTN. (2020) China's First Batch of 144 Schools Reopens in Qinghai Province. Available at: https://news.cgtn.com/news/2020-03-09/School-s-back-144-reopen-in-China-s-Qinghai-Province-OIUlUL3xaU/index.html.

Chaney S and Guilford G. (2020). Available at: https://www.wsj.com/articles/millions-of-u-s-workers-continue-to-seek-unemployment-help-amid-coronavirus-11587634201.

Channelstv. (2020) South Africa President Ramaphosa Unveils $26bn COVID-19 Relief Plan. Available at: https://www.channelstv.com/2020/04/21/south-africa-president-ramaphosa-unveils-26bn-covid-19-relief-plan/.

Chappell B. (2020) Coronavirus: WHO Head Says Nations Must Attack as 'Pandemic Is Accelerating'. Available at: https://www.npr.org/sections/coronavirus-live-updates/2020/03/23/820290984/coronavirus-who-head-says-nations-must-attack-as-pandemic-is-accelerating.

Cheng M. (2020) Europe's Hospitals Among the Best But Can't Handle Pandemic. Available at: https://www.timesofisrael.com/europes-hospitals-among-the-best-but-cant-handle-pandemic/.

Cherian D. (2020) Pakistan Extends Lockdown For 15 Days, Until May 9. Available at: https://gulfnews.com/world/asia/pakistan/pakistan-extends-lock-down-for-15-days-until-may-9-1.1587738995318.

Choon CM. (2020) South Korea Throws up Innovative Tech Solutions in Coronavirus Fight. Available at: straitstimes.com/asia/east-asia/south-korea-throws-up-innovative-tech-solutions-in-coronavirus-fight.

CNA. (2020a) China's Imported COVID-19 Cases Spike as Fears Grow of Second Wave. Available at: https://www.channelnewsasia.com/news/asia/coronavirus-covid-19-china-new-cases-imported-12569894.

CNA. (2020b) COVID-19 Tally Rises to 91 on Italian Cruise Ship in Japan. Available at: https://www.channelnewsasia.com/news/asia/covid-19-tally-rises-to-91-on-italian-cruise-ship-in-japan-12672766.

CNA. (2020c) Cruise Ship Stranded by COVID-19 Fears to Dock in Cambodia. Available at: https://www.channelnewsasia.com/news/asia/wuhan-coronavirus-covid-19-westerdam-ship-dock-cambodia-12427660.

CNBC. (2020) Spain Impose Nationwide Lockdown Due to Virus, Closes all Stores Except Groceries and Pharmacies. Available at: https://www.cnbc.com/2020/03/14/spain-declares-state-of-emergency-due-to-coronavirus.html.

Collinson S. (2020) Trump Address Sparks Chaos as Coronavirus Crisis Deepens. Available at: https://edition.cnn.com/2020/03/12/politics/donald-trump-coronavirus-europe-travel/index.html.

Connor R. (2020) Germany's Maas: Trump Coronavirus Response Took 'Too Long'. Available at: https://www.dw.com/en/germanys-maas-trump-coronavirus-response-took-too-long/a-53089068.

Crowley M, Thomas K and Haberman M. (2020) Ignoring Expert Opinion, Trump Again Promotes Use of Hydroxychloroquine. Available at: https://www.nytimes.com/2020/04/05/us/politics/trump-hydroxychloroquine-coronavirus.html.

Cullen S. (2020) Coronavirus Vaccine Won't be Ready Until End of 2021 Under "Most Optimistic" Scenario – European Expert. Available at: https://edition.cnn.com/world/live-news/coronavirus-pandemic-04-28-20-intl/h_599d6dcfa0dc6c66d271aa7c4c81e835.

Daly N. (2020) Seven More Big Cats Test Positive for Coronavirus at Bronx Zoo. Available at: https://www.nationalgeographic.com/animals/2020/04/tiger-coronavirus-covid19-positive-test-bronx-zoo/.

Davidson H. (2020a) Donald Trump Stokes Fresh Coronavirus Row as Wuhan Reopens. Available at: https://www.theguardian.com/us-news/2020/apr/08/trump-stokes-fresh-coronavirus-row-as-wuhan-reopens.

Davidson H. (2020b) Global Covid-19 cases near 2 million as Putin warns Russia faces 'extraordinary' crisis. Available at: https://www.theguardian.com/world/2020/apr/14/global-covid-19-cases-near-2-million-as-putin-warns-russia-faces-extraordinary-crisis.

DodMan B. (2020) 'Devil's dilemma': France Lifts Ban on Nursing Home Visits as Some Warn Against Relaxing Rules. Available at: https://www.france24.com/en/20200420-devils-dilemma-france-lifts-ban-on-nursing-home-visits-as-some-warn-against-relaxing-rules.

DW. (2020) Coronavirus: What Are the Lockdown Measures Across Europe? Available at: https://www.dw.com/en/coronavirus-what-are-the-lockdown-measures-across-europe/a-52905137.

Education Week. (2020) Map: Coronavirus and School Closures. Available at: https://www.edweek.org/ew/section/multimedia/map-coronavirus-and-school-closures.html.

Efrati I and Rabinowitz A. (2020) Israel Reverses the Trend: More Coronavirus Recoveries Than New Cases. Available at: https://www.haaretz.com/israel-news/.premium-israel-coronavirus-in-first-more-recoveries-than-new-cases-1.8783155.

Egypt Independent. (2020) Mosques to Remain Closed, Charity Iftar Tables Banned in Ramadan. Available at: https://egyptindependent.com/mosques-to-remain-closed-charity-iftar-tables-banned-in-ramadan/.

Erica Werner, Stein J and DeBonis M. (2020) Negotiations Intensify on Capitol Hill Over Massive Stimulus Legislation as Coronavirus Fallout Worsens. Available at: https://www.washingtonpost.com/business/2020/03/18/trump-coronavirus-economic-plan/.

Euroean Commission. (2020a) Applications Welcome From Startups and SMEs With Innovative Solutions to Tackle Coronavirus Outbreak. Available at: https://ec.europa.eu/info/news/startups-and-smes-innovative-solutions-welcome-2020-mar-13_en.

Euroean Commission. (2020b) Commission Publishes Guidance on Export Requirements for Personal Protective Equipment. Available at: https://trade.ec.europa.eu/doclib/press/index.cfm?id=2123.

Express & Star. (2020) The NHS Workers Who Have Died During the Coronavirus Pandemic. Available at: https://www.expressandstar.com/news/uk-news/2020/04/23/the-nhs-workers-who-have-died-during-the-coronavirus-pandemic/.

Folley A. (2020) McDonald's Apologizes After Store in China Displayed Sign Banning Black People. Available at: https://thehill.com/blogs/blog-briefing-room/news/492760-black-people-are-not-allowed-to-enter-mcdonalds-china.

Foran C, Raju M, Byrd H, et al. (2020) Trump Signs Historic $2 Trillion Stimulus After Congress Passes it Friday. Available at: https://edition.cnn.com/2020/03/27/politics/coronavirus-stimulus-house-vote/index.html.

France-Presse A. (2020) Senegal Bans Layoffs During Coronavirus Crisis. Available at: https://www.barrons.com/news/senegal-bans-layoffs-during-coronavirus-crisis-01586545505.

France 24. (2020a) Cuba Closes Borders to Non-residents Over Virus: President. Available at: https://www.france24.com/en/20200320-cuba-closes-borders-to-non-residents-over-virus-president.

France 24. (2020b) Lebanon Announces Two-Week Lockdown Over Coronavirus. Available at: https://www.france24.com/en/20200315-lebanon-announces-two-week-lockdown-over-coronavirus.

Gabbatt A. (2020) US Anti-lockdown Rallies Could Cause Surge in Covid-19 Cases, Experts Warn. Available at: https://www.theguardian.com/us-news/2020/apr/20/us-protests-lockdown-coronavirus-cases-surge-warning.

Gajanan M and Mansoor S. (2020) Cruise Ship Docks in Mexico, Passengers Allowed to Disembark After Being Denied Entry in Jamaica, Cayman Islands Amied Coronavirus Fears. Available at: https://time.com/5790955/cruise-ship-coronavirus-jamaica-cayman-islands/.

Galford C. (2020) CEPI Invests $620,000 into Potential COVID-19 Vaccine From University of Hong Kong. Available at: https://homelandprepnews.com/stories/46064-cepi-invests-620000-into-potential-covid-19-vaccine-from-university-of-hong-kong/.

Gaouette N, Marquardt A and Atwood K. (2020) European Union Leaders Denounce Trumps Coronavirus Travel Restrictions. Available at: https://edition.cnn.com/2020/03/12/politics/european-leaders-us-travel-coronavirus/index.html.

Garda. (2020) Liberia: President Extends Lockdown Measures for Two Weeks From April 24/Update 6. Available at: https://www.garda.com/crisis24/news-alerts/336071/liberia-president-extends-lockdown-measures-for-two-weeks-from-april-24-update-6.

Gov.UK. (2020a) Foreign Travel Advice: Italy. Available at: https://www.gov.uk/foreign-travel-advice/italy/coronavirus.

Gov.UK. (2020b) UK Helps World's Poorest Countries Withstand the Economic Disruption of Coronavirus. Available at: https://www.gov.uk/government/news/uk-helps-worlds-poorest-countries-withstand-the-economic-shock-of-corona virus.

Gresik D and Altman H. (2020) Latest Guard Update: More Than 11,400 Troops Mobilised for COVID-19 Response. Available at: https://www.militarytimes.com/news/coronavirus/2020/03/24/latest-guard-update-more-than-10000-troops-mobili zed-for-covid-19-response/.

Haaretz. (2020) A Fine for Not Wearing a Mask: These Are Israel's New Coronavirus Regulations. Available at: https://www.haaretz.com/israel-news/.premium-netanyahu-anno unced-easing-coronavirus-restrictions-here-s-what-you-nee d-to-know-1.8780064.

Harris B and Schipani A. (2020) Bolsonaro Defies Coronavirus to Rally Against Congress. Available at: https://www.ft.com/content/79fe5d26-621f-11ea-b3f3-fe4680ea68b5.

Hawkins J. (2020) Coronavirus: Iran Release 85,000 Prisoners in Bid to Tackle Spread of Virus. Available at: https://www.mirror.co.uk/news/world-news/breaking-coronavirus-iran-release-85000-21705108.

Haynes D. (2020) Trump invokes Defense Production Act to force GM to Make ventilators. Available at: https://www.upi.com/Top_News/US/2020/03/27/Trump-invokes-Defe nse-Production-Act-to-force-GM-to-make-ventilators/2851 585339926/.

Helsel P. (2020) Available at: https://www.nbcnews.com/politics/politics-news/two-members-house-test-positive-co vid-19-n1163511.

Holcombe M. (2020) Dallas County Judge Opposes Governor's Plan to Reopen and Calls for Residents to Follow Science and Stay Home. Available at: https://www.ksat.com/news/2020/04/28/texas-judge-opposes-governors-plan-to-reopen-and-calls-for-residents-to-follow-science-and-stay-home/.

Homeland Security. (2020) Fact Sheet: DHS Notice of Arrival Restrictions on China, Iran and Certain Countries of Europe. Available at: https://www.dhs.gov/news/2020/03/17/fact-sheet-dhs-notice-arrival-restrictions-china-iran-and -certain-countries-europe.

Ighobor K. (2020) Together We Can With the War Against COVID-19. Available at: https://www.un.org/africarenewal/magazine/special-edition-covid-19/together-we-can-win-war -against-covid-19.

IMF. (2020) IMF Executive Board Approves US$190.5 Million in Emergency Support to Albania to Combat COVID-19 Pandemic. Available at: https://www.imf.org/en/News/Articles/2020/04/10/pr20148-albania-imf-executive-boar d-approves-us-in-emergency-support-to-combat-covid-19-pandemic.

Kaneko K and Kim C-R. (2020) Italian Cruise Ship in Japan Has 48 Coronavirus Cases. Available at: https://www.reuters.com/article/us-health-coronavirus-japan-ship/itali an-cruise-ship-in-japan-has-48-coronavirus-cases-idUSKC N22504S.

Kayali L. (2020) Italy and Spain Announce Plans to Ease Coronavirus Lockdowns Further. Available at: https://www.politico.com/news/2020/04/26/italy-spain-coronavirus-lo ckdown-208260.

KFF. (2020) CEPI Approves $4.4M in Additional Funding For Coronavirus Vaccine Research, Bringing Total To $23.7M. Available at: https://www.kff.org/news-summary/cepi-approves-4-4m-in-additional-funding-for-coronavirus-vac cine-research-bringing-total-to-23-7m/.

Kirby J and Stewart E. (2020) How New York Became the Epicenter of America's Coronavirus Crisis. Available at: https://www.vox.com/coronavirus-covid19/2020/3/27/21 195162/new-york-coronavirus-news-andrew-cuomo-hospi tals-population-ventilators.

Klein B and Raju M. (2020) New York governor: "Ventilators Are to This War What Missiles Were to World War II". Available at: https://edition.cnn.com/world/live-news/coronavirus-outbr eak-03-20-20-intl-hnk/h_e6334d86533d447ff0efcde50d381 286.

Krisel b. (2020) UN Headquarters Closes to Public as Coronavirus Precaution. Available at: https://patch.com/new-york/midtown-nyc/un-headquarters-closes-public-coronavirus-precaution.

Lambert L. (2020) Real Unemployment Rate Soars Past 20%—and the U.S. Has Now Lost 26.5 Million Jobs. Available at: https://fortune.com/2020/04/23/us-unemployment-rate-numbers-claims-this-week-total-job-losses-april-23-2020-ben efits-claims/.

Landauro I and Keeley G. (2020) Spain Sees Slowing Coronavirus Toll, Holds Virtual Easter Parades. Available at: https://www.reuters.com/article/us-health-coronavirus-spa in/spain-sees-slowing-coronavirus-toll-holds-virtual-easter -parades-idUSKCN21S0ZJ.

Landay J and Shephardson D. (2020) U.S. Airlines Receive Extra $9.5 Billion in Payroll Support: U.S. Treasury. Available at: https://www.reuters.com/article/us-health-coronavirus-usa-airlines/u-s-airlines-receive-extra-9-5-billion-in-payroll -support-u-s-treasury-idUSKCN2270OG?il=0.

Lee Y. (2020) Singapore Stops Zoom for Home-Schooling After Hacking Report. Available at: https://www.bloomberg.com/news/articles/2020-04-10/singapore-stops-zoom-for-home-based-learning-after-hacker-breach.

Lentile G. (2020) Famotidine Trial Underway in NYC for COVID-19 Treatment. Available at: https://www.drugtopics.com/latest/famotidine-trial-underway-nyc-covid-19-treatment.

Liptak K. (2020) Trump Declares National Emergency – and Denies Responsibility for Coronavirus Testing Failures. Available at: https://edition.cnn.com/2020/03/13/politics/donald-trump-emergency/index.html.

Llyushina M. (2020) Russia Will "Face a New and Grueling Phase of the Pandemic," Putin Says. Available at: https://edition.cnn.com/world/live-news/coronavirus-pandemic-04-28-20-intl/h_14f73feb35572faea65379f3ca967ace.

Long H. (2020) U.S. Now Has 22 Million Unemployed, Wiping Out a Decade of Job Gains. Available at: https://www.washingtonpost.com/business/2020/04/16/unemp loyment-claims-coronavirus/.

Long H and Dam AV. (2020a) America is in a Depression. The Challenge Now Is to Make it Short-Lived. Available at: https://www.washingtonpost.com/business/2020/04/09/66-million-americans-filed-unemployed-last-week-bringing-pandemic-total-over-17-million/.

Long H and Dam AV. (2020b) America is in a Depression. The Challenge Now is to Make it Short-Lived. Available at: https://www.washingtonpost.com/business/2020/04/09/66-million-americans-filed-unemployed-last-week-bringing-pandemic-total-over-17-million/.

Mahmud F. (2020) Hundreds of Doctors in Bangladesh Infected With Coronavirus. Available at: http://web.archive.org/web/20200425044259/https://www.aljazeera.com/news/2020/04/hundreds-doctors-bangladesh-infected-coronavirus-200423080515266.html.

Mai J. (2020) Coronavirus: Beijing's Ban on Foreign Travellers Comes into Force Months After it Criticised Other Countries for 'Isolating China'. Available at: https://www.scmp.com/news/china/society/article/3077355/coronavirus-beijings-ban-foreign-travellers-comes-force-months.

Marchand O and Faigle N. (2020) Will Coronavirus Reduce Emissions Long Term? Available at: http://www.climateaction.org/news/will-coronavirus-reduce-emissions-long-term.

Martens J. (2020) Belgium to Gradually Ease Virus Lockdown in First Half of May. Available at: https://www.bloomberg.com/news/articles/2020-04-24/belgium-to-gradually-ease-virus-lockdown-in-first-half-of-may.

Mastercard. (2020) COVID-19 Therapeutics Accelerator Awards $20 Million in Initial Grants to Fund Clinical Trials. Available at: https://newsroom.mastercard.com/mea/press-releases/covid-19-therapeutics-accelerator-awards-20-million-in-initial-grants-to-fund-clinical-trials/.

Mayberry K, Siddiqui U and Uras U. (2020) Coronavirus Crisis 'Like No Other' as Cases Near 2m: Live Updates. Available at: https://www.aljazeera.com/news/2020/04/million-confirmed-coronavirus-live-updates-200413235036857.html.

McCabe C and Ostroff C. (2020) Stocks Plunge 10% in Dow's Worst Day Since 1987. Available at: https://www.wsj.com/articles/global-stocks-follow-u-s-markets-lower-11583975524.

McCurry J. (2020) Japan Declares State of Emergency Over Coronavirus. Available at: https://www.theguardian.com/world/2020/apr/07/japan-shinzo-abe-declares-state-of-emergency-over-coronavirus.

McIntyre N and Duncan P. Care Homes and Coronavirus: Why We Don't Know the True UK Death Toll. Available at: https://www.theguardian.com/world/2020/apr/14/care-homes-coronavirus-why-we-dont-know-true-uk-death-toll.

Meseret E and Meldrum A. (2020) As Virus Spreads, Africa Gets Medical Supplies From Chinese billionaire. Available at: https://www.theday.com/article/20200322/NWS13/200329822.

Millhiser I. (2020) The Dow Jones Had its Biggest Point Drop in History Monday. Available at: https://www.vox.com/2020/3/16/21182341/dow-jones-biggest-point-drop-coronavirus-3000.

Mischke J. (2020) Angela Merkel's First Coronavirus Test Result is Negative. Available at: https://www.politico.com/news/2020/03/23/angela-merkels-first-coronavirus-test-result-is-negative-144257.

Moreno e, Jorgic D and Nomiyama C. (2020) Panama Suspends Domestic Flights to Curb the Spread of Coronavirus: Civil Aviation Authority. Available at: https://www.usnews.com/news/world/articles/2020-03-25/panama-suspends-domestic-flights-to-curb-the-spread-of-coronavirus-civil-aviation-authority.

Morris L and Beck L. (2020) Germany to Reopen Schools, Shops After 'Fragile' Success. Available at: https://www.washingtonpost.com/world/2020/04/15/coronavirus-latest-news/.

Mourad M. (2020) Egypt Shuts Mosques and Churches Over Coronavirus Fears. Available at: https://www.reuters.com/article/us-health-coronavirus-egypt-religion/egypt-shuts-mosques-and-churches-over-coronavirus-fears-idUSKBN2180M5.

Neuman S. (2020a) China Raises Wuhan Death Stats by Half to Account for Reporting Delays and Omissions. Available at: https://www.npr.org/sections/coronavirus-live-updates/2020/04/17/836700806/china-raises-wuhan-death-stats-by-half-to-account-for-reporting-delays-and-omiss.

Neuman S. (2020b) South Africa Reports First COVID-19 Deaths, Goes into 3-Week Lockdown. Available at: https://www.npr.org/sections/coronavirus-live-updates/2020/03/27/822363982/south-africa-reports-first-covid-19-deaths-goes-into-3-week-lockdown.

Nick Miroff, Sacchetti M and Jan T. (2020) Trump to Suspend Immigration to U.S. for 60 Days, Citing Coronavirus Crisis and Jobs Shortage, But Will Allow Some Workers. Available at: https://www.washingtonpost.com/immigration/coronavirus-trump-suspend-immigration/2020/04/21/464e2440-838d-11ea-ae26-989cfce1c7c7_story.html.

Niesner L and Murphy F. (2020) Austria Reopens Thousands of Shops in First Loosening of Coronavirus Lockdown. Available at: https://www.reuters.com/article/us-health-coronavirus-austria/austria-reopening-thousands-of-shops-in-first-loosening-of-lockdown-idUSKCN21V25G.

Nottingham S. (2020) Nearly 91% of Americans Have Been Ordered to Stay at Home. Available at: https://edition.cnn.com/world/live-news/coronavirus-pandemic-04-02-20-intl/h_31be689eb8404149e126dce751d6045f.

O'Donnell T. (2020) China Says all Coronavirus Patients Been Discharged. Available at: https://news.yahoo.com/china-says-coronavirus-patients-wuhan-150411821.html.

Office of the President. (2020a) Letter From President Donald J. Trump on Emergency Determination Under the Stafford Act. Available at: https://www.whitehouse.gov/briefings-statements/letter-president-donald-j-trump-emergency-determination-stafford-act/.

Office of the President. (2020b) Remarks by President Trump and Vice President Pence at a Coronavirus Briefing with Health Insurers. Available at: https://www.whitehouse.gov/briefings-statements/remarks-president-trump-vice-president-pence-coronavirus-briefing-health-insurers/.

Office of the Texas Governor. (2020) Governor Abbott Issues Executive Order Establishing Strike Force to Open Texas. Available at: https://www.who.int/docs/default-source/coronaviruse/transcripts/who-audio-emergencies-coronavirus-press-conference-17apr2020.pdf?sfvrsn=1bd9c4cd_2.

Onishi N and Méheut C. (2020) Paris, a Magnet for the World, Becomes a Ghost City After a Lockdown Takes Effect. Available at: https://www.nytimes.com/2020/03/17/world/europe/paris-coronavirus-lockdown.html.

Oppmann P. (2020) Cuba Is Going Under Lockdown Over Coronavirus Concerns. Available at: https://edition.cnn.com/world/live-news/coronavirus-outbreak-03-24-20-intl-hnk/h_7b694d17a78f2c02d7c76570e1726508.

Orihuela R, Donahue P and Follain J. (2020) Italy Joins Germany in Prolonging Lockdown to Quell Outbreak. Available at: https://www.bloomberg.com/news/articles/2020-04-01/italy-to-extend-lockdown-to-april-13-health-minister-says.

Park JG. (2020) COVID-19: How a Phone App Is Assisting South Korea Enforce Self-Quarantine Measures. Available at: https://www.sbs.com.au/language/english/covid-19-how-a-phone-app-is-assisting-south-korea-enforce-self-quarantine-measures.

Perrigo B. (2020) Why Is Germany's Coronavirus Death Rate So Low? Available at: https://time.com/5812555/germany-coronavirus-deaths/.

Phillips t. (2020) First Yanomami Covid-19 Death Raises Fears for Brazil's Indigenous Peoples. Available at: https://www.theguardian.com/world/2020/apr/10/first-yanomami-covid-19-death-brazl-indigenous.

Picheta R. (2020) Spain to Extend Coronavirus State of Emergency as Deaths Soar. Available at: https://edition.cnn.com/2020/03/22/europe/spain-coronavirus-sunday-intl/index.html.

Pramuk J and Dzhanova Y. (2020) Connecticut Becomes Latest State to Postpone 2020 Primary as Coronavirus Spreads. Available at: https://www.cnbc.com/2020/03/19/connecticut-latest-state-to-postpone-2020-primary-as-coronavirus-spreads.html.

Press A. (2020) Iran Begins to Open its Economy Despite Fears of Second Wave of Infection. Available at: https://time.com/5824109/iran-opens-economy-coronavirus/.

Quinn C. (2020a) Brazil's Populist President Ousted His Respected Health Minister While Continuing to Downplay the Coronavirus Pandemic. Available at: https://foreignpolicy.com/2020/04/17/jair-bolsonaro-brazil-fires-heath-minister-mandetta-coronavirus-inections-grow/.

Quinn C. (2020b) Italy's Coronavirus Death Toll Surpasses China's. Available at: https://foreignpolicy.com/2020/03/20/italys-coronavirus-death-toll-surpasses-chinas/.

Ramsay G. (2020) Japanese PM and IOC Chief Agree to Postpone 2020 Olympics Until 2021. Available at: https://edition.cnn.com/2020/03/24/sport/olympics-postponement-tokyo-2020-spt-intl/index.html.

Rapperport A and Smialek J. (2020) I.M.F. Predicts Worst Downturn Since the Great Depression. Available at: https://www.nytimes.com/2020/04/14/us/politics/coronavirus-economy-recession-depression.html?action=click&module=RelatedLinks&pgtype=Article.

Razek R. (2020) 24 States Have Declared a State of Emergency Due to Coronavirus. Available at: https://edition.cnn.com/world/live-news/coronavirus-outbreak-03-11-20-intl-hnk/h_5c886c400fa63ae66fd197ec23927eca.

Regencia T, Stepansky J and Varshalomidze T. (2020) Global Coronavirus Death Toll Exceeds 100,000: Live Updates. Available at: https://www.aljazeera.com/news/2020/04/coronavirus-deaths-rise-signs-progress-live-updates-200409231002574.html.

Rein L. (2020) In Unprecedented Move, Treasury Orders Trump's Name Printed on Stimulus Checks. Available at: https://www.washingtonpost.com/politics/coming-to-your-1200-relief-check-donald-j-trumps-name/2020/04/14/071016c2-7e82-11ea-8013-1b6da0e4a2b7_story.html.

Reuters. (2020a) Austrian Joblessness Hits Record Despite Government Bit to Avoid Layoffs. Available at: https://www.reuters.com/article/austria-economy-unemployment/austrian-joblessness-hits-record-despite-government-bid-to-avoid-layoffs-idUSL8N2BP5LP.

Reuters. (2020b) Bolivia Postpones Elections, Announces Nationwide 14-Day Quarantine to Stem Spread of Coronavirus. Available at: https://www.reuters.com/article/us-health-coronavirus-bolivia/bolivia-announces-nationwide-14-day-quarantine-to-stem-spread-of-coronavirus-idUSKBN2180VG.

Reuters. (2020c) China's Coronavirus Epicenter Reports Just Five Cases, Beijing Tomb-Sweepers Urged to Stay Back. Available at: https://www.reuters.com/article/us-health-coronavirus-china/chinas-coronavirus-epicenter-reports-just-five-cases-beijing-tomb-sweepers-urged-to-stay-back-idUSKBN2100BP.

Reuters. (2020d) Dozens of Protesters Were Arrested in Berlin on Saturday for Flouting Lockdown Rules and Staging a Demonstration Against Lockdown Measures. Available at: https://www.theguardian.com/world/video/2020/apr/26/coronavirus-dozens-arrested-in-berlin-protesting-against-lockdown-video.

Reuters. (2020e) Dutch Extend Ban on Major Public Events Until Sept. 1. Available at: https://www.reuters.com/article/health-coronavirus-netherlands/dutch-extend-ban-on-major-public-events-until-sept-1-idUSS8N2AW01F.

Reuters. (2020f) Europe Restarts Car Factories Amid Uncertain Demand. Available at: https://www.nytimes.com/reuters/2020/04/27/business/27reuters-health-coronavirus-volkswagen-factory.html.

Reuters. (2020g) Global Coronavirus Cases Pass 2.5 Million as U.S. Tally Surpasses 800,000. Available at: https://www.usnews.com/news/world/articles/2020-04-21/global-coronavirus-cases-pass-25-million-as-us-tally-nears-800-000.

Reuters. (2020h) Honduras Extends Coronavirus Curfew by One Week to May 3. Available at: http://cms.trust.org/item/20200426185211-dh38h.

Reuters. (2020i) Italy's Coronavirus Lockdown Measures to be Extended to April 13: Minister. Available at: https://www.reuters.com/article/us-health-coronavirus-italy-lockdown/italys-coronavirus-lockdown-measures-to-be-extended-to-april-13-minister-idUSKBN21J4RU.

Reuters. (2020j) Kazakhstan, Uzbekistan Close Borders After First Coronavirus Cases. Available at: https://www.reuters.com/article/us-health-coronavirus-kazakhstan-emergen/

kazakhstan-uzbekistan-close-borders-after-first-coronavirus-cases-idUSKBN2120EX.

Reuters. (2020k) Lebanon Advised to Extend Coronavirus Lockdown to May 10. Available at: https://www.reuters.com/article/us-health-coronavirus-lebanon/lebanon-advised-to-extend-coronavirus-lockdown-to-may-10-idUSKCN22621J.

Reuters. (2020l) Mexico Declares Health Emergency as Coronavirus Death Toll Rises. Available at: https://www.reuters.com/article/us-health-coronavirus-mexico/mexico-declares-health-emergency-as-coronavirus-death-toll-rises-idUSKBN21I05K.

Reuters. (2020m) Nigeria Closes Land Borders to Fight Coronavirus Spread. Available at: https://www.uneca.org/stories/african-finance-ministers-call-coordinated-covid-19-response-mitigate-adverse-impact.

Reuters. (2020n) Pakistan Suspends Internationa Flights for Two Weeks. Available at: https://www.theguardian.com/world/2020/mar/21/pakistan-suspends-international-flights-for-two-weeks-to-stem-covid-19-spread.

Reuters. (2020o) Portugal to Treat Migrants as Residents During Coronavirus Crisis. Available at: https://www.reuters.com/article/us-health-coronavirus-portugal/portugal-to-treat-migrants-as-residents-during-coronavirus-crisis-idUSKBN21F0N7.

Reuters. (2020p) Saudi Top Religious Authority Recommends Home Prayers in Ramadan Amid Coronavirus. Available at: https://news.trust.org/item/20200419074210-cmru0.

Reuters. (2020q) Spain to Allow Outdoor Exercise if Coronavirus Cases Contine to Fall. Available at: https://www.usnews.com/news/world/articles/2020-04-25/spain-to-allow-outdoor-exercise-if-coronavirus-cases-continue-to-fall.

Reuters. (2020r) Vietnam in Talks to Borrow $1 Billion as Budget Deficit Seen Widening. Available at: https://www.reuters.com/article/us-health-coronavirus-vietnam/vietnam-in-talks-to-borrow-1-billion-as-budget-deficit-seen-widening-idUSKCN21S0PI.

Rich M, Ueno H and Inoue M. (2020) Japan Declared a Coronavirus Emergency. Is It Too Late? Available at: https://www.nytimes.com/2020/04/07/world/asia/japan-coronavirus-emergency.html.

Roberts W. (2020) US Senate Approves $484bn Funding for Small Businesses, Hospitals. Available at: https://www.aljazeera.com/news/2020/04/senate-approves-484bn-funding-small-businesses-hospitals-200421192959062.html.

Rockefeller Foundation. (2020) The Rockefeller Foundation Commits $20 Million in COVID-19 Assistance.

Rojas J-PF. (2020) Coronavirus: Heathrow Passenger Demand to Fall by More Than 90% in April. Available at: https://news.sky.com/story/coronavirus-heathrow-passenger-demand-to-fall-more-than-90-in-april-11972915.

Romo V. (2020) Prince Albert II of Monaco Test Positive for Coronavirus. Available at: https://www.npr.org/sections/coronavirus-live-updates/2020/03/19/818698736/prince-albert-ii-of-monaco-tests-positive-for-coronavirus.

RTVE. (2020) The Coronavirus Map in SPAIN: 23,521 Dead and More Than 209,000 Infected. Available at: https://www.rtve.es/noticias/20200427/mapa-del-coronavirus-espana/2004681.shtml.

Russell J. (2020) WWE Announces Layoffs Two Days After Florida Deems Company an 'Essential Business'. Available at: https://www.pressdemocrat.com/news/10900529-181/wwe-announces-layoffs-two-days.

Schad T. (2020) Tokyo Olympics Will be Canceled, Not Delayed, if Coronavirus Pandemic Still Poses Threat in 2021, Top Official Says. Available at: https://www.usatoday.com/story/sports/olympics/2020/04/28/tokyo-olympics-canceled-if-coronavirus-still-threat-21/3038465001/.

Schnirring L. (2020) As Italy COVID-19 Cases Soar, WHO Tackles PPE, Test Shortages. Available at: https://www.cidrap.umn.edu/news-perspective/2020/03/italy-covid-19-cases-soar-who-tackles-ppe-test-shortages.

Schreier J. (2020) Gaming Sales Are Up, But Production Is Down. Available at: https://www.nytimes.com/2020/04/21/technology/personaltech/coronavirus-video-game-production.html.

Sevastopulo D and Manson K. (2020) Donald Trump Threatens to Freeze Funding for WHO. Available at: https://www.ft.com/content/193453e3-479f-4fef-9234-d0f9f14c5a6e.

Shapiro E. (2020) New York City Public Schools to Close to Slow Spread of Coronavirus. Available at: https://www.nytimes.com/2020/03/15/nyregion/nyc-schools-closed.html.

Shear MD. (2020) Trump Extends Social Distancing Guidelines Through End of April. Available at: https://www.nytimes.com/2020/03/29/us/politics/trump-coronavirus-guidelines.html.

Shih G. (2020) China Pledges Additional $30 Million Funding for World Health Organization. Available at: https://www.washingtonpost.com/world/asia_pacific/china-pledges-additional-30-million-funding-for-world-health-organization/2020/04/23/24f9b680-8539-11ea-81a3-9690c9881111_story.html.

Shroff N. (2020) India Extends Ban on International Flights Until April 14. Available at: https://www.businesstraveller.com/business-travel/2020/03/27/india-extends-ban-on-international-flights-until-april-14/.

Sider A and Mann T. (2020) Airlines Seek $50 Billion Coronavirus Aid Package. Available at: https://www.wsj.com/articles/airlines-seek-up-to-50-billion-in-government-aid-amid-coronavirus-crisis-11584378242.

Siobhán O'Grady, O'Grady S, Rick Noack, et al. (2020a) As U.S. Coronavirus Deaths Surpass 10,000, HHS Watchdog Says American Hospitals Face 'Severe' Shortages of Equipment, Staff and Tests. Available at: https://www.washingtonpost.com/world/2020/04/06/coronavirus-latest-news/.

Siobhán O'Grady, Rick Noack, Marisa Iati, et al. (2020b) China Reports Zero New Local Coronavirus Infections; Trump Signs Bill to Ensure Paid Leave, Other Financial Benefits. Available at: https://www.washingtonpost.com/world/2020/03/18/coronavirus-latest-news/.

Smith D. (2020) Too soon': Trump Disagrees with Georgia Governor's Decision to Reopen Businesses. Available at: https://www.theguardian.com/world/2020/apr/22/trump-georgia-reopen-coronavirus-briefing-us-latest.

Snuggs T. (2020) Coronavirus Deaths in Italy up by 250 in a day to 1,266. Available at: https://news.sky.com/story/coronavirus-deaths-in-italy-rise-to-1-266-up-250-in-a-day-11957245.

Sparrow A, Campbell L and Rawlinson K. (2020) Available at: https://www.theguardian.com/politics/live/2020/mar/23/uk-coronavirus-live-news-latest-boris-johnson-minister-condemns-people-ignoring-two-metre-distance-rule-in-parks-as-very-selfish.

Spotlight. (2020) Global Death Toll From Coronavirus Tops 200,000, 813 Recovered. Available at: https://www.spotlightnepal.com/2020/04/26/global-death-toll-coronavirus-tops-200000-813000-recovered/.

Stamouli N. (2020) Greece to go into Coronavirus-Induced Lockdown. Available at: https://www.politico.eu/article/greece-to-go-into-coronavirus-induced-lockdown/.

Suleymanova R. (2020) Crash! US Crude Futures Turn Negative for First Time in History. Available at: https://www.aljazeera.com/ajimpact/crash-crude-futures-turn-negative-time-history-200420183431731.html.

Sun LH and Dawsey J. (2020) White House Expected to Urge Americans to Wear Face Coverings in Public to Slow Spread of Coronavirus. Available at: https://www.washingtonpost.com/health/2020/04/02/coronavirus-facemasks-policyreversal/.

Suneja K. (2020) Government Bans Exports of Certain Masks, Ventilators, Raw Material for Masks, Coveralls. Available at: https://economictimes.indiatimes.com/news/economy/foreign-trade/government-bans-exports-of-certain-masks-ventilators-raw-material-for-masks-coveralls/articleshow/74718029.cms.

Techakitteranun H. (2020) Available at: https://www.straitstimes.com/asia/se-asia/thailand-declares-state-of-emergency-to-curb-spread.

The Citizen. (2020) Zimbabwe Shuts Borders After First Coronavirus. Available at: https://citizen.co.za/news/news-africa/2259427/zimbabwe-shuts-borders-after-first-coronavirus-death/.

The Herald. (2020) Breaking: Air Zim Sends Workers on Unpaid Leave. Available at: https://www.herald.co.zw/air-zim-sends-workers-on-unpaid-leave/.

The Japan Times. (2020a) Japan to Declare Nationwide State of Emergency as Virus Spreads. Available at: https://www.japantimes.co.jp/news/2020/04/16/national/state-of-emergency-expansion/#.XphHTS_MxQI.

The Japan Times. (2020b) One Crew Member Tests Positive, 20 Feverish on Cruise Ship in Japan. Available at: https://www.japantimes.co.jp/news/2020/04/21/national/one-crew-member-tests-positive-20-feverish-cruise-ship-japan/#.XqQ9w8gzZPY.

The Nation. (2020) PM Announces 10pm to 4am Nationwide Curfew. Available at: https://www.nationthailand.com/news/30385290.

The New York Times. (2020a) C.D.C. Gives New Guidelines, New York to Close Restaurants and Schools and Italian Deaths Rise. Available at: https://www.nytimes.com/2020/03/15/world/coronavirus-live.html.

The New York Times. (2020b) U.S. Now Leads the World in Confirmed Cases. Available at: http://nytimes.com/2020/03/26/world/coronavirus-news.html.

The Open. (2020) Statement From The R&A/The Open in 2020 to be Cancelled. Available at: https://www.theopen.com/latest/2020/04/theopencancellation2020.

The Star. (2020) China Reports 74 Newly Imported Covid-19 Cases and One in Wuhan. Available at: https://www.thestar.com.my/news/regional/2020/03/24/china-reports-74-newly-imported-covid-19-cases.

The Straits Times. (2020a) 34 Crew Have Coronavirus on Cruise Ship Docked for Repairs in Japan. Available at: https://www.straitstimes.com/asia/east-asia/japans-nagasaki-confirms-33-coronavirus-cases-on-cruise-ship-docked-for-repairs.

The straits Times. (2020b) China Tightens Russian Border Checks, Approves Experimental Coronavirus Vaccine. Available at: https://www.straitstimes.com/asia/east-asia/chinas-heilongjiang-province-bordering-russia-reports-79-new-imported-coronavirus.

The straits Times. (2020c) China's Imported Coronavirus Cases Soar, No Local Transmission for Third Straight Day. Available at: https://www.straitstimes.com/asia/east-asia/chinas-imported-coronavirus-cases-jump-as-students-expats-flock-home.

The Straits Times. (2020d) Indian PM Modi Urges Citizens to Follow Lockdown as Coronavirus Cases Rise. Available at: https://www.straitstimes.com/asia/south-asia/indian-pm-modi-urges-citizens-to-follow-lockdown-as-coronavirus-cases-rise.

The Sun. (2020) Boris Johnson's Move From Intensive Care to a General Ward Is the Lift Britain Needed. Available at: https://www.thesun.co.uk/news/11367851/boris-johnson-move-intensive-care-lift-britain/.

The world Bank. (2020a) World Bank East Asia and Pacific Economic Update, April 2020: East Asia and Pacific in the Time of COVI-19. Available at: https://openknowledge.worldbank.org/handle/10986/33477.

The World Bank. (2020b) World Bank Group Increases COVID-19 Response to $14 Billion to Help Sustain Economies, Protect Jobs. Available at: https://www.bloomberg.org/press/releases/michael-r-bloomberg-accelerates-fight-against-global-coronavirus-pandemic/.

Thomson E. (2020) World's First Covid-19 Immunity Cards Are Coming to Chile. Available at: https://www.bloomberg.com/news/articles/2020-04-16/chile-to-start-controversial-coronavirus-immunity-card-system.

Tirrell M, Wells N and Taylor H. (2020) More Than 1 Million People Tested for Coronavirus in US, But Access Varies From State to State. Available at: https://www.cnbc.com/2020/04/03/coronavirus-testing-which-states-are-doing-the-most-covid-19-screening.html.

Today. (2020a) Georgia Proposes 10-Day Lockdown of Four Cities Including Capital. Available at: https://www.todayonline.com/world/georgia-lock-down-four-cities-including-capital-10-days-pm.

Today. (2020b) UK Not Thinking of Easing Virus Lockdown Measures Yet: Minister. Available at: https://www.todayonline.com/world/uk-not-thinking-easing-virus-lockdown-measures-yet-minister.

Tour de France. (2020) The Tour de France 2020 From August 29th to September 20. Available at: https://www.letour.fr/fr/actus/2020/le-tour-de-france-2020-du-29-aout-au-20-septembre/1283442.

Tugwell P. (2020) Greece to Gradually Start Lifting Lockdown Measures on May 4. Available at: Greece to Gradually Start Lifting Lockdown Measures on May 4.

UN. (2020) Key COP26 Climate Summit Postponed to 'Safeguard Lives'. Available at: https://news.un.org/en/story/2020/04/1060902.

UN Secretary-General. (2020) Secretary-General's remarks at launch of Global Humanitarian Response Plan for COVID-19. Available at: https://www.un.org/sg/en/content/sg/statement/2020-03-25/secretary-generals-remarks-launch-of-global-humanitarian-response-plan-for-covid-19.

UNECA. (2020) African Finance Ministers Call for Coordinated COVID-19 Response to Mitigate Adverse Impact on Economies and Society. Available at: https://www.uneca.org/stories/african-finance-ministers-call-coordinated-covid-19-response-mitigate-adverse-impact.

UNICEF. (2020) A Global Approach Is the Only Way to Fight COVID-19, the UN Says as it Launches Humanitarian Response Plan. Available at: https://www.unicef.org/press-releases/global-approach-only-way-fight-covid-19-un-says-it-launches-humanitarian-response.

Ward-Henninger C. (2020) Coronavirus: Boston Celtics Guard Marcus Smart Tests Positive for COVID-19. Available at: https://www.cbssports.com/nba/news/coronavirus-boston-celtics-guard-marcus-smart-tests-positive-for-covid-19/.

Ward M. (2020) Chinese Businessman to Donate 500,000 Test Kits and 1 Million Masks to the U.S. Available at: https://www.politico.com/news/2020/03/13/jack-ma-coronavirus-test-kits-128522.

Watts A and Simon M. (2020) World Health Organization Has Distributed 1.5 Million Coronavirus Lab Tests Around the World. Available at: https://edition.cnn.com/world/live-news/coronavirus-outbreak-03-20-20-intl-hnk/h_e6334d86533d447ff0efcde50d381286.

Wellcome. (2020) Global COVID-Zero Initiative Launched to Fill $8bn Shortfall for Coronavirus Response. Available at: https://wellcome.ac.uk/press-release/global-covid-zero-initiative-launched-fill-8bn-shortfall-coronavirus-response.

Whitcomb D. (2020a) Chicago's Largest Jail Reports 450 Inmates, Staff Positive for Coronavirus. Available at: https://globalnews.ca/news/6803935/coronavirus-chicago-jail-cases/.

Whitcomb D. (2020b) Two Los Angeles Lakers Players Have Tested Positive for COVID-19, Team Says. Available at: https://www.reuters.com/article/us-health-coronavirus-lakers/two-los-angeles-lakers-players-have-tested-positive-for-covid-19-team-says-idUSKBN21700H.

White House. (2020) President Donald J. Trump Is Beginning the Next Phase in Our Fight Against Coronavirus: Guidelines for Opening Up America Again. Available at: https://www.whitehouse.gov/briefings-statements/president-donald-j-trump-beginning-next-phase-fight-coronavirus-guidelines-opening-america/.

Whiteman H and Sharma A. (2020) Australia Bans Overseas Travel and Extends Social Restrictions. Available at: https://www.militarytimes.com/news/coronavirus/2020/03/24/latest-guard-update-more-than-10000-troops-mobilized-for-covid-19-response/.

WHO. (2020a) Coronavirus Disease 2019 (C0VID-19): Situation Report - 77. Available at: https://www.who.int/docs/default-source/coronaviruse/situation-reports/20200406-sitrep-77-covid-19.pdf?sfvrsn=21d1e632_2.

WHO. (2020b) Coronavirus Disease 2019 (COVID-1): Situation Report - 79. Available at: https://www.who.int/docs/default-source/coronaviruse/situation-reports/20200408-sitrep-79-covid-19.pdf?sfvrsn=4796b143_6.

WHO. (2020c) Coronavirus Disease 2019 (COVID-19): Situation Report -53. Available at: https://www.who.int/docs/default-source/coronaviruse/situation-reports/20200313-sitrep-53-covid-19.pdf?sfvrsn=adb3f72_2.

WHO. (2020d) Coronavirus Disease 2019 (COVID-19): Situation Report -60. Available at: https://www.who.int/docs/default-source/coronaviruse/situation-reports/20200320-sitrep-60-covid-19.pdf?sfvrsn=8894045a_2.

WHO. (2020e) Coronavirus Disease 2019 (COVID-19): Situation Report -64. Available at: https://www.who.int/docs/default-source/coronaviruse/situation-reports/20200324-sitrep-64-covid-19.pdf?sfvrsn=723b221e_2.

WHO. (2020f) Coronavirus Disease 2019 (COVID-19): Situation Report -68. Available at: https://www.who.int/docs/default-source/coronaviruse/situation-reports/20200328-sitrep-68-covid-19.pdf?sfvrsn=384bc74c_4.

WHO. (2020g) Coronavirus Disease 2019 (COVID-19): Situation Report -74. Available at: https://www.who.int/docs/default-source/coronaviruse/situation-reports/20200403-sitrep-74-covid-19-mp.pdf?sfvrsn=4e043d03_12.

WHO. (2020h) Coronavirus Disease 2019 (COVID-19): Situation Report -82. Available at: https://www.who.int/docs/default-source/coronaviruse/situation-reports/20200411-sitrep-82-covid-19.pdf?sfvrsn=74a5d15_2.

WHO. (2020i) Coronavirus Disease 2019 (COVID-19): Situation Report -97. Available at: https://www.who.int/docs/default-source/coronaviruse/situation-reports/20200426-sitrep-97-covid-19.pdf?sfvrsn=d1c3e800_6.

WHO. (2020j) Coronavirus Disease 2019 (COVID-19): Situation Report - 54. Available at: https://www.who.int/docs/default-source/coronaviruse/situation-reports/20200314-sitrep-54-covid-19.pdf?sfvrsn=dcd46351_2.

WHO. (2020k) Coronavirus Disease 2019 (COVID-19): Situation Report - 55. Available at: https://www.who.int/docs/default-source/coronaviruse/situation-reports/20200315-sitrep-55-covid-19.pdf?sfvrsn=33daa5cb_8.

WHO. (2020l) Coronavirus Disease 2019 (COVID-19): Situation Report - 56. Available at: https://www.who.int/docs/default-source/coronaviruse/situation-reports/20200316-sitrep-56-covid-19.pdf?sfvrsn=9fda7db2_2.

WHO. (2020m) Coronavirus Disease 2019 (COVID-19): Situation Report - 59. Available at: https://www.who.int/docs/

default-source/coronaviruse/situationeports/20200319-sitrep-59-covid-19.pdf?sfvrsn=c3dcdef9_2.
WHO. (2020n) Coronavirus Disease 2019 (COVID-19): Situation Report - 63. Available at: https://www.who.int/docs/default-source/coronaviruse/situation-reports/20200323-sitrep-63-covid-19.pdf?sfvrsn=b617302d_4.
WHO. (2020o) Coronavirus Disease 2019 (COVID-19): Situation Report - 66. Available at: https://www.who.int/docs/default-source/coronaviruse/situation-reports/20200326-sitrep-66-covid-19.pdf?sfvrsn=81b94e61_2.
WHO. (2020p) Coronavirus Disease 2019 (COVID-19): Situation Report - 69. Available at: https://www.who.int/docs/default-source/coronaviruse/situation-reports/20200329-sitrep-69-covid-19.pdf?sfvrsn=8d6620fa_8.
WHO. (2020q) Coronavirus Disease 2019 (COVID-19): Situation Report - 70. Available at: https://www.who.int/docs/default-source/coronaviruse/situation-reports/20200330-sitrep-70-covid-19.pdf?sfvrsn=7e0fe3f8_2.
WHO. (2020r) Coronavirus Disease 2019 (COVID-19): Situation Report - 73. Available at: https://www.who.int/docs/default-source/coronaviruse/situation-reports/20200402-sitrep-73-covid-19.pdf?sfvrsn=5ae25bc7_4.
WHO. (2020s) Coronavirus disease 2019 (COVID-19): Situation Report - 78. Available at: https://www.who.int/docs/default-source/coronaviruse/situation-reports/20200407-sitrep-78-covid-19.pdf?sfvrsn=bc43e1b_2.
WHO. (2020t) Coronavirus Disease 2019 (COVID-19): Situation Report - 80. Available at: https://www.who.int/docs/default-source/coronaviruse/situation-reports/20200409-sitrep-80-covid-19.pdf?sfvrsn=1b685d64_6.
WHO. (2020u) Coronavirus Disease 2019 (COVID-19): Situation Report - 81. Available at: https://www.who.int/docs/default-source/coronaviruse/situation-reports/20200410-sitrep-81-covid-19.pdf?sfvrsn=ca96eb84_2.
WHO. (2020v) Coronavirus Disease 2019 (COVID-19): Situation Report - 85. Available at: https://www.who.int/docs/default-source/coronaviruse/situation-reports/20200414-sitrep-85-covid-19.pdf?sfvrsn=7b8629bb_4.
WHO. (2020w) Coronavirus Disease 2019 (COVID-19): Situation Report - 86. Available at: https://www.who.int/docs/default-source/coronaviruse/situation-reports/20200415-sitrep-86-covid-19.pdf?sfvrsn=c615ea20_4.
WHO. (2020x) Coronavirus Disease 2019 (COVID-19): Situation Report - 91. Available at: https://www.who.int/docs/default-source/coronaviruse/situation-reports/20200420-sitrep-91-covid-19.pdf?sfvrsn=fcf0670b_4.
WHO. (2020y) Coronavirus Disease 2019 (COVID-19): Situation Report - 93. Available at: https://www.who.int/docs/default-source/coronaviruse/situation-reports/20200422-sitrep-93-covid-19.pdf?sfvrsn=35cf80d7_4.
WHO. (2020z) Coronavirus Disease 2019 (COVID-19): Situation Report - 95. Available at: https://www.who.int/docs/default-source/coronaviruse/situation-reports/20200424-sitrep-95-covid-19.pdf?sfvrsn=e8065831_4.
WHO. (2020aa) Coronavirus Disease 2019 (COVID-19): Situation Report -88. Available at: https://www.who.int/docs/default-source/coronaviruse/situation-reports/20200417-sitrep-88-covid-191b6cccd94f8b4f219377bff55719a6ed.pdf?sfvrsn=ebe78315_6.
WHO. (2020ab) COVID-19 Virtual Press Conference. Available at: https://www.who.int/docs/default-source/coronaviruse/transcripts/who-audio-emergencies-coronavirus-press-conference-17apr2020.pdf?sfvrsn=1bd9c4cd_2.
WHO. (2020ac) Opening Statement, COVID-19 Press Conference, 16 April 2020. Available at: https://www.afro.who.int/regional-director/speeches-messages/opening-statement-covid-19-press-conference-16-april-2020.
WHO. (2020ad) WHO Director-General's Opening Remarks at the Media Briefing on COVID-19 – 11 March 2020. Available at: https://www.who.int/dg/speeches/detail/who-director-general-s-opening-remarks-at-the-media-briefing-on-covid-19—11-march-2020.
WHO. (2020ae) WHO Director-General's Opening Remarks at the Media Briefing on COVID-19 – 13 March 2020. Available at: https://www.who.int/dg/speeches/detail/who-director-general-s-opening-remarks-at-the-mission-briefing-on-covid-19—13-march-2020.
WHO. (2020af) WHO Director-General's Opening Remarks at the Media Briefing on COVID-19 – 27 March 2020. Available at: https://www.who.int/dg/speeches/detail/who-director-general-s-opening-remarks-at-the-media-briefing-on-covid-19—27-march-2020.
Wilks A. (2020) Turkey to Free One-Third of its Prisoners to Curb Coronavirus. Available at: https://www.aljazeera.com/news/2020/04/turkey-free-prisoners-curb-coronavirus-200414062852220.html.
Williams A. (2020) EBRD Unveils €1 Billion Emergency Coronavirus Financing Package. Available at: https://www.ebrd.com/news/2020/ebrd-unveils-1-billion-emergency-coronavirus-financing-package.html.
Willsher K and Sabbagh D. (2020) Inquiry After 668 of French Aircraft Carrier's Crew Catch Coronavirus. Available at: https://www.theguardian.com/world/2020/apr/16/inquiry-french-aircraft-carrier-crew-catch-coronavirus-charles-de-gaulle.
Wimbish J. (2020) Coronavirus: Nuggets Report Member of Organization Tested Positive for COVID-19. Available at: https://www.cbssports.com/nba/news/coronavirus-nuggets-report-member-of-organization-tested-positive-for-covid-19/.
Wise J. (2020) WHO Chief Warns Against 'Politicizing' Coronavirus Unless 'You Want to Have More Body Bags'. Available at: https://thehill.com/policy/international/491805-who-chief-warns-against-politicizing-coronavirus-unless-you-want-to-have.
Woodward A. (2020) US Coronavirus Death Toll Now Higher Than American Fatalities in Vietnam War. Available at: https://www.independent.co.uk/news/world/americas/us-coronavirus-death-toll-vietnam-war-american-fatalities-a9489241.html.
World Food Programme. (2020) Statement From WFP Executive Director David Beasley. Available at: https://insight.wfp.org/statement-from-wfp-executive-director-david-beasley-11da6cef2a10.

Worldometer. (2020) Report Coronavirus Cases. Available at: https://www.worldometers.info/coronavirus/.

Wu H. (2020) Remote Chinese City Hit by Coronavirus After Weeks of Feeling Safe. Available at: https://www.reuters.com/article/us-health-coronavirus-china-border/remote-chinese-city-hit-by-coronavirus-after-weeks-of-feeling-safe-idUSKCN21Y0J2.

Xinhua. (2020a) Africa's COVID-19 Death Toll Hits 1,080, as Confirmed Cases Rise to 21,317: Africa CDC. Available at: https://www.chinadaily.com.cn/a/202004/20/WS5e9c8adaa3105d50a3d173cf.html.

Xinhua. (2020b) Czech Parliament OKs Extending State of Emergency Until May 17. Available at: http://www.xinhuanet.com/english/2020-04/29/c_139016349.htm.

Xinhua. (2020c) Except Wuhan, China's Hubei Reopens Domestic Flights. Available at: http://www.xinhuanet.com/english/2020-03/29/c_138928281.htm.

Yamey G. (2020) What the U.S. Needs to do Today to Follow South Korea's Model for Fighting Coronavirus. Available at: https://time.com/5804899/u-s-coronavirus-needs-follow-s-korea/.

Yun M. (2020) How Taiwan is Containing Coronavirus Despite Diplomatic Isolation by China. Available at: https://www.theguardian.com/world/2020/mar/13/how-taiwan-is-containing-coronavirus-despite-diplomatic-isolation-by-china.

Zagoria A. (2020) Three Members of the Philadelphia 76ers Organization Test Positive for Coronavirus. Available at: https://www.forbes.com/sites/adamzagoria/2020/03/19/three-members-of-the-philadelphia-76ers-organization-test-positive-for-coronavirus/#adb4766dfd70.

Zhang L and Munroe T. (2020) China Sees Rise in Asymptomatic Coronavirus Cases, to Tighten Controls at Land Borders. Available at: https://www.reuters.com/article/us-health-coronavirus-china/china-sees-rises-in-new-coronavirus-cases-asymptomatic-patients-idUSKBN21O01M.

Zhang LM. (2020) Available at: https://www.straitstimes.com/politics/ban-on-social-gatherings-of-any-size-in-homes-or-public-areas.

CHAPTER 4

Actualizing Big Data Through Revised Data Protocols to Render More Accurate Infectious Disease Monitoring and Modeling

INTRODUCTION

The novel coronavirus epidemic (previously identified as the 2019-nCoV, the later officially named COVID-19) led to complete lockdown of entire cities globally, starting with the city of Wuhan in China. In areas of partial closure, the restrain on people's movement was effected by instituting stringent measures, and such measures, together with high levels of alertness, are seen to be adopted in high-risk countries. In perspective, in cities such as Wuhan, Hong Kong, Beijing, and Hubei Province among others, institutions such as schools, public markets, roads, and transport sectors have been shut down (Allam, 2020d) to ensure a reduction of human-to-human infection, which is the primary means through which the virus spread is minimized. Such steps have been tagged as being the most appropriate and timely to allow authorities to establish and gain concrete and accurate information on the virus (Buckley and May, 2020). On the global context, the spread and uncertainties prompted by this new virus captured the attention of the World Health Organization (WHO), which on January 30, 2019 declared the virus outbreak a "Global Public Health Emergency." However, the body was careful not to declare the outbreak a "Public Health Emergency of International Concern" (PHEIC) yet. This is understandable as PHEIC, in definition, is argued to be

> An extraordinary event which is said to have the potential to constitute a public health risk to other regions through the international spread of disease; hence, requiring a coordinated international response whose scope may be; serious, sudden, unusual or unexpected; carries implication for public health beyond the affected State's national border; may require immediate international action *(WHO, 2020b)*.

Following past experiences with some notable influenza pandemics, a Global Initiative on Sharing all Influenza Data (GISAID) platform (Wang et al., 2020) was instituted, and it became key in helping with the speedy sharing of information by Chinese scientists and officials about the emergence of the coronavirus. The platform became instrumental in helping other scientists drawn from different regions to access valuable data and information about the virus. For instance, scientists from Australian-based Virus Identification Laboratory were able to use the information from the platform to develop similar virus in their labs (Scott et al., 2020). Numerous other online tracking services also became very popular among the larger public, as shown in Fig. 4.1.

The COVID-19 virus not only serves as a live case study for pandemic preparedness and response but also provides an opportunity to address the thematic of urban health. In the case of a viral outbreak and spread, it has been observed how technological tools, equipment, and facilities (Allam, 2020a, 2020b) across the globe have been put to practice in a bid to come up with vaccines and cures. Such concerted and collaborative efforts can serve as pointers to smart cities professionals and stakeholders on how they can work together to actualize the public safety concept on such and similar scenarios. The advantage that smart city professionals have is the availability of invariable technological tools and products that they can be exploited in areas like early detection of outbreaks. On this, concerted discussions on all matters of potential

Surveying the Covid-19 Pandemic and Its Implications. https://doi.org/10.1016/B978-0-12-824313-8.00004-8

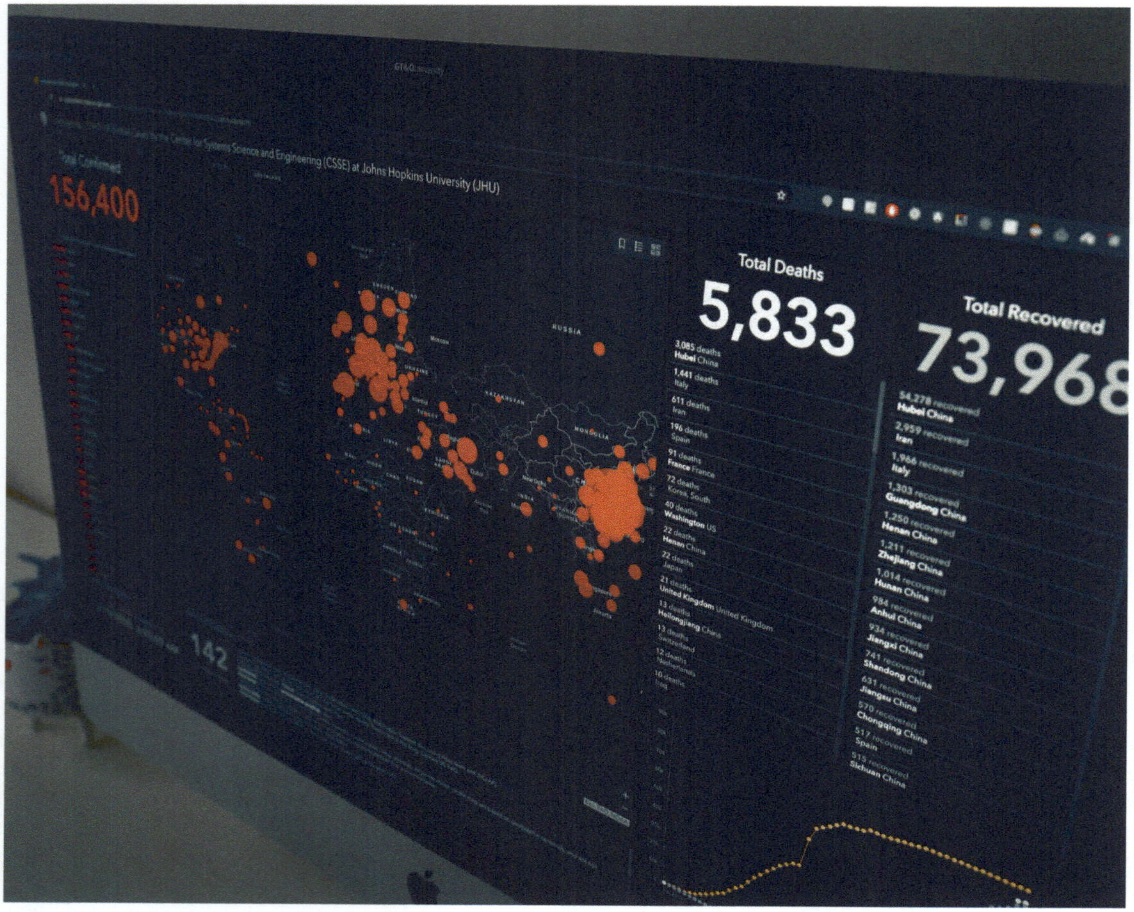

FIG. 4.1 COVID-19 tracking platform.

outbreaks, coupled with the maximum utilization of products such as the Internet of things (IoT)–powered devices and sensors and use of artificial intelligence (AI) (Kamel Boulos et al., 2019), could help put a stop to outbreaks earlier before they spread. This would lead to creation of fool-proof health databases that could guarantee accuracy of data, efficiency, scalability, and real-time information on outbreaks and eventual dispersal of virus. With such, therefore, cities would be assured of unquestionable urban risk management decisions.

To achieve the aforementioned improvement in the healthcare realm, there is need for an urgent address of existing standards, frameworks, and protocols that guide smart city products to make them uniform and seamless (Boué et al., 2018). On this, open protocols for all IoT devices is required, placing emphasis on data integrity, privacy, and safety. Such would help overcome the problem of proprietary technology (Vermesan and Friess, 2014) that is synonymous with most smart city products. By ensuring that there is a standardization of protocols, urban managers would have unrestricted access to data and information on emerging trends; hence, they would manage to make concrete and informed decisions. It is with this background that this chapter, which is also inspired by the scenarios surrounding the COVID-19 virus, seeks to explore how urban resilience can be further improved, especially if communication between different smart cities can become possible by generating larger datasets.

THE RISING IMPORTANCE OF URBAN HEALTH DATA

The digital revolution, characterized by an increase of IoT devices, has resulted to an unprecedented increase in data from diverse sectors (Allam et al., 2019), and

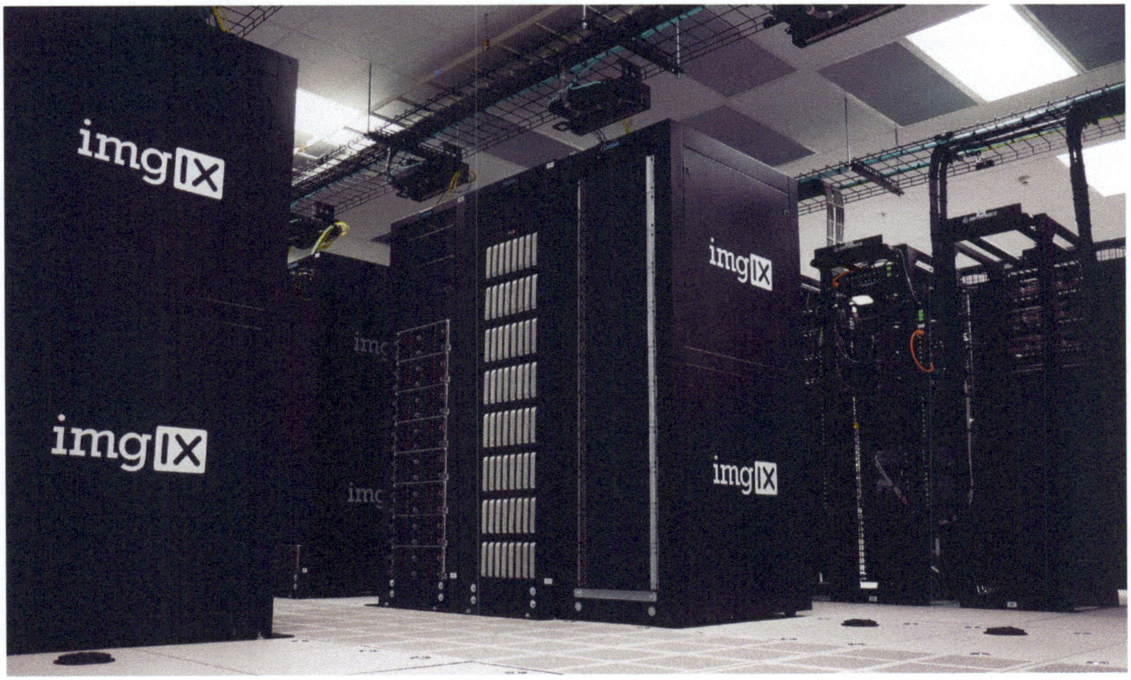

FIG. 4.2 Data servers.

the end on this is not even nigh. On this, it is expressed by Stanford Medicine (2017) that by the end of 2020, those devices will have generated data amounting to over 2314 exabyte (EB) where IEB = 1 billion GB from the health sector alone, requiring immense data servers to store such, as shown in Fig. 4.2.

These medical data will not only be gathered from medical records alone, but also there is a general agreement that most of such will be generated from smart, health devices such as wearable devices that are increasing exponentially. This increasing in adoption, as noted by Grand View Research (2019), is being driven by the enlarging global healthcare market, which is expected to reach a value of more than USD 543.3 billion by 2025. Such lucrativeness is attracting numerous startups to invest in the healthcare sector. As more of these startups join the healthcare market, attention is being shifted to how data generated by those devices adhere to security and privacy concerns, data protection and sharing protocols, and others. Such concerns come to life, especially in the current scenario where the world is battling COVID-19, and any mishap on those protocols may be disastrous to steps already made globally. In particular, noting that the data on COVID-19 are cut across different cultural and geographical boundaries, where there are different unique laws and regulations concerning data access and management, it becomes critical to ensure that such devices adhere strictly to laid-down procedures, frameworks, and protocols. But, with so many and divergent views, laws, and regulations, it would still be impossible to have the devices that are strictly adherent; hence, the discourse to have uniform, standardized, and universally agreed and acceptable approaches and protocols that would guarantee open access of data.

The significance of having an open access dataset, as noted earlier, is to ensure that critical data, as that on COVID-19, are not managed only by a fragmented, small group of users, who have the potential to capitalize on it for financial or private gains. If that happens, some regions would be at a disadvantaged as most of the startups and corporations with potential to collect, store, manage and distribute such data are, unfortunately located in specific geographies (Allam, 2018; Allam, 2019a; Allam, 2020a; Allam, 2020c; Allam and Dhunny, 2019). And, from some past experiences, it is possible that such control could be used to settle some geopolitical tag-of wars that powerful economies have playing against each other. This argument, as it were, is not far-fetched, as just we have already witnessed the "push and pull" involving China and some powerful economies such as US economy concerning the use of 5G Internet (Kharpal, 2018). Unfortunately, those geopolitical "battles" have denied the world the chance to have the 5G Internet finally rolled out, and such would go a long way in ensuring speedy sharing of data and other services. Likewise, if the COVID-19 data are to be subjected to similar geopolitical struggles, and national loyalty, instead looking at bigger picture that entails the welfare of humanity, it would be relatively hard to overcome the pandemic. Therefore, while the large corporations have the right to pursue their agendas, and safeguard their property rights, when it comes to issues touching on the welfare of human kind, they need to willingly allow for open access to big data such that efforts to come up with solutions can involve all and sundry (Allam, 2019b; Allam, 2020e; Allam, 2020f).

A BRIEF UNDERSTANDING OF THE CORONAVIRUS (COVID-19) OUTBREAK AND DATA

The fight against the COVID-19 pandemic is not only bound to be complicated by issues of nationalisms, but, as is evident from the time of the outbreak, also the challenge of movement of people into different parts of the globe has been a thorny one. With the ease, spread, and reduced costs of travel, it has been found that the spread of the virus has been extremely enhanced. To put this in perspective, since the first case was reported in Wuhan on December 31, 2019, China, in a matter of 3 weeks (by January 17, 2020), the case had increased to over 300. Ten days later, the reported cases had increased to 2,014, with 684 positively confirmed. Of those confirmed, 29 were reported outside China, and all these were exported via air travel. Following the seriousness of the disease, as of January 26, 2020, 56 individuals had succumbed (DW, 2020). As of March 31, 2020, the virus had spread to 136 countries, with 693,334 confirmed cases and, out of those, 33,106 deaths (WHO, 2020a). Among those regions that were first to have reported the outbreak outside China include Taiwan, South Korea, Japan, Thailand, France, the United States, Singapore, and Vietnam (Tierney et al., 2020). The complication in this case is based on the fact that health-related data on those found to be positive with the virus not only are based on local database but also would require access to data from other regions; thus, restriction on data access would make it had especially to establish whether the victim has had an existing health condition.

One common factor about COVID-19 is that symptoms are the same regardless of the geographical location. Nevertheless, while that is the case, and while it is also true that major cities are known to have some levels of preparedness against potential outbreaks, such are always divergent and different from each other. But, in the case of COVID-19, as highlighted by the WHO, the best approach to overcome it is to have international collaboration. In such a way, countries can benefit from the approaches taken by others, like China, which was the first to be affected, and which took drastic measures to address the outbreak. On this, during an emergency meeting held in Geneva by WHO health officials on January 22, 2020, China was lauded for its action on sharing the data, unlike in 2002 during the severe acute respiratory syndrome (SARS) outbreak where it was accused of withholding crucial information (WHO, 2020b). The delay in sharing information made the identification of the disease to drag (from November 2002 to April 2003) (Ren, 202). The same case was experienced in 2013 when Ebola virus outbreak occurred, and it took months to identify, thus causing death of over 11,000 people in West Africa. The Zika virus outbreak is also another classical case of how delayed sharing of information can impact the progress in finding medical solutions. It is reported that the virus was first reported in 2014 but was successfully identified only in 2015.

On COVID-19, following quick data sharing, it only took around 17 days (December 31, 2019—January 17, 2020) to identify the virus (Allam et al., 2020). With that information, and with availability of latest technological tools in cities, information about the virus spread has been shared in real time from different regions. This shows how the world has changed and moved away from the traditional epidemiological approaches that called for months for a successful identification and sharing of information (Grubaugh, 2020). While the information was shared in time, the impacts on cities and countries exposes how lack of international collaboration on such matters can have far reaching consequences. For instance, it has been observed that some cities and countries are overstretched in securing basic personal protective equipment, including for the health workers, thus exposing them to the virus. Wetsman (2020) posits that such are experienced since some vital information especially on issues such as how the virus was passed from person to another took time to establish; hence, cities took longer to come up with both soft and hard infrastructures. Therefore, when the information became clear, some of the countries were already overwhelmed. On this, it is the position of this chapter that such mishaps can be rectified, in the future, if there is transparency and speedy sharing of information, under the aegis of international collaboration.

URBAN ECONOMY AND HEALTH SAFETY

The outbreak of pandemics, or even diseases, either locally or internationally brings about numerous challenges, in different sectors. The economic sector is among those that are severely impacted. To put this in perspective, back in 2002 when SARS broke, the entire Asian region was observed to have shouldered a heavy burden in various sectors, with an overall impact estimated to have reached between USD 12 and 18 billion (Qiu et al., 2018). The Zika virus is estimated to have caused a loss of approximately USD 7–18 billion in the equator belt where it was experienced (UNDP, 2017). The Ebola virus that broke in 2014 in West Africa led to an economic loss of approximately USD 2.2 billion in three countries: Guinea, Liberia, and Sierra Leone in 2015 alone (Wojda et al., 2015).

Presently, although it is still early to quantify or project how much the global economy will suffer, the prelude on the economic frontier can serve as pointers as to what is coming. The expected losses will be unprecedented and immense as to what was experienced in the previous cases, as some actions taken globally were not instituted in those earlier cases. For instance, as of now, the travel industry, especially air travel and use of cruise ships, has been grounded in almost all countries of the world. Even before this happened, when COVID-19 broke in Wuhan, it was reported that more than 400 million people were expected to travel in or out of China for the Chinese New Year celebration (DW, 2020). The cancellation of travel spiraled to other industries such as the hotel industry, the hospitality industry, the art and entertainment industry, and others that rely on the opulence of the New Year celebration (BBC, 2020). Besides that, other sectors such as the manufacturing industry, the clearing and forwarding industries, the wholesale, and retail industries among others across the globe were also put on limbo by the lockdown in Chinese provinces.

This background information thus points to the fact that the impact of COVID-19 transcends the thinking that it is only an urban safety concern. It has now spilled over to all other realms within the urban and rural fabric, and each of these is experiencing unprecedented negative consequences. This means that things cannot be assumed to be normal anymore but demand that drastic and urgent decisions need to be made to ensure that the global economy does not sink to alarming levels. When this happens, the vulnerable societies and communities, especially within the global south, may find it rough to recover when the COVID-19 issues are finally behind us. On this end, therefore, the emphasis on the need for global measures that transcend nationalist agenda needs to be pursued. For instance, this would involve making the issue of data management and sharing open to all so that all those with potential to come up with solutions to the virus outbreak and spread can get fully involved. On this, Lawpoolsri et al. (2018) emphasizes that issues, such as transparency, timelessness of sharing, and access and quality of data, should be given maximum attention so that continuous monitoring and assessment can be achieved across the globe.

SHARING AND STANDARDIZATION OF DATA THROUGH URBAN NETWORKS

In the recent past, the availability of advanced technologies has made it possible to gather data from assorted sources. This has been enabled by the digitization of urban fabrics. In the same spirit, this digitization has made it possible for data on COVID-19 to be collected right from points of entries such as airports and seaports. This was enabled by the availability of numerous smart devices such as sensors installed in these establishments, such that everyone entering a region via these is screened and monitored in real time. A case in point here is the happening in the United States where it was observed that over 20 airports (Buckley and May, 2020) have had mandatory early screening and monitoring to ensure all verifiable positive cases are identified there and then. In Chinese cities, similar trends have been adopted in bus terminals, marketplaces, and subway stations in addition to health facilities.

Besides the physical monitoring and screening, it has been observed that other methods such as the use of terminal tracking systems are also being used, especially in smart cities. With such, as is highlighted by Li et al. (2020), it has become possible to distribute collected data in real time to the already installed digital infrastructures. With these infrastructures connected in a web to form a complex urban network, it becomes practically possible to provide real-time updates on different issues, thus warranting speedy reaction by the department or sector concerned. This interconnectedness is particularly important as it allows data from the ever-increasing health sensors such as wearables to be sent, stored, analyzed, and processed in record time, thus helping the health personnel within the system to derive valuable insights on the health condition of the people in the area. Such devices as expressed by Loncar-Turukalo et al. (2019) have been instrumental in the formation of Connected Health (CH) care, and this is paramount in monitoring the health status of specific areas. In addition, such approaches in the health sector are said to allow for features such as spatiotemporal mapping, remote monitoring and management, and others, all focusing on bettering urban health management (Vashist et al., 2015).

In view of the previous information, although there is a general understanding that the basic sources of healthcare data are medical labs, clinics, hospitals, and general practitioners, it is without doubt that currently it is possible to secure such data from other sources. In particular, as is evident with the current epidemic, the urban arena is a rich source of medical data. As noted in the earlier sections, it has been established that different cities and countries have set up screening and monitoring tools in the point of entry, and these have yielded a massive amount of medical data that are sufficient to enrich existing health-related databases. As more and more people transit through those points of entry or exist, the amount of data is expected to continue growing, and this has been very instrumental in identifying those individuals who need extra medical attention. The emphasis in this chapter is to consider the urban areas as sources of data for COVID-19 case are also based on the fact that a majority of the isolation and mandatory quarantine centers are located there, and these too are contributing greatly in enriching the amount of COVID-19 data. Another valid reason that makes urban areas a valid source of data is the fact that most of the advanced technologies, especially those that facilitate the application of smart cities concept, are simulated here, and these include those that help in anonymizing of data, which is a critical consideration in the management of medical data. Those urban fabrics are already well connected to vital digital infrastructures (Fig. 4.3), and technologies like blockchain technologies (Naz et al., 2019) and quantum cryptography (Zhou et al., 2018) can help in anonymizing data.

While it is evident that the technologies will transform different sectors including the health sector significantly, there are some issues that need to be sought out to streamline data collection, storage, analysis, and distribution. One such issue is the communication factor where it is evident that barely any device sourced from different corporations integrates those freely (Van den Abeele et al., 2015). This is intentionally done by manufacturers who are always in competition for market shares, and by ensuring that their devices are unique and are incompatible with networks of their competitors, they are able to secure such competitions (Allam, 2020a, Allam, 2020b). The other aspect of communication is based on the geographical restriction, where most devices are unable to communicate with their likes installed in a different geographical location. Such strategies are adopted to allow for control, maintenance, and safety of the data collected. While both reasons noted here are valid, the risk is that such only helps to cement the aspects and difficult of data sharing and open access, which are critical if different urban challenges are to be won effectively. Therefore, as the pursuit to ensure that health data are sourced from urban areas, via the different technologies, it is also paramount to simultaneously pursue the need for standardization of protocols and network as is the clarion call in this chapter. This way, it will be possible to guarantee the volume, quality, accuracy, and complexity of the data that are collected. Such pursuits are not insurmountable, as it has already been done in the United States where it is reported that all the surveillance and monitoring of healthcare are combined into a singular network—dubbed National Healthcare Safety Network (NHSH) (Tokars et al., 2004).

Having a singular global network, especially for the present case of COVID-19, would be paramount as this would enhance the efforts undertaken to bring the situation into manageable levels. This global network would allow for the creation for a universal data sharing, including allowing for the adoption of volunteered geographic information (VGI), thus making the public feel part and parcel of this global fight. These strategies would not only serve in the current case but also guarantee that future outbreaks and pandemics would be handled effectively and in a timely manner to prevent their widespread (Allam and Jones, 2020). This would be facilitated by having an enriched database, and with the employment of modern technologies such as AI tools, the combat of outbreaks would be further enhanced, and by including early detection, this would allow for improved diagnosis methods and facilitate better and quality decision-making (Jiang et al., 2017). An example of how an elaborate data sharing and collaboration strategy can work is pointed by how it was done during the 2014 Ebola outbreak in West Africa. Bockarie (2019) expresses how different health professionals collaborated, by engaging in an open data sharing program, and this allowed them to contain the virus before it spread to more countries. By the time it was contained, it had only affected three countries. One takeaway from this collaboration is how the different stakeholders maintained high levels of trust and transparency and ensured speedy sharing of all that information generated and shared (Waithira et al., 2019).

The earlier case demonstrates that it is possible to overcome emergencies like the present one and others

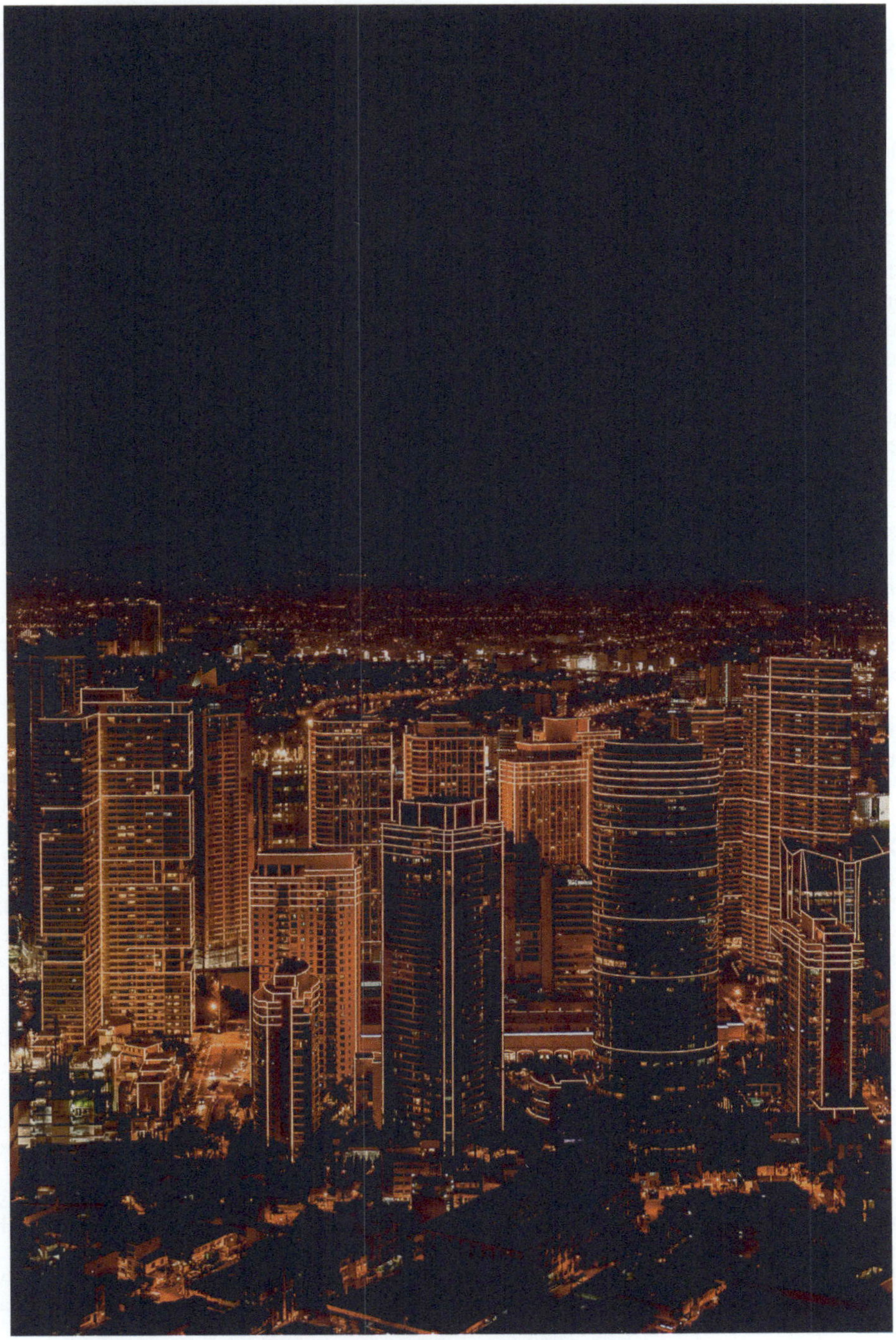

FIG. 4.3 Digitally connected urban fabric.

that may be experienced in the future by ensuring sound, regulatory practices and international healthcare guidelines are formulated and strictly adhered to. This would be even very effective if they are complimented by relying on modern technologies. With such, it would be possible to not only address health risks but also ensure its consequences are reduced to the minimum as pointed by the WHO (2019). And, the emphasis is to ensure that the application of smart devices and technologies is not overlooked, because these have potential to bring a tangible transformation.

CONCLUSION

As different urban managements and governments across the globe continue to pursue and heavily invest in the smart city concept, all geared toward achieving high levels of liveability, they should be conscious of the need to emphasis on the thematic of urban health. This is affirmed by the scenario that the present case of COVID-19 has plunged the world and even the smartest of cities around the globe, on a standstill. Therefore, this call for attention on the need for standardization of different issues appertaining to smart city technologies is topical. In particular, those in charge of cities should emphasize on having data platforms that have the capacity to communicate with each other; thus, in times of distress, like the current one, it would be practical to access the required data and information without going through the limitation of having to rely on solely specific and limited technology suppliers. Such emphasis should also be stressed in all other sectors, such that cities will be held together in a complex technological backbone that is well knit such that any uncertainty will be addressed without hitches and in record time.

REFERENCES

Allam Z. (2018) Contextualising the Smart City for Sustainability and Inclusivity. New Design Ideas 2: 124–127.

Allam Z. (2019a) The Emergence of Anti-Privacy and Control at the Nexus between the Concepts of Safe City and Smart City. Smart Cities 2.

Allam Z. (2019b) The Emergence of Anti-Privacy and Control at the Nexus between the Concepts of Safe City and Smart City. Smart Cities 2: 96–105.

Allam Z. (2020a) Cities and the Digital Revolution: Aligning Technology and Humanity: Springer International Publishing.

Allam Z. (2020b) Data as the New Driving Gears of Urbanization. In: Allam Z (ed) Cities and the Digital Revolution: Aligning technology and humanity. Cham: Springer International Publishing, 1–29.

Allam Z. (2020c) Digital Urban Networks and Social Media. In: Allam Z (ed) Cities and the Digital Revolution: Aligning technology and humanity. Cham: Springer International Publishing, 61–83.

Allam Z. (2020d) How Cities and Architecture Respond to the Wuhan Coronavirus. Available at: https://www.archdaily.com/932840/how-cities-and-architecture-respond-to-the-wuhan-coronavirus.

Allam Z. (2020e) Privatization and Privacy in the Digital City. In: Allam Z (ed) Cities and the Digital Revolution: Aligning technology and humanity. Cham: Springer International Publishing, 85–106.

Allam Z. (2020f) Theology, Sustainability and Big Data. In: Allam Z (ed) Theology and Urban Sustainability. Cham: Springer International Publishing, 53–67.

Allam Z, Dey G and Jones DS. (2020) Artificial Intelligence (AI) Provided Early Detection of the Coronavirus (COVID-19) in China and Will Influence Future Urban Health Policy Internationally. A&I 1: 156–165.

Allam Z and Dhunny ZA. (2019) On Big Data, Artificial Intelligence and Smart Cities. Cities 89: 80–91.

Allam Z and Jones DS. (2020) On the Coronavirus (COVID-19) Outbreak and the Smart City Network: Universal Data Sharing Standards Coupled with Artificial Intelligence (AI) to Benefit Urban Health Monitoring and Management. Healthcare 8: 46.

Allam Z, Tegally H and Thondoo M. (2019) Redefining the Use of Big Data in Urban Health for Increased Liveability in Smart Cities. Smart Cities 2: 259–268.

BBC. (2020) China's Travel Industry Counts Cost of Coronavirus. Available at: https://www.bbc.com/news/business-51232374.

Bockarie MJ. (2019) Sharing Data Can Help Prevent Public Health Emergencies in Africa. Available at: https://theconversation.com/sharing-data-can-help-prevent-public-health-emergencies-in-africa-119672.

Boué S, Byrne M, Hayes AW, et al. (2018) Embracing Transparency Through Data Sharing. 37: 466–471.

Buckley C and May T. (2020) Effects of Coronavirus Begin Echoing Far From Wuhan Epicenter. Available at: https://www.nytimes.com/2020/01/25/world/asia/china-wuhan-coronavirus.html.

DW. (2020) China: Coronavirus fears put damper on Lunar New Year. Available at: https://www.dw.com/en/china-coronavirus-fears-put-damper-on-lunar-new-year/a-52146076.

Grand View Research. (2019) IoT in Healthcare Market Worth $534.3 Billion by 2025 | CARG 19.9%. Available at: https://www.grandviewresearch.com/press-release/global-iot-in-healthcare-market.

Grubaugh N. (2020) Rapid Data Sharing and Genomics Vital to China Virus Response. Available at: https://medicine.yale.edu/news-article/22389/.

Jiang F, Jiang Y, Zhi H, et al. (2017) Artificial intelligence in healthcare: past, present and future. Stroke and Vascular Neurology 2: 230.

Kamel Boulos MN, Peng G and VoPham T. (2019) An overview of GeoAI applications in health and healthcare. International Journal of Health Geographics 18: 7.

Kharpal A. (2018) China 'Has the Edge' in the War for 5G and the US and Europe Could Fall Behind. Available at: https://www.cnbc.com/2018/03/07/china-has-the-edge-in-the-war-for-5g-us-and-eu-could-fall-behind.html.

Lawpoolsri S, Kaewkungwal J, Khamsiriwatchara A, et al. (2018) Data quality and timeliness of outbreak reporting system among countries in Greater Mekong subregion: Challenges for international data sharing. PLoS Neglected Tropical Diseases 12: e0006425.

Li W, Batty M and Goodchild MF. (2020) Real-time GIS for smart cities. International Journal of Geographical Information Science 34: 311-324.

Loncar-Turukalo T, Zdravevski E, Machado da Silva J, et al. (2019) Literature on Wearable Technology for Connected Health: Scoping Review of Research Trends, Advances, and Barriers. 21: e14017.

Naz M, Al-zahrani FA, Khalid R, et al. (2019) A Secure Data Sharing Platform Using Blockchain and Interplanetary File System. 11: 7054.

Qiu W, Chu C, Mao A, et al. (2018) The Impacts on Health, Society, and Economy of SARS and H7N9 Outbreaks in China: A Case Comparison Study. International Journal of Environmental Research and Public Health: 2710185.

Ren G. (202) As Coronoavirus Outbreak Surges in China, WHO Call for Emergency Meeting. Available at: https://www.healthpolicy-watch.org/as-coronavirus-outbreak-surges-in-china-who-calls-for-emergency-meeting/.

Scott S, Timms P and Florance L. (2020) Australian Lab First Outside of China to Copy Coronavirus, Helping Vaccine Push. Available at: https://www.abc.net.au/news/2020-01-29/wuhan-coronavirus-created-in-australian-lab-outside-of-china/11906390.

Stanford Medicine. (2017) Harnessing the Power of Data in Health. Stanford Medicine.

Tierney L, Meko T and Fox J. (2020) Mapping the Spread of the New Coronavirus. Available at: https://www.washingtonpost.com/world/2020/01/22/mapping-spread-new-coronavirus/?arc404=true.

Tokars JI, Richards C, Andrus M, et al. (2004) The Changing Face of Surveillance for Health Care—Associated Infections. Clinical Infectious Diseases 39: 1347-1352.

UNDP. (2017) Social and Economic Costs of Zika Can Reach up to US$18 Billion in Latin America and the Caribbean. Available at: https://www.undp.org/content/undp/en/home/presscenter/pressreleases/2017/04/06/social-and-economic-costs-of-zika-can-reach-up-to-us-18-billion-in-latin-america-and-the-caribbean.html.

Van den Abeele F, Hoebeke J, Moerman I, et al. (2015) Integration of Heterogeneous Devices and Communication Models via the Cloud in the Constrained Internet of Things. International Journal of Distributed Sensor Networks 11: 683425.

Vashist SK, Luppa PB, Yeo LY, et al. (2015) Emerging Technologies for Next-Generation Point-of-Care Testing. Trends in Biotechnology 33: 692—705.

Vermesan O and Friess P. (2014) Internet of Things—From Research and Innovation to Market Deployment, Gistrup, Denmark: River Publishers.

Waithira N, Mutinda B and Cheah PY. (2019) Data management and sharing policy: the first step towards promoting data sharing. BMC Medicine 17: 80.

Wang C, Horby PW, Hayden FG, et al. (2020) A novel coronavirus outbreak of global health concern. The Lancet 395: 470—473.

Wetsman N. (2020) Rapid Global Response to the New Coronavirus Shows Progress Made Since SARS. Available at: https://www.theverge.com/2020/1/22/21077214/coronavirus-rapid-global-response-progress-sars-unknown-virus-china-public-health.

WHO. (2019) Health Emergency and Disaster Risk Management Framework. Geneva: World Health Organisation.

WHO. (2020a) Coronavirus Disease 2019 (COVID-19) Situation Report -70. World Health Organisation.

WHO. (2020b) Statement on the Meeting of the International Health Regulations (2005) Emergency Committee Regarding the Outbreak of Novel Coronavirus (2019-nCoV). Available at: www.who.int/news-room/detail/23-01-2020-statement-on-the-meeting-of-the-international-health-regulations-(2005)-emergency-committee-regarding-the-outbreak-of-novel-corona virus-(2019-ncov.

Wojda TR, Valenza PL, Cornejo K, et al. (2015) The Ebola Outbreak of 2014-2015: From Coordinated Multilateral Action to Effective Disease Containment, Vaccine Development, and Beyond. Journal of Global Infectious Diseases 7: 127—138.

Zhou T, Shen J, Li X, et al. (2018) Quantum Cryptography for the Future Internet and the Security Analysis. Security and Communication Networks: 1—7.

CHAPTER 5

The Emergence of Voluntary Citizen Networks to Circumvent Urban Health Data Sharing Restrictions During Pandemics

INTRODUCTION

After the past three industrial revolutions, the fourth one, where use of information and communication technologies (ICT) technologies is emphasized, has accelerated our global transformation. Today, it is not unusual for different institutions and agencies to use a wide range of computing technologies in their decision-making and operations. Technologies such as artificial intelligence, big data, blockchain technologies, machine learning, cloud computing, and others such as natural language processing have become very popular. One sector that has greatly benefitted from such is health, where through the use of the said technologies, it is now possible to collect and process massive datasets, thus leading to advanced surveillance and monitoring, diagnosis, treatment, and drug manufacturing among other benefits. These have been even more instrumental in the present days when the whole world is experiencing one of its lowest moment, courtesy of COVID-19 pandemic. Use of these technologies allowed for quicker identification of the virus strand and for faster sharing of information on the virus to various global agencies for quicker actions to be taken. On the same, the use of these technologies, especially AI, machine learning, and natural language processing, through some startups, BlueDot—based in Canada, and Metabiota—based in California, the United States, was able to an earlier prediction of the next location where the virus would spread after Wuhan (Metaboita, 2020; Heaven, 2020; Allam et al., 2020). Furthermore, these technologies have become particularly handy in helping various stakeholders involved in the fight against the coronavirus in making decisions on issues such as quarantine, self-isolation, preventive measures, screening, and many others (Pringle, 2020).

With all these technologies, the common denominator is the availability of data, and without these, or when such are unreliable, low scale, compromised, or delayed, the analysis, insight derived and decision made, would undoubtably be less impactful. But, while this is the case, there is evidence that the world is amass with data from different sources, especially with the infiltration of smart phones, and availability of numerous social media platforms. There are some open databases that allow free access to data. With all these, in the case of COVID-19, startups engaged in providing more insights are observed to access data from those sources, including airline ticketing and from governments of different countries, and with these, they are able to run simulation and predictive algorithms to come up with conclusions guiding policy orientations. On this, while the outcomes from such computations are impressive and with far reaching impacts on the health frontier, the numerous challenges with data collection, storage, management, access, and distributions still linger. In the present case of COVID-19, for instance, it has become clear that some crucial data such as the actual number of those affected, the trends of spread and the number of those in self-isolation and quarantine are not available to the extent desired. Thereby, it would be a daunting task to quantify or predict the number of those who are to be infected by the virus and in which geographical location. In such circumstances, it has become relatively hard for authorities to pursue watertight preventive measures that would see the spread reduced.

These obstacles on data need to be rectified urgently if substantial steps on the fight against the virus are to be won. On this front, this chapter proposes a paradigm shift where data collection and sharing will not follow

Surveying the Covid-19 Pandemic and Its Implications. https://doi.org/10.1016/B978-0-12-824313-8.00005-X

the traditional models that are mired with the shortcomings but proposes an alternative one. In this case, the model being fronted is the volunteered geographic information (VGI), which emphasizes on having open data banks, with the public being allowed to freely share data. On this, Langley et al. (2017) note that with VGI, it increases the propensity for collaboration in matters relating to data, including with nonscientists like the general public who usually share massive amount of data via social media platforms. With the model gaining popularity, it would be easy to capitalize on the increasing popularity and numbers of smart devices and hence end up with an enriched database that can enhance the information and insights concerning the pandemic.

While VGI has the potential to positively influence the global health database, it would be significant to ensure that the restriction in data sharing is overcome such that the data can be shared in real time. This has not been the case as reported by Hamade (2020), and when that happens, there has been the challenge of lack of granularity making it hard for one jurisdiction to comfortably access and use data from a different jurisdiction. This is observed as among one of the hindrances that need to be addressed while recalibrating the standards and protocols that guide data sharing (Allam, 2019a, Allam, 2020a, Allam, 2020b, Allam, 2020c, Allam, 2020d; Allam and Jones, 2020). But even before this, there is a discourse on how that standardization can be done. It is worth noting that in the case of emergencies, as in the present case of COVID-19, one cannot wait as the situation is dire with far reaching impacts. Therefore, there is need for goodwill from all stakeholders and governments to voluntarily allow unsolicited data sharing, by overriding existing restrictions. This way, as is expressed by Romm et al. (2020), it will be possible to urgently track and trace suspected cases of the virus and, thereafter, initiate the most appropriate medical approach; whether quarantine, isolate, or hospitalize individuals depending on their health status. In view of this background, this chapter is dedicated to the exploration of whether it is feasible to adopt the VGI model during times of disaster like now, especially in this current era where the advanced computational technologies are ubiquitous.

DATA SHARING CONCERNS

The idea of data sharing, especially in the present scenario when COVID-19, has caused havoc across the globe that cannot be overemphasized. But such efforts need to be complimented by reactionary approaches aimed at helping to overcome some deep-rooted challenges that have curtailed free sharing, use, and distribution of data. In view of this, there is a substantial amount of literature dedicated to discussing primary challenges that are associated to data. Among those challenges identified include those of privacy, security, ethics, transparency, volume, and storage to name a few. The concern over those challenges is even further accentuated by the increasing technological advancement, where with some modern technologies, it has become increasingly possible for different agencies and individuals to unlawfully access private data. Tiell (2016) of Accenture affirms this and further expresses that as the amount of data increases, and the means to generate and collect such also in inexpensive ways, the privacy concerns become live. In this case, it becomes relatively hard to convince potential sources to freely share their data, as they fear that such would be compromised, especially for-profit gains. The fear also arises as it is evident that in most cases, such are stored by third parties, especially large ICT corporations that have the technological capacity to collect and store large amounts of data (Allam, 2018a, Allam, 2019b, Allam, 2020d, Allam, 2020e; Allam and Newman, 2018). The fears are compounded by the fact that these parties can, in some instances, share the data in their possession for their own selfish interest, or as tools for target marketing. Such would go against the letter and spirit of VGI, which is based on the principle of transparency and ethical use of collected data (Blatt, 2015). This fear often results in artistic manifestations, as shown in Fig. 5.1.

While those challenges persist, in the recent past, there have been spirited efforts to reverse the situation, especially through the formulation of a series of legal frameworks, standards, and protocols that would guide data management, access, and sharing. In this regard, it is possible to point some practical examples. For instance, in the European region, there is a legal framework dubbed Nordic Data Sharing Framework (Salokannel, 2013) aimed at ensuring that certain procedure, rules, and laws are followed while sharing data. Another example is the Cyber Security Information Sharing Act (CISA) (2015) that was passed in 2015 by the US Senate. Other such frameworks include the General Data Protection Regulation (GDPR) (2016), Trusted Data Sharing Framework, and the Data Sharing Code of Practice that borrows from section number 121 of the Data Protection Act passed in 2018 by the European Parliament (2018). With these, plus a myriad other based on different parts the world, those are observed to provide some reprieve when it comes to sharing of data, especially which has the potential to expose private information. With adequate safeguards and platforms, it has become possible to

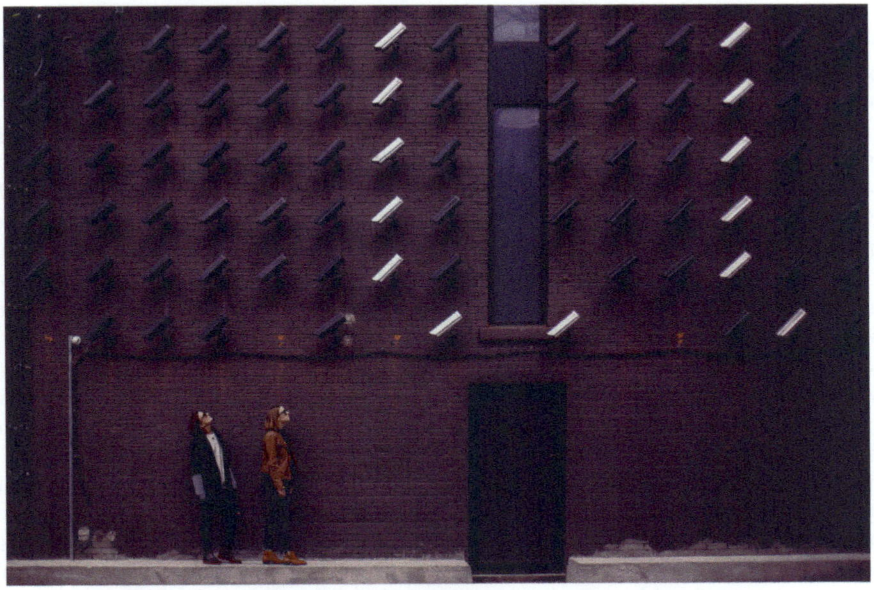

FIG. 5.1 Artistic manifestation showing unease over constant scrutiny.

overcome data silos, which most existing databases have maintained, with a bid to overcome existing restriction and filter any unauthorized communication. With such frameworks and protocols, it is a daunting task to allow for free data sharing and leave alone open access of the databases.

Besides overcoming the silos, reworking on the existing standards and protocols allows existing databases to be enriched, and this is affirmed by the quality of insight derived after analyzing the data. This does not imply that they are insufficient in their current form, but eliminating silos is the surest way of enhancing them. This is true as most of the information being sought, in most cases, especially those related to health need to be diversified, regarding issues such as geographical location and demography. For instance, in the current case of COVID-19, compelling insights can only be achieved if analysis is done with data that capture details from different geographical locations—countries, cities, and establishments. But, still, the existing frameworks are not enough; as already, due to their divergence in relation to different issues, it has become hard to have an agreement on the conclusion being drawn in different countries. For instance, China, which was the first to experience the outbreak of the coronavirus, has been accused, especially by the United States, of giving falsified data and information, especially about the emergence of the virus, the spread, and its impact (Crowley et al., 2020). According to Moorthy et al. (2020), the fight against COVID-19 needs to be addressed from a point of sincerity and transparency, especially in regard to data sharing; hence, they emphasize that all concerned agencies and governments need to ensure the authenticity and urgency of sharing the data. By doing this, the world would prevent a repeat of the 2002 severe acute respiratory syndrome (SARS) outbreak, where China was accused of delaying information on the outbreak, thus making it hard for identification and subsequent diagnosis and control of the virus (Cao et al., 2019). The World Health Organization recommends the approach taken during the 2016 Ebola virus outbreak where there were concerted efforts from different agencies and government and, thus, saw the virus contained before it could spread further beyond the three affected Western African countries (Wojda et al., 2015). With that, the current case of COVID-19 requires an open database where all participating institutions, governments, and other stakeholders can easily access the data. However, as of now, this protocol has not yet been established or communicated, but the severity of the virus demands that protocols be adopted and communicated in a clear fashion such that a solution on the virus can be formulated before the global health, society, and economy reach a tipping point.

OVERCOMING DATA SHARING AS A PSYCHOLOGICAL TRAIT

Through the numerous technological advancement that the world has been experiencing since the turn of the fourth industrial revolution, the amount of data being generated has continued to increase. There before, due to scarcity and complexity of technological tools, and the exorbitant costs of collecting, storing, analyzing, and distributing data, researchers and other data users had to face numerous challenges. Similarly, during those periods, the need for data was not as expounded as it is today; hence, people, organization, institutions, and even government could comfortably survive without data. But today, things have changed, and it has become paramount to have access to data to position oneself as a key player in this competitive world. Luckily, the infiltration and accessibility of mobile devices such as phones, cameras, and wearables have come in handy in ensuring that massive amount of data is available. Similarly, the availability of these devices has been complimented by the availability of diverse social media platforms, and fast Internet has made the generation and sharing of data even more ubiquitous. But, as has been shared comprehensively in the sections earlier, these advancements have attracted substantial challenges, especially those related to privacy, security, transparency, and ethics that have been seen to curtail the freedom, the scale, and volume of data sharing. Indeed, Bezuidenhout and Chakauya (2018) highlight that most people are now apprehensive to share their data for fear that such would be exploited to disfranchise and disadvantage them. Even in high ranking government levels, there is apprehension that some of the technologies that have been developed are maliciously crafted to enable agencies and governments to extract private data from individuals and institutions without their consent.

Some of the issues that have brought about this apprehension range from the profit value that has been attached to data, with large ICT organisations seen to be increasing their activities, including heavy investments in R&D to come up with cutting-edge technologies and devices to help them collect and store data. With such technologies, those are observed to seek increasing revenues, as most governments and institutions are constantly contracting startups with capacity to collect and store massive data on different issues. Such data have also become very popular for target marketing and those with capacity to collect gain financially by sharing insights with marketing institutions. But, further from that, the main concerns with access to data are increasing incidences of terrorism activities such as recruitment and planning. There are also fears of extortion and sabotage of personal privacy among other issues. Such have been seen to sometimes overshadow the original intents such as prevention of crime, increased efficiency in service delivery, medical purposes, improvement of liveability and resiliency of cities, and reduction in some bureaucracies and bottleneck in service delivery to mention a few. While in such scenarios, the existing data sharing frameworks and protocols have been seen to be adequate by proposing data anonymization and encryption, technology advancement is seen to enable reidentification, thus warranting the need for even more stringent measures. When all these challenges are compounded, as noted by Waithira et al. (2019), it becomes relatively hard to convince people to freely share their data, as already the levels of mistrust on agencies handling data are high and thus are seen to create psychological barriers to data sharing. This reality is not conducive for a world that is prone to numerous challenges like the present case of COVID-19, which urgently requires any available data to be analyzed to help in manufacturing vaccines, drugs, and relevant preventive tools and measures.

Though such psychological barriers may exist, it is now possible to talk through and win the public confidence on data sharing. This would be achieved by employing emerging technologies such as blockchain technologies and quantum cryptography, which have shown to be reliable in safeguarding the anonymity of individuals (Allam, 2018b; Allam and Jones, 2019; Naz et al., 2019; Shahab and Allam). As shared by Hölbl et al. (2018), blockchain technology is particularly popular currently due to its qualities such as scalability, immutability, decentralized, secure, reliable, and transparent. Such qualities are sought by those willing to share their data through trusted platforms. Therefore, while these technologies are relatively in their infancy stages and are being tested in different areas, they give a glimpse of hope in overcoming the apprehension caused by the increased leakage of data and the challenge of being traced back.

Availability of such technologies, especially in moments like now when the challenge of COVID-19 is stressing and disrupting the core of the global systems, may inspire some paradigm shift in people and encourage them to voluntarily share data. This is pegged on the fact that even in times of distress, people are not readily prepared to share their data if they are not assured of its privacy and security. This is well recognized in the General Data Protection Regulation (GDPR) (Ketola et al., 2020), which emphasizes that data especially that with potential to directly or indirectly lead to identification of a natural person need to be handled with extra care. Doing this prevents scenarios where data are traced back to their source. That is, using technologies such as machine learning and reversing the process of data sharing such that one can identify individuals involved in the designing, generating, and sharing of the data. The Imperial College London (2019) calls that process the "reverse engineering" of data, and it shows how much progress the technology has brought in the global arena and, thus, increases the apprehension that people have on sharing data, as such new technologies have the capacity to override the anonymizing and encrypting ones that have been relied upon to prevent identification of persons. Therefore, as is the view of Crutzen et al. (2019), institutions and agencies and any stakeholder involved in data need to restrict themselves to only the data they require to conduct their research work. This strategy of data minimization ensures that as much as possible, only little data that can be utilized to identify an individual are available. Such strategy of data minimization needs to be enhanced with advanced data sharing protection mechanisms, thus inspiring data handlers to share data they have ownership of.

ON VOLUNTEERED GEOGRAPHIC INFORMATION AND CITIZEN SCIENCE

While there are diverse viewpoints on data sharing and the need for stringent measures to safeguard the same, especially to overcome the psychological barriers that is created by the public not trusting the whole system of data management, some cases are different. For instance, the present case of COVID-19—its spread, infectiousness, and havoc it is causing on the health sector, the social fabric and the economy have triggered an urgency on the citizen to voluntarily share data, with a hope that it could warrant the survival of people. On this, it has been observed that a majority of people in different parts of the world are willingly presenting themselves to health facilities, and in some countries, they are willingly collaborating with government agencies (UNHCR, 2020) to voluntarily share information on the coronavirus. Same trends of voluntary data sharing have been observed with popular celebrities drawn from different backgrounds who are sharing their coronavirus health status with the world. Promising enough, these are also willingly complying with the medical requirement for quarantine and self-isolation, so that they can not only safeguard themselves but also cut the spread link, thus, protecting potent contact they would infect. On the government level, similar cases of citizen science are being demonstrated. On this, it is unusual for high-ranking government officials to disclose their health status to the public, but with the coronavirus, traditional knowledge is being shattered. For instance, in different jurisdictions, top officials such as the German's Chancellor Angela Merkel publicly shared their coronavirus status and voluntary submitted to the self-quarantine rule (Delfs and Donahue, 2020). In another case, the Prime Minister of Canada was unhesitant to disclose that his wife had tested positive, leading both of them in self-quarantine (Gillies, 2020). Same case with the British Prime Minister, Boris Johnson, who made a video to share the unfortunate news that he had contracted the virus and was henceforth working from his isolation room (BBC News, 2020) and later hospital.

In view of the earlier background and examples, it then verifies that the VGI model of data sharing can become a strong approach that can be used to enrich the available datasets, more so to overcome global, modern challenges. In the case of COVID-19 pandemic, availability of an open access dataset enriched with data from the length and breadth of the world would enhance steps being made in finding a short-term and long-term solution to the health crisis. From such a dataset, anyone now has the potential to track how the virus is spreading and areas, or regions that require concerted efforts such as supply of test kits, personal protective equipment, food and medical supply, and other essentials. Similarly, information from such datasets can inform governments on steps to take regarding travel ban, lockdowns, and other necessary measures that can prevent the spread of the virus. Likewise, similar approaches could be used in the future to address other global challenges such as terrorism and future pandemics.

The advantage on this is that with modern technologies, and availability of smart devices, it is possible for data to be sourced from different quarters in real time and in an inexpensive fashion. This is perhaps well represented in the rich assortment of wearable tech available today, represented in Fig. 5.2.

But, on this, there also need to be systems and mechanisms in place to ensure that the data shared are filtered such that only factual, time-sensitive, and comprehensive ones are admitted into those datasets. This way, the quality of insight drawn from analyzing such data would be assured. And, while this is pursued, issues such as privacy and security that hold backs voluntary data sharing need to be fully addressed to assure the public of the trust and transparency.

DISCUSSION AND CONCLUSION

The discussion in the previous section, in an expounded way, demonstrates that most of the urban challenges can be, in a larger margin, solved by analyzing the massive

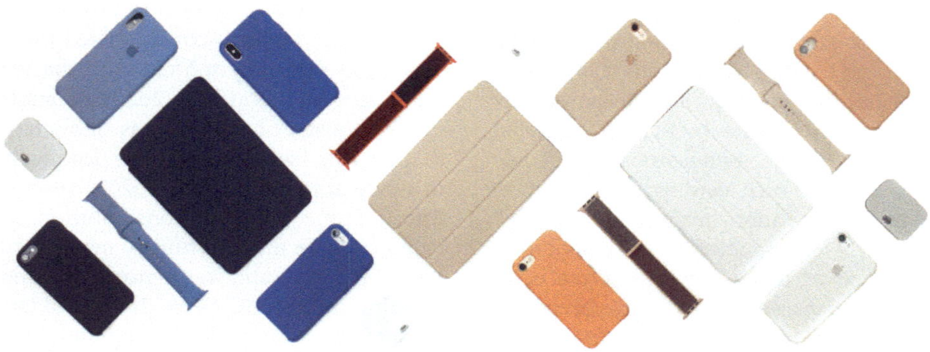

FIG. 5.2 Common wearable technology and portable devices.

data being generated from different quarters. In particular, with the increasing penetration of smart mobile devices, sensors, and other smart devices, which has the potential to link to an existing network, the amount of data being generated and shared is massive, and such can be exploited to develop long-lasting solutions. One such scenario where data have been handy is the present case of COVID-19 pandemic, where through data, its spread, its infectiousness, and its impacts have been made known to the public. Such were shared by BlueDot and Metabiota, some of the modern startups that use data, and through advanced technologies, such as natural language processing and machine learning, they were able to predict some of the geographical location that the virus would spread next from Wuhan, days before first cases were reported in those regions. In addition, it is through availability of data from different locations and sources that health officials, governments, and researchers and other stakeholders are able to establish the manifestation and impacts of the coronavirus in respect to demographic factors such as age, gender, preexisting health condition, neighborhoods, and others. But, from the global happening, where despite spirited efforts and measures like quarantine, self-isolations, lockdowns, and others that have been instituted have not been successful in preventing the virus from spreading. This means that more data require to be collected and analyzed, especially in laboratories and in other medical fields to comprehensively come up with a solution that can help in containing the outbreak.

Regarding the earlier call for more data, there are now some steps that have already been made, especially in coming up with smartphone applications that have the potential to track and report on the infected people. With these Apps, and relying on the concept of citizen science, there is optimism that people can voluntarily continue to share more data, which would ultimately be very useful in advancing research on how to contain the virus. In this front, some of the Apps that are already in use include the COVID-19 tracker that is dedicated to tracking all aspects of COVID-19 with the perimeters of the United Kingdom (Wakefield, 2020). In China, where the virus broke first, giant companies such as Alibaba Group and Tencent are said to have taken the challenge of fighting the virus spread by incorporating coronavirus trackers in their existing Apps. For instance, Alibaba incorporated a color QR code in Alipay App dedicated to identifying those suspected to have contracted the virus. Those whose color turns red after the QR code is scanned then can use the company's messaging App (DingTalk) to seek medical services (Li, 2020). The same approach of using QR code is also available in WeChat App (owned by Tencent) (Voa Student Union, 2020), and such are said to be playing a significant role in ensuring the virus is contained in the country. In the United States, the government is discussing with social media giants such as Facebook, Twitter, and Google to help track whether people are maintaining social distance (Porterfield, 2020). The emergence of these, and many other, Apps dedicated to track the virus across the globe is aimed at enhancing data collection mechanism, especially focusing on the voluntary sharing. The success of such Apps will help in complimenting the existing data collection mechanism, with the main goal focusing on having enriched databases that can be used to give insights on the global virus status.

While those efforts geared toward increasing voluntary data sharing are necessary, the need to strengthen data security and privacy should simultaneously be enhanced, thus assuring those sharing their data, including private ones that such would not land in hands of malicious people, will not in any way be used beyond their intended purpose. Such efforts would not only help in breaking the psychological barrier but would also increase the confidence and trust that the public has with data-oriented institutions and agencies, and ultimate effect would be increased volumes of data shared. This, coupled with modern technologies, as is discussed above would in turn lead to improved service delivery, lead to improved liveability status, and increase urban digital solutions. The same, especially sourced from health devices and wearable technologies, would help in formulating solutions for medical problems such as pandemics, help in improving diagnosis, and help in surveillance and monitoring to name a few. Availability of big data would also help in optimal use of resources, reduction in pollution, and speeding up efficiency in service delivery.

While there is evidence that there are some emerging, positive changes in the data landscape scene, more study is still necessary to explore how such changes are impacting different sectors, especially on social and economic frontiers. The need for this is based on the fact that, in the recent past, data are argued to be the "new oil" of this modern time, and wide scale acceptance of the concept of VGI would only lead to an increased amount; thus, it would be expected that social and economic sectors would change for the good. But, while that is the same, it is also known that some organizations have been increasing their investments in the ICT so that they can profit from data management (Yigitcanlar and Bulu, 2016); hence, the expected positive changes in the aforementioned sectors may not be actualized, or in the scale commensurate with amount of data shared. With further study, it would be possible to establish such and recommend some of the proactive actions that can be taken to ensure the public truly benefit from their actions to accept the call to voluntary share their data.

REFERENCES

(2018) Data Protection Act. *12*. United Kingdom: Legislation. gov.uk.

Allam Z. (2018a) Contextualising the Smart City for Sustainability and Inclusivity. New Design Ideas 2: 124–127.

Allam Z. (2018b) On Smart Contracts and Organisational Performance: A Review of Smart Contracts through the Blockchain Technology. Review of Economic and Business Studies 11: 137–156.

Allam Z. (2019a) Achieving Neuroplasticity in Artificial Neural Networks through Smart Cities. Smart Cities 2.

Allam Z. (2019b) The Emergence of Anti-Privacy and Control at the Nexus between the Concepts of Safe City and Smart City. Smart Cities 2: 96–105.

Allam Z. (2020a) Biometrics, Privacy, Safety, and Resilience in Future Cities. In: Allam Z (ed) Biotechnology and Future Cities: Towards Sustainability, Resilience and Living Urban Organisms. Cham: Springer International Publishing, 69–87.

Allam Z. (2020b) Biotechnology to Render Future Cities as Living and Intelligent Organisms. In: Allam Z (ed) Biotechnology and Future Cities: Towards Sustainability, Resilience and Living Urban Organisms. Cham: Springer International Publishing, 1–15.

Allam Z. (2020c) Data as the New Driving Gears of Urbanization. In: Allam Z (ed) Cities and the Digital Revolution: Aligning Technology and Humanity. Cham: Springer International Publishing, 1–29.

Allam Z. (2020d) Digital Urban Networks and Social Media. In: Allam Z (ed) Cities and the Digital Revolution: Aligning Technology and Humanity. Cham: Springer International Publishing, 61–83.

Allam Z. (2020e) Privatization and Privacy in the Digital City. In: Allam Z (ed) Cities and the Digital Revolution: Aligning Technology and Humanity. Cham: Springer International Publishing, 85–106.

Allam Z, Dey G and Jones DS. (2020) Artificial Intelligence (AI) Provided Early Detection of the Coronavirus (COVID-19) in China and Will Influence Future Urban Health Policy Internationally. AI 1: 156–165.

Allam Z and Jones DS. (2019) The Potential of Blockchain within Air Rights Development as a Prevention Measure Against Urban Sprawl. Urban Science 3: 38.

Allam Z and Jones DS. (2020) On the Coronavirus (COVID-19) Outbreak and the Smart City Network: Universal Data Sharing Standards Coupled with Artificial Intelligence (AI) to Benefit Urban Health Monitoring and Management. Healthcare 8: 46.

Allam Z and Newman P. (2018) Redefining the Smart City: Culture, Metabolism & Governance. Smart Cities 1: 4–25.

BBC News. (2020) Coronavirus: Prime Minister Boris Johnson Tests Positive. Available at: https://www.bbc.com/news/uk-52060791.

Bezuidenhout L and Chakauya E. (2018) Hidden concerns of Sharing Research Data by Low/Middle-Income Country Scientists. Global Bioethics 29: 39–54.

Blatt AJ. (2015) Data Privacy and Ethical Uses of Volunteered Geographic Information. In: Blatt AJ (ed) Health, Science, and Place: A New Model. Cham: Springer International Publishing, 49–59.

Cao W, Fang L and Xiao D. (2019) What we have learnt from the SARS epdemics in mainland China? Global Health Journal 3: 55–59.

Crowley M, Wong E and Jakes L. (2020) Coronavirus Drives the U.S. and China Deeper Into Global Power Struggle. Available at: https://www.nytimes.com/2020/03/22/us/politics/coronavirus-us-china.html.

Crutzen R, Ygram Peters G-J and Mondschein C. (2019) Why and How We Should Care About the General Data Protection Regulation. Psychology and Health 34: 1347–1357.

Delfs A and Donahue P. (2020) Merkel Quarantine Puts Another Crack in Europe Virus Defense. Available at:

https://www.bloomberg.com/news/articles/2020-03-22/merkel-in-quarantine-at-home-after-contact-with-infected-doctor.

Gillies R. (2020) Canadian Prime Minister's Wife Sophie Grégoire Trudeau Tests Positive for Coronavirus. Available at: https://time.com/5802290/canada-prime-minister-justin-trudeau-wife-coronavirus/.

Hamade MA. (2020) COVID-19: How to Fight Disease Outbreaks With Data. Available at: https://www.weforum.org/agenda/2020/03/covid-19-how-to-fight-disease-outbreaks-with-data/.

Heaven WD. (2020) AI Could Help With The Next Pandemic-But Not With This One. Available at: https://www.technologyreview.com/s/615351/ai-could-help-with-the-next-pandemicbut-not-with-this-one/?set=615328&set&=615328.

Hölbl M, Kompara M, Kamišalí A, et al. (2018) A Systematic Review of the Use of Blockchain in Healthcare. Symmetry 10: 1–22.

Imperial College London. (2019) Anonymizing Personal Data 'Not Enough to Protect Privacy,' Shows New Study. Available at: www.sciencedaily.com/releases/2019/07/190723110523.htm.

Ketola A, Kleemola M, Kuula-Luumi A, et al. (2020) Data Management Guidelines. Available at: https://www.fsd.tuni.fi/aineistonhallinta/en/anonymisation-and-identifiers.html.

Langley SA, Messina JP and Moore N. (2017) Using Meta-Quality to Assess the Utility of Volunteered Geographic Information for Science. International Journal of Health Geographics 16: 40.

Li C. (2020) Alibaba Unveils Technologies to Empower Partners in Fight Against Coronavirus. Available at: https://www.alizila.com/alibaba-unveils-technologies-to-empower-partners-in-fight-against-coronavirus/.

Metaboita. (2020) Confronting the Risk You Can't See. Available at: http://metabiota.com/.

Moorthy V, Restrepo AMH, Preziosi M-P, et al. (2020) Data Sharing for Novel Coronavirus (COVID-19). Bulletin of the World Health Organization 98.

Naz M, Al-zahrani FA, Khalid R, et al. (2019) A Secure Data Sharing Platform Using Blockchain and Interplanetary File System. 11: 7054.

Porterfield C. (2020) Surge of Smartphone Apps Promise Coronavirus Tracking, But Raise Privacy Concerns. Available at: https://www.forbes.com/sites/carlieporterfield/2020/04/01/surge-of-smartphone-apps-promise-coronavirus-tracking-but-raise-privacy-concerns/#7c9191a72681.

Pringle D. (2020) Computer science versus COVID-19. Available at: https://sciencebusiness.net/news/computer-science-versus-covid-19.

Romm T, Dwoskin E and Timberg C. (2020) U.S. Goverment, Tech Industry Discussing Ways to Uses Smart Phone Location Data to Combat Coronavirus. Available at: https://www.washingtonpost.com/technology/2020/03/17/white-house-location-data-coronavirus/.

Salokannel M. (2013) Nordic Data Sharing Framework: A Legal Perspective. Stockholm.

Shahab S and Allam Z. Reducing Transaction Costs of Tradable Permit Schemes Using Blockchain Smart Contracts. *Growth and Change* n/a.

Tiell SC. (2016) Security and Data Ethics: Best practices for Data Security. Available at: https://www.accenture.com/us-en/blogs/blogs-security-data-ethics-best-practices-data-sharing.

UNHCR. (2020) Coronavirus (COVID-19) Update. Available at: https://www.unhcr.org/ke/coronavirus-covid-19-update.

Voa Student Union. (2020) Phone Apps in China Track Coronavirus. Available at: https://www.voanews.com/student-union/phone-apps-china-track-coronavirus.

Waithira N, Mutinda B and Cheah PY. (2019) Data Management and Sharing Policy: the First Step Towards Promoting Data Sharing. BMC Medicine 17: 80.

Wakefield J. (2020) Coronavirus: Tracking App Aims for One Million Downloads. Available at: https://www.bbc.com/news/technology-52033210.

Wojda TR, Valenza PL, Cornejo K, et al. (2015) The Ebola Outbreak of 2014–2015: From Coordinated Multilateral Action to Effective Disease Containment, Vaccine Development, and Beyond. Journal of Global Infectious Diseases 7: 127-138.

Yigitcanlar T and Bulu M. (2016) Urban Knowledge and Innovation Spaces. Journal of Urban Technology 23: 1–9.

CHAPTER 6

The Rise of Machine Intelligence in the COVID-19 Pandemic and Its Impact on Health Policy

INTRODUCTION

The fourth industrial revolution has brought numerous transformations in the world, catalyzed by the advent and rapid adoption of digital tools. One notable disruption that this revolution has brought is the advent of novel computing methodologies and technologies, which are seen to be transforming all spheres of the global economies. These are observed to be the basis for the unquestionable improvements and quality risk assessments that each sector within the global fabric is experiencing. On this note, one sector that has truly been transformed is the medical sphere, which now prides itself of enriched databases following novel application of different technologies such as artificial intelligence (AI), machine learning, natural language processing, big data, and Internet of things (IoT) and others. With the increased data, and the technology, those working in the sector have access to advanced predictive modeling and computing tools that have transformed areas such as personal medicine and epidemiology, medical operations, diagnosis, and drug manufacturing (Allam et al., 2019). In addition, as noted by Watson (2019), the technologies are helping the medical fraternity to draw variable predictions by comparing historical and present medical data. For instance, it is now possible to use such predictions to assess the healthcare labor force and subsequently use the results to initiate recruitment processes in areas that are most deserving in a meritocratic way. Even if AI tools are observed to sometimes extend biases, those are being addressed, a hiring authority can manage to effect the concept of inclusivity and streamline some lingering workforce challenges among other things.

While these computing technologies and tools have already given a glimpse of how they can transform the health sector, it is worth appreciating that most of them are still a "work-in-progress" in the medical field and hence need to continue evolving and streamlined. Therefore, in that regard, it is understandable that some teething problems and challenges are inevitable, but such need to be addressed with time. Additionally, it has been found that some medical professionals and stakeholders in this field are yet to fully embrace the computing tools as part of the advancement in the medical realm; hence, they continue to rely on human-based interpretation, including in life-threatening situations. And, from records, such decisions sometimes tend to be time-consuming and are at times, far from being correct. Therefore, to ensure that such scenarios are minimized, there is a need for frameworks to guide the usage of those technologies so that they can be widely accepted and ultimately lead to saving more lives. In particular, the issues of data collection, storage, management, and sharing require to be urgently addressed, as it is seen as the primary source of the apprehension that some in the health community have against them. On this, for a start, the challenge of standardization of protocols needs to be sorted as this hosts issues such as limiting the scope of data, is associated with incompatibility of devices and networks, and exposes the field to extra costs to name a few.

Addressing such challenges would be key, especially in a period of emergencies like now, when the entire world is hurting from the impacts of COVID-19 pandemic. For instance, despite the challenges raised earlier, some startup companies were able to use the available data from social media, airline ticketing, and medical institutions to identify that the world is experiencing a new virus outbreak days before those in medical fraternity had made similar findings (Gaille, 2019). With these technologies, it also took less time to identify the outbreak, unlike in other previous outbreaks like in the

Surveying the Covid-19 Pandemic and Its Implications. https://doi.org/10.1016/B978-0-12-824313-8.00006-1

case of the severe acute respiratory syndrome (SARS) outbreak in 2002 that took relatively 4 months to identify (Qiu et al., 2018). In the case of COVID-19, initially known as 2019-nCoV, it only took 7 days (WHO, 2020b). These breakthroughs in the medical field, therefore, need to be encouraged, and one way of doing this is the streamlining all available obstacles. In support of this, this chapter surveys how AI processes, aided by availability of data managed to allow for early detection of the coronavirus outbreak, and through the findings, showcase that enhanced data sharing protocols hold the key to improved future urban health policies.

THE EARLY DETECTION OF THE CORONAVIRUS

The first official confirmation of novel coronavirus (now known as the COVID-19) was made public by the World Health Organization (WHO) on January 9, 2020, after its officials based in China received reports from the Chinese health official of a new type of infectious virus (WHO, 2020a). But from records, before this actual confirmation, there were reports that some people had started to show signs like those of the virus as early as December 8, 2019, in Wuhan. Of these, six had presented themselves to the hospital in where they were treated and later discharged. But, the cases of similar symptoms continued, and this raised an alarm among health officials who embarked on a fact-finding mission to establish whether they were dealing with a commonly known virus outbreak or a new type altogether. It was after this that, on December 31, 2019, Chinese officials liaised with the WHO officials to establish that this was truly a new strait of coronavirus. This prompted concerted efforts that lead to the official confirmation of the virus on January 9, 2020, which later became widespread worldwide (Fig. 6.1) and classified as a pandemic.

In view of this historical perceptive, it is true that there was a time lag between when the first symptoms were reported and when the confirmation was done (WHO, 2020b); thus, since it is now clearly known how the virus is transmitted (from person-to-person), there must have been a sizable number of people contracted the virus. This prompted Chinese health officials to place the entire region of Wuhan city under a total lockdown as from January 23, 2020, to prevent further spread (Li et al., 2020). But, unfortunately, noting that this is a busy city, people from other regions, and countries, as was

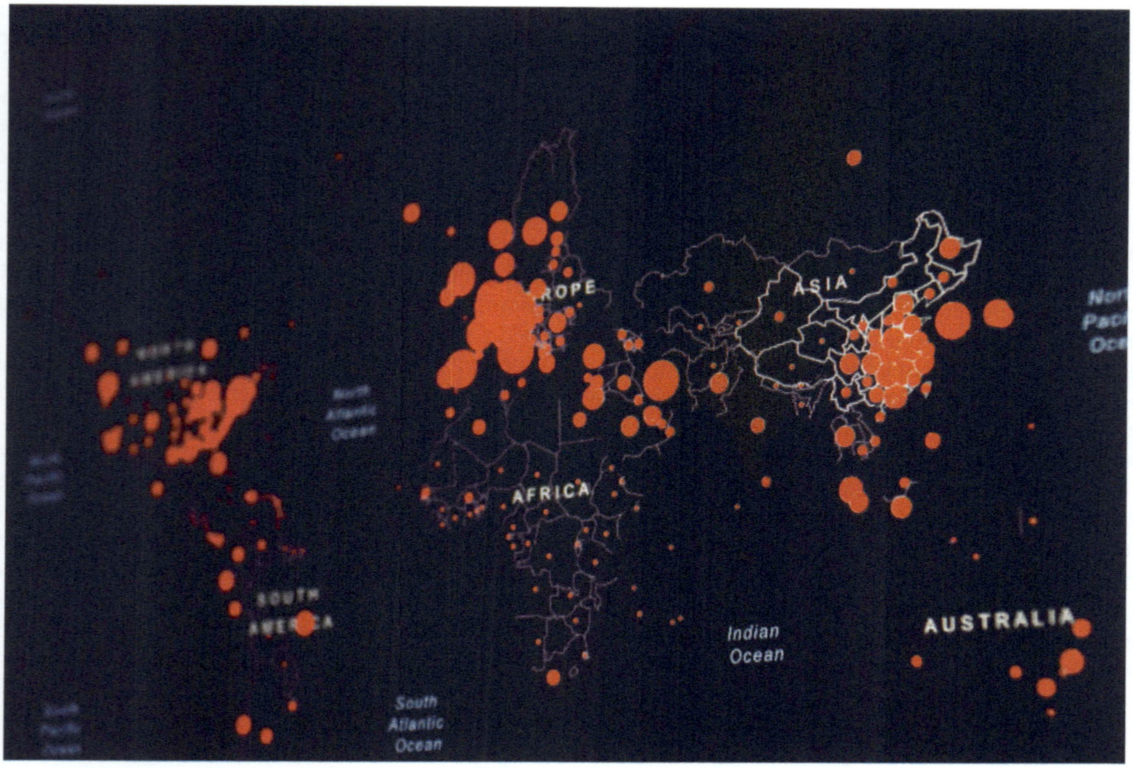

FIG. 6.1 Representation of the COVID-19 global spread.

later established by BlueDot, who may have contracted the virus had already traveled back to their countries, and this opened the door for further spread across regions and finally into the breadth and length of the world.

In respect to the actual origin of the virus, for now, only theories have been advanced. But, reports to date (Retamal, 2020) support that the first victims of this virus contracted it from the Huanan Seafood Wholesale Market in Wuhan city. And as noted earlier, being a new virus, the tests were initially being conducted only in China, specifically in Wuhan, with the health officials suspecting it to be SARS virus, but this was ruled out on January 5, 2020. This raised alarms, and when it was officially identified and provisionally named "2019-nCoV" on January 7, 2020, and the data subsequently shared to public, an Australian Virus Identification Laboratory based at the Peter Doherty Institute for Infection and Immunity immediately embarked on its research and by January 25, 2020, it was able to clone the virus (Nature, 2020). But this is not the only institution that took the virus outbreak seriously. According to Niiler (2020), BlueDot, whose profile is shared in the following, was able to employ the services of AI-driven algorithms, to analyze data gathered from sources such as new reports, air ticketing, and animal disease outbreaks to predict that the world is facing a new type of virus outbreak. Besides the prediction of the new virus outbreak, this startup and another called Metabiota (both profiles shared in the following) were able to predict (independently) correctly some of the areas that would experience the virus spread next. Among regions and countries predicted by each of these startups that turned to be true include Japan, Taiwan, South Korea, Singapore, Thailand, and Hong Kong (Heilweil, 2020). Such predictions came days earlier before any of the said country reported their first case.

The information from these different quarters became instrumental in combating the virus. It was through the spread prediction mapped by BlueDot and Metabiota that the rest of the world and concerned institutions and agencies came to learn that the world is confronting a highly infectious virus that was spreading at alarming rates. On the same, after successfully cloning the virus, the Virus Identification Laboratory shared the data in an open database where authorized researchers and labs can access and conduct further research on cures and vaccines (Nature, 2020). All these efforts prove that with technologies, it is now possible to confront pandemics of global magnitude. But such drive needs to be backed by concerted efforts aimed at eliminating data sharing obstacles associated with different advanced computing technologies and tools.

A BRIED SURVEY ON INFECTIOUS DISEASE OUTBREAK IN A 20-YEAR PERIOD

The current case of COVID-19 is not the most devastating nor the only virus that the world has had to struggle with. Indeed, looking at the historical fact, there have had some more contagious, devastating, and widespread pandemics experienced before. In the early 14th century, it is documented that a deadly plague dubbed the *Black Death* (Bubonic plague) struck the world and killed approximately 50 million people in a span of 5 years (Duncan and Scott, 2005). Fast forward, in 1918, another deadly pandemic was the *Spanish flu* (H1N1 influenza virus) struck. This is a type of influenza that is believed to have originated in Étaples, France, and it went on to infect over 500 million people, killing around 50 million of these globally (Martini et al., 2019). Between 1957 and 1958, another type of influenza (A subtype H2N2) also known as *Asian flu* broke in China, and by the time it was contained, it had claimed the lives of 1.1 million people. Ten years later (1968), the world suffered another outbreak; this time influenza A (H3N2) first reported in Hong Kong, killing over 1 million people. Later on, in 2009, the swine flu (H1N1 influenza virus) killed 12,469 people in the United States alone (CDC, 2019). Before this, in 2002, there was an outbreak of SARS in China that killed 774 people (Song et al., 2019). There was also Ebola (Zaire Ebola Virus) that was first reported in Democratic Republic of Congo that claimed approximately 11,315 people, followed by the Zika Virus in 2015 that infected approximately 500,000 people, killing 18 people. In 2020, the world is now confronting the coronavirus, which has spread to over 200 countries, and the end to it is not predictable at the time of writing of this chapter.

In all the examples cited earlier, the common denominator is that the success of containing any of these viruses depends on detection and identification. That said, it is worth noting that these pandemics were caused by different types of viruses. These include the influenza virus, Henipavirus (Nipah virus), Filoviruses like those responsible for Ebola, and Flavivirus that is responsible for Zika (Aris-Brosou et al., 2017; Madhav et al., 2018) to name a few. This process usually equates to extensive laboratory testing, as illustrated in Fig. 6.2.

Regarding their detection, it is dependent on the type of technology use; hence, from the emergence of the digital revolution, things are seen to be changing in respect to amount of time taken for detection. However, here too, other factors such as the availability of data, quality of the same, and sharing methods are critical. For instance, despite having some levels of modern technology, it took approximately 4 months to identify the SARS

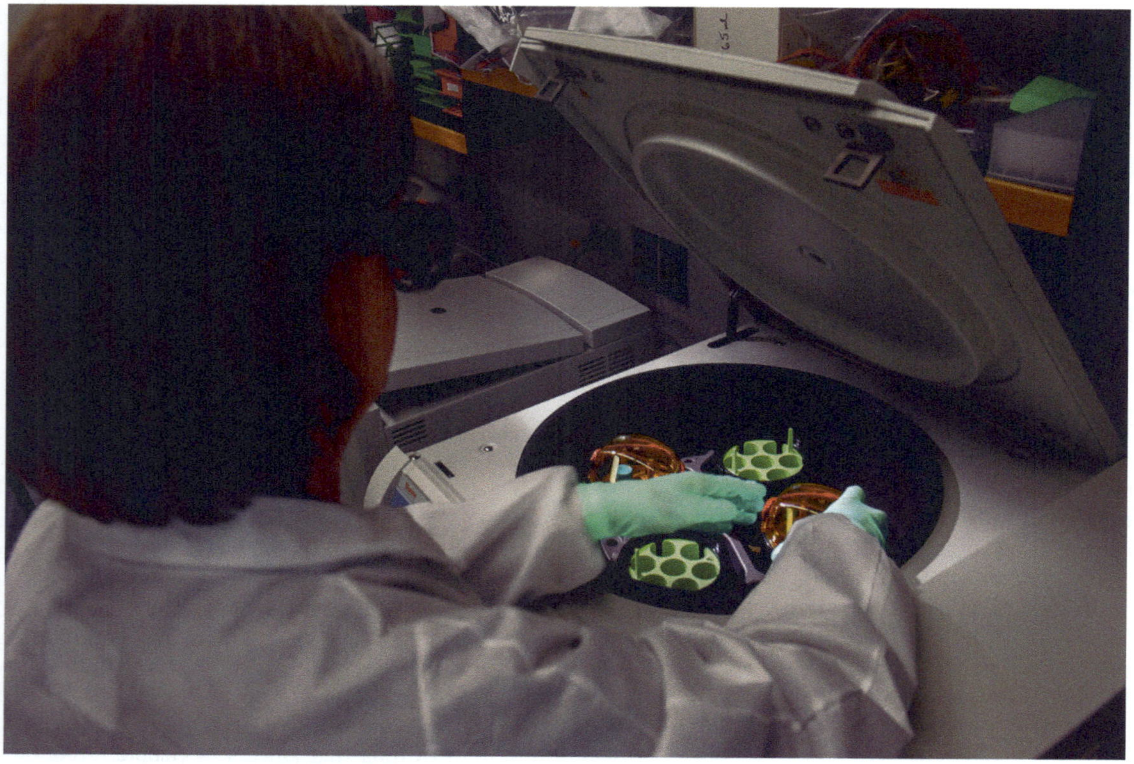

FIG. 6.2 Laboratory testing at the Centers for Disease Control and Prevention (CDC).

virus. Such delays, however, are credited to the action or inaction of the Chinese health officials to withhold information concerning the virus outbreak. In cases where there were concerted efforts between different players, like in the case of 2014 Ebola outbreak in West Africa, it is reported that the virus was identified in a record time, and this prevented its spread beyond the three countries (Liberia, Sierra Leone, and Guinea) that it was first reported (Wojda et al., 2015). In the current case of COVID-19, as noted earlier, it only took only 7 days to detect and identify the virus and to also predict how it would spread from the original epicenter (Wuhan). This was possible due to availability of technologies such as AI (Bini, 2018), machine learning, and natural language processing; the aforementioned startups were able to use to gather and analyze the data. In particular, the advancement in AI-based infectious disease-surveillance algorithms is understood to reduce the amount taken to detect a virus outbreak. It is evident that since the emergence of the AI-based surveillance, there is a notable level of improvement and efficiency. This is particularly important noting that technological advancements in other sectors such as transport have made movement of people relatively cheaper, quicker, and comfortable; thus, importation of virus and diseases from regions of high concentration to those with little or no virus or disease has become relatively high. This is the reality with the COVID-19, which was first imported from China and then later from some European countries such as Italy to the rest of the world.

In this regard, it is true that there are ongoing works and discussion aimed at revising existing policies to ensure the loopholes that have existed, thus allowing that spread of diseases and other outbreaks to nonendemic regions have been sealed. But, with the current happening, it is true that much effort is still needed. The amount of emerging computing literature on infectious diseases demonstrates that substantial research, supported by development of AI-based algorithms, has been increasing exponentially supporting an incline in use of AI technologies involved in diseases and virus surveillance.

The increased use of AI-based tools to monitor and survey outbreaks in different regions, through a forward step toward early prevention, needs to be complimented by the availability of substantial data. Therefore, as has been stamped in this chapter, it is paramount to have a framework that clearly outlines how specific data need to be shared with the public. In particular, this would help to overcome challenges of insufficient data that are instigated by the act of withholding information by some entities or countries surfing on private interest. On this, a positive step toward its actualization was made in 2016 by the WHO after the Zika virus outbreak where through unfettered sharing of data, different agencies and stakeholders were able to utilize advanced technologies to prevent the spread of the virus. And, as noted earlier, such efforts were fruitful in that, unlike other previous virus outbreaks, this had the least number of casualties (18). Henceforth, the use of technologies is seen to be gaining traction with use of analytical tools such as AI algorithms becoming popular as it allows for data scouring from diverse targets (Lau et al., 2019) and it is also compatible with other technologies such as machine learning and natural language processing. Such technologies, as noted earlier, are what allowed BlueDot and Metabiota to obtain the correct predictions they made about the outbreak and spread of COVID-19 to different regions. The use of these modern tools is also hailed for they have the potential to lead to quick diagnosis, help in development of vaccines and cures of outbreaks, and also would prompt development of raft of preventive strategies in areas that would be predicted to be of high risk of experience an outbreak (Martins, 2019). This is what the two aforementioned companies, whose description is given in the next section, achieved in the current case of COVID-19.

THE TWO COMPANIES THAT PROVIDED EARLY DETECTION OF COVID-19

This section highlights some briefs on how BlueDot and Metabiota were able to utilize modern computing technologies to accurately, and in record time predict coronavirus outbreak, and the target countries that were at risk of experiencing the outbreak.

BlueDot

BlueDot is a web-based startup that was pioneered in 2003 by Dr. Kamran Khan after the SARS outbreak. Initially, it was known by the trade name of Bio-Diaspora, but in 2014, it seeded round with a Sri Lankan private venture (Horizons Ventures) prompting its renaming to BlueDot. The startup came into limelight in 2009 when the H1N1 influenza pandemic broke, where it was able to correctly predict that global pathway of the virus by relying on worldwide air travel data. It cemented its authority in the use of modern computing technologies in 2014, where it developed risk assessment models that allowed it to predict the spread of Ebola virus outbreak that struck three West Africa countries (Allen, 2016). In the current predicament of COVID-19 pandemic, BlueDot was among the first to predict (9 days before official announcement) that the world was experiencing a new outbreak and also correctly identified countries that were at high risk of being next target of the outbreak (Bowles, 2020).

The answer to the success of this startup in making correct predictions lies on their reliance on modern, advanced, computing technologies and availability of data from different spheres. In respect to technologies, the company is observed to heavily rely on AI-based tools, machine learning technology, and natural language processing technologies. Using different models and algorithms, the company managed to scour valuable data from different sources such as diverse, global news outlets, global airline ticketing data (Heaven, 2020), population density data, global infectious disease alert, climate report, and Insect Vectors and Animal Diseases Reservoirs. In its website (2020b), it is clearly noted that it relies on over 10,000 official and media sources drawn from over 60 languages each day. It also queries reputable databases such as World Factbook and national statistics reports from different regions. With the available technologies, the company is able to employ filters on information from the different sources to narrow the results to the issue at hand (BlueDot, 2020a). On the same, the technologies also allow the use of modern clustering tools that allow it to quickly, and in real time, identify areas or regions with the potential to become hot spots, cold spots, and/or spatial outliers. It also relies on the power of machine learning to train its system using the assorted dataset, and in turn, the systems are able to generate real-time and regular alerts on issues of interest to the company's clients. It is through this that it was able to flag out coronavirus as an outbreak that had potential to spread to other regions quickly.

Metabiota

The history of Metabiota takes us back to 2009 when it was initiated. During those early days, its main engagements were in research focusing on how human and animal health were linked, especially in the African context. In 2014, when the Ebola virus broke in West Africa, the company was already active, and through its work attracted the attention of the US government, which at the time was actively involved in combating this outbreak (Rossi, 2019). Having experience on the African context, Metabiota was requested to assist, and it did a remarkable job, but after the Ebola situation was contained, the US government withdrew the funding to the company. The reduction of the funds took a toll on the company, hence prompting a paradigm shift, which entailed the company expanding its operation scope to enable it to serve more clients. In this regard, its target market was insurance companies, who would benefit from information concerning disease outbreaks. Henceforth, the company embarked on enriching its disease database, which today is among the most comprehensive ones (Rossi, 2019). To achieve this, the company embarked on investing and utilizing advanced computation and predictive technologies, and such included AI, machine learning, big data, and natural language processing (NLP) algorithms. Through this, the San Francisco—based company serves a wide range of clients including government agencies, insurance companies, contractors, diverse non—profit-making organizations, NGOs, and others that, in one way or the other, depends on information of infectious diseases outbreaks to enhance their decision-making.

With these technologies, it has become among the leading startups in rendering predictions about infectious diseases outbreaks, spread, interventions, and event severity (Heaven, 2020). It uses NLP algorithms to scour data from diverse sources (both official and unofficial sources). From its website (Metaboita, 2020), it sources range from biological, political, socioeconomic, environmental, and social media among others. The data gathered from these are analyzed and categorized using reputable analytical and visualization technologies into clusters such as frequencies, severity, and time (duration of outbreaks), and these are shared with its clients depending on information being sought. In the recent case of COVID-19, Metabiota was in the forefront to analyze the outbreak, and during the analysis of the data, some even sourced from social media, the company was able to predict which neighboring countries were at high risk of being the next target of the virus spread, more so because the panic in Wuhan had stated to trigger some fear, forcing people to flee. By relying on AI, machine learning, and NLP, the company analyzed human predictive behaviors and scare levels, thus managing to correctly make the predictions a week earlier before any of the said countries (Japan, Thailand, Hong Kong, and others) had reported any case of the virus (Tong, 2020).

THE INCREASING ROLE OF BIOINFORMATICS

When it comes to pandemics, one sure way of protecting the masses and averting related negative impacts on the social fabric, the economy and human lives to name a few are providing early detection. Today where there are enough digital tools and technologies with capacity to allow for real-time data collection, fast and comprehensive computation, and prediction, early detection ought to be emphasized. But even with these technologies, any lapses, especially in data sharing, are bound to delay the detection and identification of the outbreak and that can prove to be fatal. For instance, in 2002, when SARS (SARS-CoV) broke in Guangdong local market in China, health officials and Chinese authorities withheld information on the outbreak, and this prompted the identification of the virus to drag for around 4 months. While the fatalities from this virus outbreak were only 774 reported across 17 countries where the virus had spread, such could have been avoided. By the time the virus was contained, it had already spread to 29 countries. In a totally different case, as reported earlier, due to collaborative measures taken in 2016 when Ebola virus broke in West Africa, the virus was identified in a reasonable time, and this prevented further spread of the virus beyond Liberia, Guinea, and Sierra Leone. Though this virus is very infectious and tends to have high casualties, it leads to the unfortunate death of 11,310 people. If the outbreak here was to take the same route that SARS, it could have been disastrous and would have spread to numerous countries.

In the present case of coronavirus (COVID-19) pandemic that originated in Wuhan city, China, the response was totally different from the 2002 SARS incident. This time round, the Chinese authorities were quicker and forthright in their reporting, and also in sharing subsequent information and data. Nevertheless, some quarters continue to accuse the Chinese authorities for the global spread of the virus. But while mistrust exists, the steps taken by Chinese authorities have been lauded. Additionally, as noted earlier, when the WHO officials were notified of this outbreak, they were also quick to identify the virus and to take decisive measures in ensuring that the spread was contained. It only took 7 days for the identification, but as noted earlier, it had taken approximately 23 days (from December 8, 2019—31 December 2019) to detect that the world was confronting a new type of coronavirus.

The breakthrough in the early detection being witnessed in these recent years can be credited to several factors. First, the reasons learnt from previous occurrences may have prompted some changes on how governments and stakeholders perceive the issue of pandemic outbreak. Secondly, and more importantly, the emergence and subsequent acceptability of a wide range of computational technologies has made it possible for faster data collection, data sharing, and advanced computation and analysis. The availability of data from different sources, including smart devices and health-wearable devices, social media, and existing health database, has also been handy and influential in determining the detection period and tracking of outbreaks. For this reason, Gaille (2019) notes that besides technologies, availability of data in large quantities is now seen as the world's new "gold rush" of this century. The availability of these not only influences health outcomes but is also seen to determine geopolitical standing, with those in position to collect, store, and control most of the data seen to be positioned as a global power house and, hence, the push and pull on the 5G Internet between power economies (Allam, 2019a; Allam and Dhunny, 2019; Allam and Jones, 2019; Allam and Newman, 2018; Kharpal, 2018). In addition, even in lower levels of governance, the control of data is seen to be raising heat with large ICT corporations competing to control the market share such that they can have exclusive control of data, thus increasing their profit standing (Allam and Jones, 2020). But, beyond selfish interests, it is possible for corporations and governments and organisations with capacity to manage large quantities of data to work together for the sake of the economic landscape, the welfare of the social fabric, and the improvement in the health sector (Allam, 2019b; Allam, 2020c; Allam, 2020d). Such calls are valid in a time like now when the entire global economy, the health sector, and societies are in limbo due to the impacts of COVID-19.

To achieve such noble goals, however, as noted in the previous sections, there are several things that need to be addressed to streamline the data usage landscape. Among these include addressing some notable challenges with computing technologies used in analyzing big data. First, there needs to be a framework that guides how data have for long been highly guarded, collected, shared, and accessed in such a way that it does deem to be compromising the security and privacy of individuals. By doing this, it would be possible to increase personal data even further as the ethical and moral issues associated with data sharing would be lifted (Allam, 2020a; Allam, 2020b). In particular, this would be important when it comes to accessing and using data comprising personal genome, personal demographic information, and other personal identifying details (Vayena and Blasimme, 2018). In cases where such must be accessed, the use of strategies like k-anonymity (i.e ensuring that datasets have no combination of user identifying attribute) (Sweeney, 2002) to anonymise data, or the use of technologies such as blockchain or quantum cryptography must be made to ensure total anonymization of data. The framework should also address issues to do with standardization of protocols and networks, which have for long been seen to reduce communication of systems, especially in urban areas. On this, as shared by Allam and Jones (2020), standardization would then support seamless flow at an urban, regional, and international scale.

Besides streamlining on the use of technologies, and data-related issues, as has comprehensively been shared earlier, the war against COVID-19, as has been done already in different countries, needs to be supported by strengthening instituted quarantines, self-isolation, and lockdowns. These actions are in their part enough in enriching health databases, as it is from these that data on people contracting, recovering, and succumbing from the virus are being collected, in addition to those already sourced in medical facilities.

CONCLUSION

This work has candidly explored the role of various technologies, especially AI, machine learning, and NLP and big data in early detection of COVID-19, especially by exploring how such were instrumental in assisting BlueDot and Metabiota companies make their groundbreaking predictions for rendering early detection of the coronavirus. The exploration has demonstrated that the future of the health sector, among others, is promising, if such predictive achievements are to continue. To make this even better, it is the position in this paper that data sharing practices need to be encouraged by adopting best practices such as standardization of protocols, enhancing anonymization, and employing modern technologies such as blockchain and quantum cryptography, which have proven to be novel in such fields. There is also needed to emphasize cooperation between different agencies, institutions, and corporations to ensure that corporate monetary interest on data does not overshadow work aimed toward improving global health, economic equity, and social welfare.

REFERENCES

Allam MZ. (2019a) Urban Resilience and Economic Equity in an Era of Global Climate Crisis. University of Sydney.

Allam Z. (2019b) The Emergence of Anti-Privacy and Control at the Nexus between the Concepts of Safe City and Smart City. Smart Cities 2: 96–105.

Allam Z. (2020a) Cities and the Digital Revolution: Aligning Technology and Humanity: Springer International Publishing.

Allam Z. (2020b) Data as the New Driving Gears of Urbanization. In: Allam Z (ed) Cities and the Digital Revolution: Aligning Technology and Humanity. Cham: Springer International Publishing, 1–29.

Allam Z. (2020c) Privatization and Privacy in the Digital City. In: Allam Z (ed) Cities and the Digital Revolution: Aligning Technology and Humanity. Cham: Springer International Publishing, 85–106.

Allam Z. (2020d) Theology, Sustainability and Big Data. In: Allam Z (ed) Theology and Urban Sustainability. Cham: Springer International Publishing, 53–67.

Allam Z and Dhunny ZA. (2019) On Big Data, Artificial Intelligence and Smart Cities. Cities 89: 80–91.

Allam Z and Jones DS. (2019) The Potential of Blockchain within Air Rights Development as a Prevention Measure against Urban Sprawl. Urban Science 3: 38.

Allam Z and Jones DS. (2020) On the Coronavirus (COVID-19) Outbreak and the Smart City Network: Universal Data Sharing Standards Coupled with Artificial Intelligence (AI) to Benefit Urban Health Monitoring and Management. Healthcare 8: 46.

Allam Z and Newman P. (2018) Redefining the Smart City: Culture, Metabolism & Governance. Smart Cities 1: 4-25.

Allam Z, Tegally H and Thondoo M. (2019) Redefining the Use of Big Data in Urban Health for Increased Liveability in Smart Cities. Smart Cities 2: 259-268.

Allen K. (2016) How a Toronto Company Used Big Data to Predict the Spread of Zika. Available at: https://www.thestar.com/news/insight/2016/02/22/how-a-toronto-company-used-big-data-to-predict-the-spread-of-zika.html.

Aris-Brosou S, Ibeh N and Noël J. (2017) Viral Outbreaks Involve Destabilized Evolutionary Networks: Evidence From Ebola, Influenza and Zika. Scientific Reports 7: 11881.

Bini SA. (2018) Artificial Intelligence, Machine Learning, Deep Learning, and Cognitive Computing: What Do these Terms Mean and How will they Impact Health Care? The Journal of Arthroplasty 33: 2358-2361.

BlueDot. (2020a) Better Public Health Surveillance for Infectious Diseases. Available at: https://bluedot.global/products/explorer/.

BlueDot. (2020b) BlueDot protects people around the world from infectious diseases with human and artificial intelligence. Available at: https://bluedot.global/about/.

Bowles J. (2020) How Canadian AI Start-Up BlueDot Spotted Coronavirus Before Anyone Else Had a Clue. Available at: https://diginomica.com/how-canadian-ai-start-bluedot-spotted-coronavirus-anyone-else-had-clue.

CDC. (2019) Influenza (Flu). Available at: https://www.cdc.gov/flu/pandemic-resources/2009-h1n1-pandemic.html.

Duncan CJ and Scott S. (2005) What Caused the Black Death? Postgraduate Medical Journal 81: 315.

Gaille B. (2019) 29 Wearable Technology Industry Statistics, Trends & Analysis. Available at: https://brandongaille.com/29-wearable-technology-industry-statistics-trends-analysis/.

Heaven WD. (2020) AI Could Help With The Next Pandemic-But Not With This One. Available at: https://www.technologyreview.com/s/615351/ai-could-help-with-the-next-pandemicbut-not-with-this-one/?set=615328&set=615328.

Heilweil R. (2020) How AI is Battling the Coronavirus Outbreak. Available at: https://www.vox.com/recode/2020/1/28/21110902/artificial-intelligence-ai-coronavirus-wuhan.

Kharpal A. (2018) China 'Has the Edge' in the War for 5G and the US and Europe Could Fall Behind. Available at: https://www.cnbc.com/2018/03/07/china-has-the-edge-in-the-war-for-5g-us-and-eu-could-fall-behind.html.

Lau AYS, Staccini P, Section Editors for the IYSoE, et al. (2019) Artificial Intelligence in Health: New Opportunities, Challenges, and Practical Implications. Yearbook of medical informatics 28: 174–178.

Li S, Areddy Jt and Deng C. (2020) China Locks Down City at Center of Coronavirus Outbreak. Available at: https://www.wsj.com/articles/china-virus-cases-pass-400-11579670877.

Madhav N, Oppenheim B, Gallivan M, et al. (2018) Risks, Impacts, and Mitigation. In: Jamison DT, Gelband H, Horton S, et al. (eds) Disease Control Priorities: Improving Health and Reducing Poverty. 3rd ed. Washington DC: The International Bank for Reconstruction and Development/The World Bank.

Martini M, Gazzaniga V, Bragazzi NL, et al. (2019) The Spanish Influenza Pandemic: a Lesson From History 100 years After 1918. Journal of preventive medicine and hygiene 60: E64-E67.

Martins N. (2019) How Healthcare is using Big Data and AI to Cure Disease. Available at: https://www.forbes.com/sites/nicolemartin1/2019/08/30/how-healthcare-is-using-big-data-and-ai-to-cure-disease/#7ebe957645cf.

Metaboita. (2020) Confronting the Risk You Can't See. Available at: http://metabiota.com/.

Nature. (2020) Coronavirus latest: Australian Lab First to Grow Virus Outside China. Available at: https://www.nature.com/articles/d41586-020-00154-w.

Niiler E. (2020) An AI Epidemiologist Sent the First Warnings of the Wuhan Virus. Available at: https://www.wired.com/story/ai-epidemiologist-wuhan-public-health-warnings/.

Qiu W, Chu C, Mao A, et al. (2018) The Impacts on Health, Society, and Economy of SARS and H7N9 Outbreaks in China: A Case Comparison Study. International Journal of Environmental Research and Public Health 2018: 2710185.

Retamal H. (2020) Where it all Began: Wuhan's Virus Ground-Zero 'Wet Market' Hides in Plain Sight. Available at: https://www.timesofisrael.com/wuhans-virus-ground-zero-market-hides-in-plain-sight/.

Rossi B. (2019) The Metaboita Story. Available at: https://medium.com/@billrossi/the-metabiota-story-d553f41d03bd.

Song Z, Xu Y, Bao L, et al. (2019) From SARS to MERS, Thrusting Coronaviruses into the Spotlight. Viruses 11: 59.

Sweeney L. (2002) k-Anonynity: A Model for Protecting Privacy. 10: 557–570.

Tong S. (2020) Big Data Predicted the Coronavirus Outbrea and Where it Would Spread. Available at: https://www.marketplace.org/2020/02/04/big-data-predicted-coronavirus-outbreak-where-it-may-go-next/.

Vayena E and Blasimme A. (2018) Health Research with Big Data: Time for Systemic Oversight. 46: 119–129.

Watson K. (2019) Predictive Analytics in Health Care: Emerging Value and Risks. In: Leo E, Allen S and Bhat R (eds). Deloitte Development LLC.

WHO. (2020a) Emergencies Preparedness, Response. Available at: https://www.who.int/csr/don/12-january-2020-novel-coronavirus-china/en/.

WHO. (2020b) Novel Coranvirus (2019-nCoV) Situation Report. World Health Organisation.

Wojda TR, Valenza PL, Cornejo K, et al. (2015) The Ebola Outbreak of 2014-2015: From Coordinated Multilateral Action to Effective Disease Containment, Vaccine Development, and Beyond. Journal of Global Infectious Diseases 7: 127–138.

CHAPTER 7

Vital COVID-19 Economic Stimulus Packages Pose a Challenge for Long-Term Environmental Sustainability

INTRODUCTION

The COVID-19 epicenter is moving from east to west and sparking, as it moves, the lockdown of entire cities, regions, and countries. The global economy is taking a blow as supply chains are impacted. The future looks uncertain. However, one recent good news among all this chaos is that emissions have been on the decline. This was expected as factories and airports are closed, and mobility is reduced due to lockdowns. For instance, consumption of coal in China plummeted 36% compared with the same period last year. NO_2 levels in Italy have been noted to be on the decline with industries shutdown, an activity that represents 24% of their gross domestic product (GDP). A similar story playing out in Spain, the United Kingdom, and other parts of the world. The question that everybody is now asking is: how long will the good news last and will it sustain postvirus?

A clear answer is tricky, as we are yet to see how, and for how long, the COVID-19 story will unfold and how deep we will be scarred. But the certainty is that the situation in least developed, and developing, economies will be dire. Health infrastructure in those places is not as developed as their western counterparts. Africa, for instance, for its 1.2 billion population, has 1 doctor for 2000 people versus Europe which has 1 doctor for 500 people for a population of 741 million. The numbers are just not comparable, and this aligns with essentials such as ventilators, testing capacity, and others. While it is expected that the outbreak may be slower in hotter climates, scientific evidence is yet to be produced to support this claim. So, policy-makers are preparing for the worst and equipping cities and countries to face lockdowns, but this decision has severe consequences on their socioeconomic fabric.

While Europe and China have deep pockets and are economically equipped to finance lockdowns, developing economies are not. Last week, Africa called for a $100 billion loan to combat the impact of the coronavirus pandemic; this will add on to their existing $350 billion debt. While a "V" or even "U" shape recovery may be possible for the former, Africa and other developing economies will face a very different future, leading to increased north/south inequality. The solution that many governments are now turning to is the modeling of aggressive stimulus economic packages, supported through external loans, a necessary, but expensive, move. One issue will be the rush to restart economic wheels postvirus in the hopes to get back to business as usual, so as to repair economic damages and retain political and economic mileages. On this, an injection of capital in existing activities may have a devastating consequence on the long term as it may tie the country toward longer fossil fuel–based activities, hence exploding previous commitments for reducing carbon emissions.

An analysis of CO_2 emissions after the financial crisis of 2008 provides an interesting precedent on this, showing that emissions dropped during the crisis and the economic policy responses that followed led to a quick rebound in emissions, where it rose faster than they had before. So, while stimulus packages will have a key role to play internationally within the next months, we must remember that their intended role will be to jump start economies in short timelines, but those, if not properly framed, can have long-term negative impacts on both environment and economy.

Another challenge will be that the drop in oil pricing we are currently experiencing will create a difficult competitive arena for renewable energy, and this will be more difficult with all the policy efforts geared on pandemic preparedness plans. The implementation of new solar energy power plants is thus expected to take a hit this year in favor of continued fossil fuel–based

Surveying the Covid-19 Pandemic and Its Implications. https://doi.org/10.1016/B978-0-12-824313-8.00007-3

energy sources, which will be extended to absorb the current oil competitive edge and gain from the COVID-19 stimulus packages. This will push us back on our global CO_2 emissions target.

On this, the COP26, the next most important event since the Paris Agreement, initially set in November this year may now be reported due to the uncertainty of how the pandemic will unfold, coupled with the fact that governments are realigning efforts from environmental agendas toward health emergency policies. So, even if the COP26 is kept on track or postponed to early 2021, the question whether governments will be prepared to further environmental conversations in a significant fashion remains. The conversation, however, should not be sidetracked, and supporting the continued global emissions rise will further negatively impact on us.

One opportunity on this, pre-COP26, is that COVID-19 provided us the opportunity of testing a number of green alternatives that the world was previously reluctant to try. For example, ZOOM, the video conferencing platform, noted a surge of 1,270% downloads from February 22 to March 22. While we are yet to see the quantitative studies on emissions decline that ZOOM users contributed to, this creates a precedent for reinforced discussions that alternatives do work and that a different lifestyle is possible.

We are yet to see how the complete COVID-19 story unfolds, but there is certainty that we will see a short-term drop in emissions in 2020. If bailouts are geared toward supporting fossil fuel–based heavy industries, we will then see a similar trend as post-2008 recession, leading to a rapid rise in emissions. A balancing act will be required to shape "transition" stimulus packages, and how governments play their role during the next few months will be decisive to guide sustainability agendas.

This chapter explores the need for crafting those transition stimulus packages to ensure long-term sustainability.

THE WORLD IS RUNNING A REGENERATIVE COURSE DUE TO THE COVID-19

Even before COVID-19 was declared an international emergency of concern on January 30, 2020, leave alone a pandemic on March 11, 2020, Wuhan, the initial epicenter of the virus and other regions in the country were already placed under lockdown (Buckley and May, 2020). Italy also initiated a total lockdown before even the virus outbreak was declared a global pandemic by the World Health Organization (WHO) following the speed of its spread in the country and subsequent consequences. After, the announcement to date, cases of lockdown across the globe have amassed, with approximately 3 billion people, which translates to approximately 40% of the global population being immobilized and have had their social and economic lifestyles disrupted. The closure of Chinese borders and cities as an immediate result of the outbreak sent strong signals to the global community and economies that moving forward global systems would be different—and relatively difficult on the immediate short term. Locally, the liveability status of the population was immediately impacted. On the global economic perspective, the lockdown of parts of China which is taunted as the "global factory and supplier" meant that different regions of the world would have their economic terrains disrupted. On this, it is expected that the global economic growth will drop by approximately 2.4% in the first quarter of this year (OECD, 2020). This is a substantial decline noting that by the end of the past year (2019), the global GDP growth saw an increase of 2.9%. This drop is partly influenced by the 17.2% decline in China's export within the first 2 months (January and February) after the outbreak (Segal and Gerstel, 2020). Also, the toll the pandemic is having on other global economies is going to influence the negative spiral of this global economic growth.

While the social and economic landscapes continue to bear subsequent blows, the environmental frontier is seen to be somehow gaining from this situation. In particular, the reduced economic activities—global reduction of air and water travels, reduced vehicular activities across different cities due to lockdown, and reduction in activities in factories and manufacturing sectors—have helped to achieve reductions in levels of emissions across the globe, to the advantage of the environment. For instance, in the first quarter of this year, it is reported that China's emissions have already reduced by 25% (equivalent to 200 million metric tons of CO_2) (Myllyvirta, 2020). In New York City, the emissions are observed to have reduced by approximately 50% in the same period (Henriques, 2020). In Europe, satellite images have shown that already, there is substantial reduction in emissions, with expert approximating that to be in the range of 5% in the 1 month most of the countries across the regions have been put under lockdown (Boyle, 2020). According to Global Data Energy (2020), as reduction in the use of coal (estimated to have reduced by 40% in this first quarter), it is reported that demand for renewable energy especially in some regions such as the United Kingdom and the United States is increasing and is expected to increase even further in the second quarter of this year. All these reductions are being hailed and seen as blessings in disguise to the global environmental, as pointed by the increasing air and water qualities in different parts of the world. For instance, in China, it is reported that air quality is improved by approximately 83%, leading to clear skies, a new normal that has not been witnessed in a long time (Stephanie and Gerstel, 2020).

Besides the environmental benefits, there are further positive outcomes observed in the natural landscape. In different parts of the globe, there are signs of natural regenerative activities, especially regarding organisms "reclaiming" some of their habitats impacted, and taken over, by humans. From a conservation perspective, the presence of human beings and the required activities sustaining our economic systems in land, air, and water have been a hindrance to wildlife—noting that such produces different pollution like noise, emits effluent and other harmful substances in water and air, and impacts on wildlife. The constant movement of people, irrespective of periods across the year, is also a nuisance on both the health and liveability of people. But with the lockdown and the restrained economic activities, there are reports of wild animals in cities and near shores of water bodies (Ball, 2020; Frishberg, 2020; Singh, 2020). In Chile, Ball (2020) reports that Pumas have occasionally been spotted in Santiago. In Paris, families of ducks were spotted freely wondering and crossing the usually busy highways, streets, and even airport. In busy canals of Venice, it is reported that the water quality has greatly improved, and this has attracted swarms of silver fish and sea birds (swans) that have long deserted the area (Bressan, 2020). In Nara, Japan, Sika deer were spotted roaming the usually busy streets and subway stations, whereas in Oakland, California, wild turkeys were observed to freely explore the streets (Singh, 2020).

The aforementioned happenings showcase that amid the COVID-19 outbreak, and its subsequent impacts on the global economy and social fabric, all is not lost, and in future, human decisions could lead to further natural regeneration. This could spark discussions on the need to control human activities threatening the environment and endangering wildlife. On this, as has been discussed in some quarters (Eaubien, 2020), the case of COVID-19 outbreak, especially with claim that the virus may have originated from bats, or other wild animals, would enhance calls on ending animal trafficking. It would also lead to strengthening of policies toward abolishment of consumption of some of these animals.

However, there are fears that the reduction in emissions and the natural regeneration may not continue post-COVID-19, as will be described in detail in the next section. Such fears are not far-fetched, as there is enough evidence that after such global crisis, governments, and economies tend to concentrate on restarting economic engines and neglect or overlook the plight of the environment and the natural ecosystems. This is further discussed in the succeeding section.

THE PAST SHOWS THAT A SPIKE IN EMISSIONS HAPPENS POSTRECESSION

While governments, different agencies, and institutions are actively working to contain and eradicate the virus, and mitigate the impacts of COVID-19, there are indicators supporting that the global economy is headed toward a recession. One such indicator, as noted, is the unprecedented reduction in emissions due to a stop in economic activities, especially in geographies, that for the past years have been recording some levels of increase on the same. On this, a historical perspective of previous recessions showcases that before this happens, different economies are seen to increase their emissions, but as the impacts of recessions start to be felt, emissions tend to slow down. That is, with recession, economic activities in areas such as construction, manufacturing sectors, and other industries reduce significantly; hence, burning of fossil fuels and excessive energy consumption are reduced, along with the impacts on natural resources, which is often characterized by prolonged scenes of coal-fired power plants, as illustrated in Fig. 7.1.

For instance, in the 2008–09 global recession, it is reported that developed economies, which were in most cases high emitters, were significantly impacted, leading to a global reduction in emissions by approximately 3% (Vidal, 2009). In these developed economies, they experienced a 1.3% reduction in 2008 and an impressive 7.6% drop in emissions in 2009 (Connor, 2011; Ritchie and Roser, 2017). But before these drops, it was reported that industries such as cement production and consumption of fossil fuels, especially in generation of energy, were on the rise, especially in China and the United States (Liu et al., 2015). As noted by The World Bank (2019a), CO_2 emissions, immediately after the 2002 recessions, were on upward swing and only halting in 2008–09.

In most cases of recessions experienced, such reduction in emissions has benefited the environment and the natural ecosystem. For instance, between 1970 and 1975, the recession caused a reduction of CO_2 emissions by approximately 3% (100 million tons) and in 1980–1981, reductions were approximated at 1 billion tons of greenhouse gases (GHGs), whereas in 2009, the reductions of approximately 300 million tons were experienced (Ambrose, 2020). In 2020, already, following the lockdowns and the slowed economic activities prompted by COVID-19, it has already been projected that the drop in emissions globally may reach a low of 5%, equivalent to 2.5 billion tons of GHGs (Ambrose, 2020). While it is true that some of these reductions may be attributable to adoption of some forms of renewable energy, Slini et al. (2014) note that such moves can be attributed prerecession,

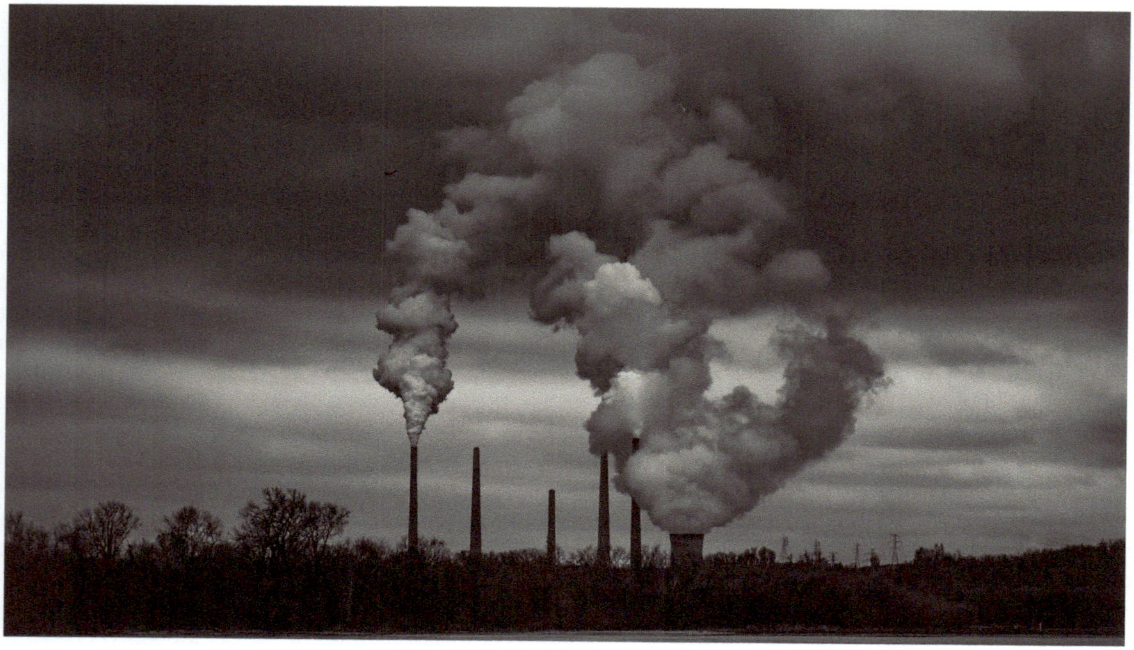

FIG. 7.1 Coal-fired power plant.

in particular, regarding the increased oil prices supporting renewable energy transitions. Such high prices cause reduced importation, thus causing shortages that in turn have been seen to force the use of renewable energies. Secondly, the high price becomes unattractive compared with those of renewable sources.

Recessions do not only prompt reduction in emissions, but in fact, in most cases, emissions also reduce due to contraction in the growth of GDPs of different economies. For instance, during the 1975 recession, the reductions in emissions were prompted by the reducing global GDP growth, which dropped from 6.5% to 0.603% between 1973 and 1975, respectively (United Nations, 1976). In the 1981–82 recession, the GDP growth plummeted 1.908% (1981) to a low of 0.431% (1982) (The World Bank, 2019c). The astounding decline in growth in global GDP was experienced between 2007 and 2010, where it fell from a high of 4.319% to a record low of −1.679% (WorldoMeter, 2019). Such reduced rates are prompted by factors such as increased oil prices, high rates of unemployment, unprecedented inflation rates, and increased debt crisis, which hinders any tangible investments with a potential to reverse the situation.

However, as is evident from the different past recessions, the declining GDP rate is succeeded by spirited growth, following diverse intervention measures that different governments put in place. For instance, after initiating different economic stimulus and fiscal mechanisms, it was observed that the growth of global GDP grew from 0.603% (1975) to 5.272% in 1976 (United Nations, 1976). The same trend was observed between 1982 and 1984 where growth increased from 0.431% to 4.506% respectfully (WorldoMeter, 2019). The growth rose from 1.427% in 1991 to 3.001% in 1994, with the most dramatic turnaround witnessed between 2010 and 2011. During this period, the recovery prompted a rise of over 5 points (−1.679%–4.299%) (The World Bank, 2019c). The bulk of the economic interventions that different governments initiate postrecessions are those that attract high influx of both foreign and local investments, especially in sectors like the construction industry, which has a potential to both retain and spark employment.

While the said interventions as shown earlier spark economic growth, they, however, reverse the environmental gains experienced during the recessions. This happens as most of the sectors receiving economic boosts are those known to have high emissions capacities. For instance, after the 2009 recession, in 2010, emissions in China rose by approximately 10.4% following increased activities in cement production and in other areas of the construction industry (Zheng et al., 2019). During the same period, India is reported to have increased its emissions by 9.4%, and in the European Union, emissions increased by 2.2%. Globally, Peters et al. (2011) report that the emissions increased by approximately 5.9%, especially due to increased global demands for fossil fuel–generated energy, and also by activities in the construction industry, in particular

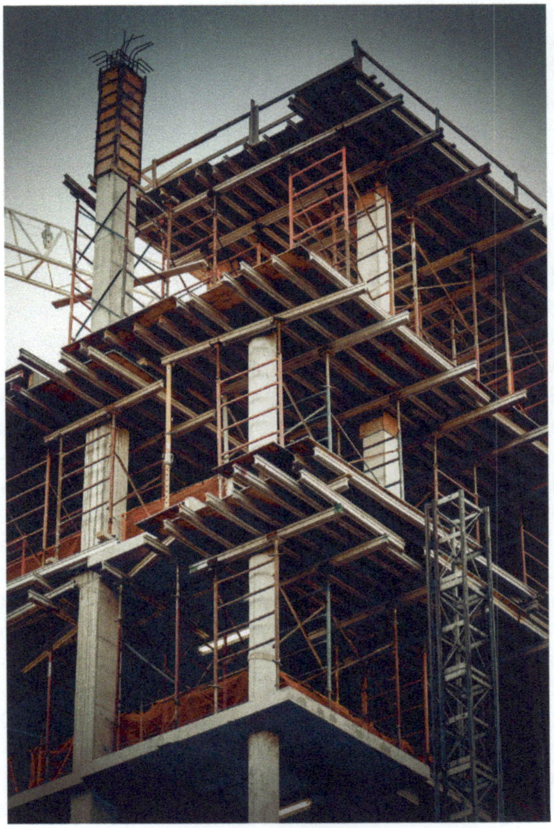

FIG. 7.2 Closed construction site.

cement production, a key product to restart construction sites on hold due to COVID-19 lockdowns around the world. A locked-down construction site is represented in Fig. 7.2.

In the United States, Klein and Staal (2017) report that the government initiated a robust economic stimulus backed by $800 billion proposed in the American Recovery and Reinvestment Act (ARRA) of 2009. While this move was envisioned to promote job creation and enhance economic recovery, the move also saw the country increased its emissions from 5388 million tons to 5586 million tons between 2009 and 2010. The 10.4% emissions rise in China was as a result of $586 billion stimulus package that the local government had announced as a fiscal response to prevent the economy from plummeting further after the recession. Such stimulus packages have been common with governments in developed economies, and as demonstrated here, their impacts have been to the detriment of environmental sustainability. Even in the looming recession post-COVID-19, signs are clear that emissions may rise, as economies, especially developed ones, are highly impacted by lockdowns that will try to aggressively rebound back. A pointer to this is the stimulus packages already advanced by some governments to caution businesses against the impact of coronavirus. For instance, at the time of writing this chapter, there was already a $2 trillion available, while in the United Kingdom, $ 33.786 bn (£30bn) has been proposed (Chan, 2020). If such trends are to be observed postcoronavirus, the emissions are bound to continue increasing.

EARLY (JANUARY TO APRIL) ECONOMIC RESPONSE TO COVID-19

The COVID-19 pandemic has brought numerous and unprecedented disruptions across the globe, along with the sudden stop of the world's economic engines. It started in China after the confirmation of the virus, and thereafter, as the virus continued to spread and cause havoc, more and more economies followed the lead. Only necessary and essential factories are left performing to ensure that the health sectors remain afloat and that the entire world does not succumb to this virus. But even while those few engines continue to grind, the majority, and equally important, especially regarding economic growth, job creation, revenue creation for governments and those that sustain the general population, have been silenced. In fact, even in the most developed economies like the United States, and those in Europe, the general population is largely depending on the goodwill of the local government even on basic activities, such as food supply through reliefs and such. However, in some developing and least developed economies, the situation is different, where most of the population are struggling to get enough food supply and leave alone medical supplies and shelter.

Before the outbreak of COVID-19, China's top officials had made it clear that they would steer the country's economic growth to 6% in 2020 and, by doing so, double the economy to what it was in 2010 (Wang, 2020a). Such optimism was hinged on the promising 6.1% economic growth that the country had achieved in 2019 (Wang, 2020a). But, with COVID-19, and the subsequent stringent measures such as lockdown and closure of industries, factories, and external actions taken by different governments, such targets are hard to achieve now. For instance, in the first 2 months of this year (January and February), the country was observed to have had its GDP growth plummet to a low of 2.6% (Cheng, 2020). This drop was prompted by 13.5% reduction in its manufacturing sector, a 24.5% and 20.5% drop in fixed assets investment and retail sales, respectively (Bermingham, 2020). Beside these, the lockdown and air travel bans impacted heavily on the tourism sector, especially in January, when the country usually has a cocktail of tourism activities warranted by the Chinese's Lunar year celebrations. It is estimated that in the first quarter of this year (2020), the number of domestic tourists in China reduced by 56%, resulting to a 15.5% reduction on the visitors for the entire year compared those that were recorded in 2019 (Thomala, 2020). In terms of earnings, in the first quarter, the tourism industry in China lost 69% in revenue, compared with similar period 2019. Overall, the earning from the sector in 2020 is expected to plummet by 20.6% compared with 2019 (Thomala, 2020). Such drops result from the ban in local travels, closure of hospitality facilities such as restaurants, and entertainment joints and from reduced consumption on tourist's goods among other things.

In other economies that continue to institute lockdowns as the spread of the virus escalates, economies are continuing to experience severe blows. For instance, in the first quarter and the second quarter of this year (2020), Italy's economic growth dropped to −3% and −5% (Statista, 2020b), respectively, following total lockdown on the entire country. The closure of sectors such as transport, the sport industry, air travel, hotels, and tourism industry is also contributing to such unprecedented negative growth. In France, the economic growth has reduced to −0.3% in the first quarter and is projected that, postcoronavirus, it would only increase to 0.9% (Statista, 2020a). In the United States, it is expected that in the first quarter of 2020, the economy will reduce by 0.4% and 12% drop in the second quarter (Shwartz, 2020). In Africa, it is projected that the continent's economic growth will reduce by approximately 2%−3.2% equivalent to $65 billion following the impacts such as disruption of world's supply chain (China in particular, being the main trading partner) and plummeting oil prices (Africa Renewal, 2020). The case of most countries in this continent is dire noting that most of them usually rely on external financial support to run most of their activities, and with the pandemic forcing them to lockdown, internal revenue generation will be limited. For this reason, they have been reported to plead with international financial agencies such as International Monetary Fund (IMF) and World Bank for stimulus packages to bailout their economies (Muchira, 2020).

On a global scale, sectors such as tourism, which contributes to over 10% of the global GDP, are highly hit by the spread of the pandemic. According to a report by Faus (2020) of World Economic Forum, it is projected that by the time the virus is contained, the tourism industry would have cut 50 million jobs globally. It is also projected that it will take at least 10 months for the sector to recover. The World Tourism Organization (WTO) project that this year (2020), the sector will incur a loss of approximately $300 to $450 billion that could have been spent by international travelers in travel tickets, in restaurants, and in buying different goods and services, among others (UNWTO, 2020). On this, it is estimated that it could even exceed the projected figure, as there is no clear estimate on when the virus would end. Similar challenges are experienced in other sectors such as global trade where it is reported a significant reduction in exports and imports following reduced activities in the manufacturing industries, in the retail industry, and in other related supply chains.

Following the aforementioned impacts on both local and global economies, different governments as noted earlier have taken emergency steps to bailout various economic sectors, just like had been done in cases of previous recessions. For the current crisis, America has advanced a $2 trillion stimulus package (Pramuk, 2020), whereas Germany announced an $810 billion package for companies (Nienaber and Stonestreet, 2020). France announced a $49 billion package, whereas South Korea extended a $9.8 billion package (Alpert, 2020), and Canada has a $20 billion to cushion its economy and the population from the impact of the virus. Italy has a $28 billion plan for same purpose (Sirletti et al., 2020). As noted earlier, even African countries are not left behind and are seeking aid to cushion their economy against the virus and also from the impacts of external debts. Such bailout plans are expected to continue post-COVID-19 and during the recession that has already been seen to be looming as a result of the current pandemic.

THE NEED FOR (RE)ALIGNING EMERGENCY ECONOMIC RESPONSES TO SUPPORT LONG-TERM SUSTAINABILITY

As the impacts of COVID-19 continue to be felt in over 210 countries worldwide, disrupting social fabric—how people live, interact and relate, conduct their daily business and behave, and also prompt unprecedented blows on the economies—the hope of many is now pegged on how their governments react. In many economies as noted earlier, there are diverse responses that different governments have initiated. Some of these are aggressive, while in some, one can lead the desperation of the government. On this, it has been found out that the most developed and some developing economies, which have been experiencing some levels of balanced balance sheet in respect to their GDP, have been able to propose robust economic and social stimulus packages to cushion both the economies and the population from the fierce impacts of the pandemic. In least developed economies, as has also been discussed earlier, most of them still rely on external financial aid, and they have urgently requested for emergency bailout packages to shield their economies and their population. On the two-case scenarios noted here—that of developed economies with capacity to finance themselves and those relying on external assistance—the common objective is the need to support their economies and livelihood of communities therein. Therefore, while such objectives are being pursued, it has been argued that such need to capture both the immediate and long-term effects of the bailout plans.

In pursuant of those objectives, relating and putting to mind the historical experiences of similar scenarios, especially those posed by several major economic recessions that the world has endured before, is paramount. With such, it has been argued that responses instituted, and the policies that have been enacted postrecessions in the past, have all proven to dictate the short-run and long-run effects on both the economy and climate. For instance, as noted in the previous section, the United States enacted an $800 billion stimulus package after the 2008–09 recession to kick start the economy and shield the population again job loss and also stimulate environmentally friendly investments (Klein and Staal, 2017). During the same period, Spain proposed €11 billion ($16.17bn) (Burnett, 2009) to reignite its economic activities, and of these, €800 million ($1.176bn) were earmarked for environmental sustainability (Burnett, 2009). China introduced a 4-trillion Yuan ($585bn) stimulus package with sectors such as the economy, environment, and the social fabric being the target (Plafker, 2009). Other such budgets include the $38 billion in Republic of Korea and AU$42 billion ($26.5bn) by the Australian government (Taylor, 2009; Wenning, 2009). In the bulk of these and many others that were set after the 2009 recession, on the face value, they all had all sectors of the economies covered. However, some years later, even to date, though most of the economies responded and recovered strongly from the scars of past recessions, the environment did not benefit from the proposed packages. Instead, it has continually been compromised with increasing emissions, prompting global communities to turn toward measures such as the Paris Agreement to urge economies to reduce their emissions.

As shown earlier, US emissions have been seen to be increasing steadily after the 2009 recession, though the stimulus package had a provision to ensure these are lowered. This is supported through the rise in emissions as observed in 2009, where emissions were at 5.388 million metric tons, and by 2015, they had risen to 5.411 million metric tons (Wang, 2019). Such rise occurred despite the country embarking on gradually shifting to alternative energy, starting at an introduction of new 6 GW in 2010, and adding new 9.6, 18.4, 8.9, 12.7, and 16.4 GW of renewable energy in 2011, 2012, 2013, 2014, and 2015, respectively (Wang, 2020b). This demonstrates that bulk of the economic stimulus was injected in heavy industries such as steel manufacturing and the construction industry to stimulate economic growth. In China, the stimulus packages lead to unprecedented economic growth of above 6% (CEIC, 2020) but at the same time led to a steeper increase of emissions from a low of 6.01 million metric tons in 2009 to a high of 7.544 million tons in 2014 (The World Bank, 2019b). Like in the case of the United States, the increase in emissions is credited to the robust investment in China embarked on in manufacturing industry to continue supply the insatiable global market.

The current scenario of COVID-19 and the responses it has triggered in different parts of the globe may eventually prompt a repeat of what the world has been experiencing after every recession. That is, the problem of paving way for unsustainable economic practices, which, at the least ties most economies, especially those of developing, least developed, and SIDS (small island developing states) to unsustainable fossil fuel use. In the current scenario, the setback would be that already, following the Paris Agreement and the subsequent ratification of the same by many countries, it was clear that the world was on the right track to actualize environmental sustainability. Similarly, the world would have achieved the Sustainable Development Goals (SDGs), but the commitment on these now lies in limbo as most economies will look to reignite their economies in urgency, and sustainability issues may come in second. Additionally, in the least developed economies, and those incurring new debts as a result of COVID-19, it will also be daunting for them to consider investing in infrastructural developments that target the promotion of environmental sustainability.

Another challenge that has the potential to draw back economies to unsustainable practices is that most decisions on stimulus packages are being championed by politicians. On this, with the looming political contestations such as the upcoming presidential election in the United States, the BREXIT negotiation in Europe and political push and pull in other parts of the globe, the policies crafted to shield economies and societies may be populist in nature and meant for short-termed political mandates. But such will have long-term impacts on how the global spheres such as environment and economies fight against climate change and achievement of SDGs will pan out. Therefore, while there is an emergent need for aligning short-term and long-term policies against the impact of COVID-19 and the looming recession, there is a need to redefine economic systems to ensure that there is accountability and continuity postvirus. This way, target policies may be computed and weighted against both the short-term and long-term impacts on the economy, both at local and global levels.

REFERENCES

Africa Renewal. (2020) ECA Estimates Billions Worth of Losses in Africa Due to COVID-19 Impact. Available at: https://www.un.org/africarenewal/news/coronavirus/eca-estimates-billions-worth-losses-africa-due-covid-19-impact.

Alpert G. (2020) Government Stimulus Efforts to Fight the COVID-19 Crisis. Available at: https://www.investopedia.com/government-stimulus-efforts-to-fight-the-covid-19-crisis-4799723.

Ambrose J. (2020) Carbon Emissions From Fossil Fuels Could Fall by 2.5bn Tonnes in 2020. Available at: https://www.theguardian.com/environment/2020/apr/12/global-carbon-emisions-could-fall-by-record-25bn-tonnes-in-2020.

Ball S. (2020) Pumas in Santiago: Wildlife Takes to Cities Amid Coronavirus Lockdown. Available at: https://www.france24.com/en/20200403-pumas-in-santiago-wildlife-takes-to-cities-amid-coronavirus-lockdown.

Bermingham F. (2020) Coronavirus: World Faces 'similar Economic Shocks' to China as the Global Lockdowns Escalate. Available at: https://www.scmp.com/economy/china-economy/article/3075414/coronavirus-world-faces-similar-economic-shocks-china-global.

Boyle L. (2020) Satellite Images Show Emissions Drops Over European Cities Amid Coronavirus Lockdown. Available at: https://www.independent.co.uk/environment/satellite-images-emissions-climate-crisis-coronavirus-europe-map-a9426436.html.

Bressan D. (2020) Animals Roam Freely in Italian Cities with Humans in Lockdown. Available at: https://www.forbes.com/sites/davidbressan/2020/03/20/animals-roam-freely-in-italian-cities-with-humans-in-lockdown/#ca4882879565.

Buckley C and May T. (2020) Effects of Coronavirus Begin Echoing Far From Wuhan Epicenter. Available at: https://www.nytimes.com/2020/01/25/world/asia/china-wuhan-coronavirus.html.

Burnett V. (2009) Spain Unveils €11 Billion Economic Stimulus Package. Available at: https://www.nytimes.com/2008/11/27/business/worldbusiness/27iht-peseta.4.18215053.html.

CEIC. (2020) China Real GDP Growth. Available at: https://www.ceicdata.com/en/indicator/china/real-gdp-growth.

Chan j. (2020) Stimulus Packages Outlined by UK Government in Response to Coronavirus. Available at: https://www.financialdirector.co.uk/2020/04/06/stimulus-packages-outlined-by-the-uk-government-in-response-to-coronavirus/.

Cheng E. (2020) 'Not Unreasonable' for China's Economy to Shrink 10% in the First Quarter, Independent Survey Shows. Available at: https://www.cnbc.com/2020/03/24/china-beige-book-q1-contraction-in-chinas-economy-from-coronavirus.html.

Connor SA. (2011) Recession Did Not Lower CO_2 Emissions. Available at: https://www.independent.co.uk/environment/climate-change/recession-did-not-lower-c02-emissions-6272333.html.

Eaubien J. (2020) Why They're Called 'Wet Markets' — and What Health Risks They Might Pose. Available at: https://www.npr.org/sections/goatsandsoda/2020/01/31/800975655/why-theyre-called-wet-markets-and-what-health-risks-they-might-pose.

Faus J. (2020) This is How Coronavirus Could Affect the Travel and Tourism Industry. Available at: https://www.weforum.org/agenda/2020/03/world-travel-coronavirus-covid19-jobs-pandemic-tourism-aviation/.

Frishberg H. (2020) Wild Animals Are Exploring Cities During the Coronavirus Lockdowns. Available at: https://nypost.com/2020/03/23/wild-animals-are-exploring-cities-during-the-coronavirus-lockdowns/.

Global Data Energy. (2020) Carbon Neutrality and Covid-19 Impact. Available at: https://www.power-technology.com/comment/carbon-neutrality-covid-19-impact/.

Henriques M. (2020) Will Covid-19 Have a Lasting Impact on the Environment? Available at: https://www.bbc.com/future/article/20200326-covid-19-the-impact-of-coronavirus-on-the-environment.

Klein B and Staal K. (2017) Was the American Recovery and Reinvestment Act an Economic Stimulus? International Advances in Economic Research 23: 395—404.

Liu Z, Guan D, Wei W, et al. (2015) Reduced Carbon Emission Estimates From Fossil Fuel Combustion and Cement Production in China. Nature 524: 335—338.

Muchira N. (2020) Finance Ministers seek $100b Cushion Against Coronavirus. Available at: https://www.theeastafrican.co.ke/business/Finance-ministers-seek-usd100b-cushion-against-coronavirus/2560-5507014-140jey5/index.html.

Myllyvirta L. (2020) Analysis: Coronavirus Temporarily Reduced China's CO_2 Emissions by a Quarter. Available at: https://www.carbonbrief.org/analysis-coronavirus-has-temporarily-reduced-chinas-co2-emissions-by-a-quarter.

Nienaber M and Stonestreet J. (2020) Factbox: Germany's Anti-Coronavirus Stimulus Package. Available at: https://www.reuters.com/article/us-health-coronavirus-germany-measures-f/factbox-germanys-anti-coronavirus-stimulus-package-idUSKBN21C26Y.

OECD. (2020) Coronavirus: The World Economy at Risk. OECD.

Peters G, Marland G, Le Quéré C, et al. (2011) Rapid Growth in CO_2 Emissions After the 2008–2009 Global Financial Crisis. Nature Climate Change 2: 2–4.

Plafker T. (2009) A Year Later, China's Stimulus Package Bears Fruit. Available at: https://www.nytimes.com/2009/10/23/business/global/23iht-rglobalchin.html.

Pramuk J. (2020) Trump Calls for $2 Trillion Infrastructure Package as Part of Coronavirus Response. Available at: https://www.cnbc.com/2020/03/31/coronavirus-stimulus-trump-calls-for-2-trillion-infrastructure-plan.html.

Ritchie H and Roser M. (2017) CO_2 and Greenhouse Gas Emissions. Available at: https://ourworldindata.org/co2-and-other-greenhouse-gas-emissions.

Segal S and Gerstel D. (2020) The Global Economic Impacts of COVID-19. Available at: https://www.csis.org/analysis/global-economic-impacts-covid-19.

Shwartz ND. (2020) Coronavirus Recession Looms, Its Course 'Unrecognizable'. Available at: https://www.nytimes.com/2020/03/21/business/economy/coronavirus-recession.html.

Singh M. (2020) Emboldened Wild Animals Venture into Locked-Down Cities Worldwide. Available at: https://www.theguardian.com/world/2020/mar/22/animals-cities-coronavirus-lockdowns-deer-raccoons.

Sirletti S, Follain J and Rotondi F. (2020) Italy Announces $28 Billion Plan to Cushion Virus-Hit Economy. Available at: https://www.bloomberg.com/news/articles/2020-03-10/conte-calls-on-ecb-to-do-whatever-it-takes-against-coronavirus.

Slini T, Giama E and Papadopoulos A. (2014) The Impact of Economic Recession on Domestic Energy Consumption. International Journal of Sustainable Energy 34.

Statista. (2020a) Coronavirus (COVID-19) Impact on GDP Growth in France 2020. Available at: https://www.statista.com/statistics/1103142/impact-coronavirus-gdp-france/.

Statista. (2020b) Forecasted Impact of Coronavirus (COVID-19) on GDP in Italy Q1-Q2 2020. Available at: https://www.statista.com/statistics/1101019/forecasted-impact-of-coronavirus-covid-19-on-gdp-in-italy/.

Stephanie S and Gerstel D. (2020) The Global Economic Impacts of COVID-19. Available at: https://www.csis.org/analysis/global-economic-impacts-covid-19.

Taylor R. (2009) Australia Unveils $26.5 bln Second Stimulus. Available at: https://www.reuters.com/article/us-australia-economy-stimulus/australia-unveils-a42-bln-second-stimulus-idUSTRE5120DU20090203.

The World Bank. (2019a) CO_2 Emissions (kt). Available at: https://data.worldbank.org/indicator/en.atm.co2e.kt.

The World Bank. (2019b) CO_2 Emissions (metric tons per capita) – China. Available at: https://data.worldbank.org/indicator/EN.ATM.CO2E.PC?locations=CN.

The World Bank. (2019c) GDP Growth (Annual %). Available at: https://data.worldbank.org/indicator/NY.GDP.MKTP.KD.ZG.

Thomala LL. (2020) COVID-19 Coronavirus Impact on Domestic Tourism in China 2020. Available at: https://www.statista.com/statistics/1109554/china-coronavirus-covid-19-pandemic-impact-on-domestic-tourism/.

United Nations. (1976) Supplement to World Economy Survey, 1976. ST/ESA/74 ed.: United Nations.

UNWTO. (2020) Tourism and COVID-19. Available at: https://www.unwto.org/tourism-covid-19.

Vidal J. (2009) Carbon Emissions Will Fall 3% Due to Recession, Say World Energy Analysts. Available at: https://www.theguardian.com/environment/2009/oct/06/carbon-cuts-recession-iea.

Wang O. (2020a) China may Adjust 2020 GDP Growth Target Due to Coronavirus, Goverment Policy Adviser Says. Available at: https://www.scmp.com/economy/china-economy/article/3051200/china-may-adjust-2020-gdp-growth-target-due-coronavirus.

Wang T. (2019) U.S. Carbon Dioxide Emissions 1975–2018. Available at: https://www.statista.com/statistics/183943/us-carbon-dioxide-emissions-from-1999/.

Wang T. (2020b) U.S. Capacity of Renewable Energy Build 2009–2019. Available at: https://www.statista.com/statistics/189421/renewable-and-total-electricity-net-summer-capacity-in-the-us/.

Wenning RJ. (2009) Economic Stimulus and the Environment. Integrated Environmental Assessment and Management 5: 185.

WorldoMeter. (2019) Global GDP This Year. Available at: https://www.worldometers.info/gdp/.

Zheng J, Mi Z, Coffman DM, et al. (2019) Regional Development and Carbon Emissions in China. Energy Economics 81: 25–36.

CHAPTER 8

The Forceful Reevaluation of Cash-Based Transactions by COVID-19 and Its Opportunities to Transition to Cashless Systems in Digital Urban Networks

INTRODUCTION

COVID-19 is impacting, at the time of writing, over 210 countries, and the number of those confirmed to be positive globally exceeds 2.4 million people (WHO, 2020a). The increase in the number of these cases is unprecedented, since, by the end of January, those confirmed globally were only 9826 people, with only 106 cases reported outside China (WHO, 2020b). This high rate of infection has prompted increased attention and research as scientists, and those in the medical sphere, try to establish how the virus evolves and the various ways infections can be passed to one another. On this, numerous theories and hypothesis have been developed, with some being rejected and others confirmed (Chunshan, 2020; Molten and Webster, 2020). For instance, it took scientists and the medical fraternity across the globe to almost a month to ascertain that, truly, the virus is transmittable from human to human (WHO, 2020c). There before, agencies, including the World Health Organization (WHO), were adamant that the virus could not be passed from one person to the other.

Following those developments, the most surprising medium through which the virus may spread is through monetary transactions (banknotes and coins) (Gardner, 2020). This is extremely astonishing as in all economies, people are accustomed to using hard currencies. This is true though in the recent past, there has been some steps toward the introduction of digital currencies aimed at promoting cashless economies. On the issue of money being a conducive medium for the COVID-19 virus, there is research showing that beyond money, there are other surfaces such as plastics and other hard surfaces that may have the potential to allow for the spread of viruses. According to van Doremalen et al. (2020), the COVID-19 virus may survive at least 24 h on cardboards, and even longer in nonporous materials such as plastics and stainless steel. But, on money, a study done by Thomas et al. (2008) highlights that some viruses, especially those associated with human flu, have the potential to persist for days on banknotes. Therefore, while nonporous surfaces have higher propensity to spread the virus, the frequency of touching money makes it more "dangerous" as a medium for infection and propagation, as virus can be there for longer. In particular, this would be more pronounced in case of smaller denominations that circulate faster by changing hands and are more common with people in remote rural areas (Auer et al., 2020). When hard currencies are handled by asymptomatic individuals, it is understood that they have the potential to spread the virus even more.

The revelation that hard currency could spread the virus has led to some panic as people, especially in the beginning, were not sure how they would transact, especially for basic amenities and items that only require small valued currencies. Some reprieve was, and is still is, on those countries with established digital transaction practices, such as the use of mobile money, use of card swipes, card taps, or even through mobile phones (Fig. 8.1).

The greatest challenge, in such circumstances, is on the banking sector, which has been facing stiff competition from the digital platforms and are forced to establish strategies allowing them to preserve their ecosystem and retain their customer base. Among some of the strategies that have been observed in different economies is the widespread disinfection (sterilization) of banknotes and coins by some banks (The Financial, 2020). In other cases, central banks of countries such as Kuwait,

Surveying the Covid-19 Pandemic and Its Implications. https://doi.org/10.1016/B978-0-12-824313-8.00008-5

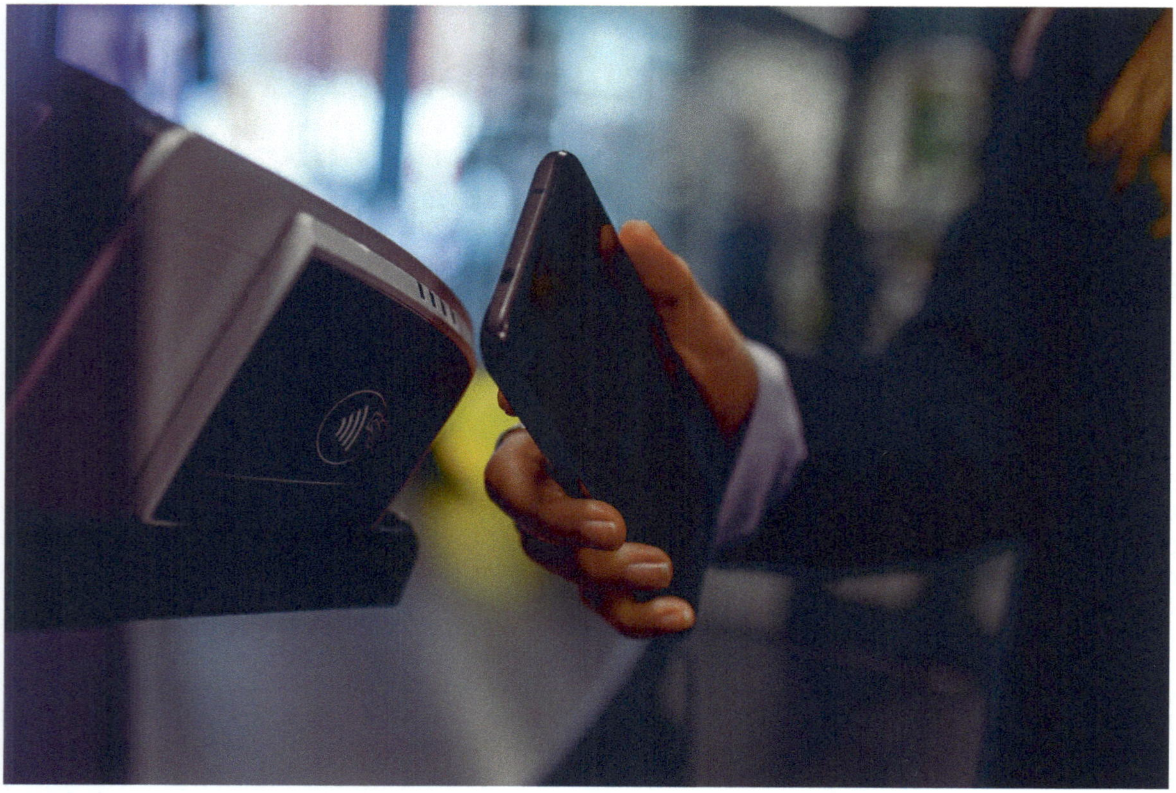

FIG. 8.1 Mobile phone payment wireless tap.

China, Kenya, South Korea, and other economies have been observed to emphasize the quarantine of banknotes to ensure that any currency released to the public is free from the viruses (France-Presse, 2020).

In addition, banks are also seen to be partnering with digital money service providers and other Fintech companies to continue servicing their customers, while also delivering a wide scope of options (Crowder et al., 2020). Such include digital banking opportunities that allow customers to access financial services from their banks via the Internet without having to be physically present in banking halls. Such a strategy aligns well with calls for social distancing and "stay-at-home" protocols that are emphasized as a strategy to reduce human-to-human infection. Therefore, it is true that the emergence of COVID-19 led to disruptions on how businesses operate, especially with a majority of them opting for online payment or cashless payments options.

However, while this paradigm shift in payment behavior is playing a critical role in the fight against COVID-19, the question that remains is whether postpandemic, the financial institutions, in particular, banks, will revert back to the traditional way of doing business and traditional payment options. From a historical perspective, it is apparent that the banking sector in different economies has been bracing for digital opportunities, and the emergence of the pandemic may be a perfect springboard to actualize such an unprecedented move. For instance, in Singapore, before the emergence of COVID-19, banks had already started embracing digital solutions, with most of them providing digital cards to their clients. Therefore, during the COVID-19 outbreak, Wong (2020) reported that it only accelerated their resolve to move to cashless options, as their customers have already taken the lead by maximizing the digital transaction option for their daily transactions. This option of using digital platforms for daily transactions is also being encouraged in least developed economies such as in Africa, and going forward, it would be emphasized in most economies as it not only presents better financial solutions, but it is also seen as a platform that could increase opportunities for investors and corporations alike. In addition, especially where partnership between traditional financial institutions such as banks and insurances and modern startups such as Fintech is emphasized, this will provide opportunities, even to the unbanked in the society to have opportunities to access financial services at reach. Opening the financial doors for this segment of the population will not only provide them with the opportunities to grow economically but also act as a tool that can be used to fight pandemics, even in the future, as use of hard currency will slowly fade away.

In view of the aforementioned background, this chapter explores how this "forced" transition (from hard currency to digital and cashless payments) may impact future digital cities and explore the opportunities that may emerge from this trend, if pursued.

INFORMATION AND COMMUNICATION PAYMENTS TRENDS IN CITIES

As the global population continue to increase toward the projected figures of 8.5 and 9.7 billion people by 2030 and 2050, respectively, it is prompting several global phenomena in view of the increasing pressures on urban infrastructures. For instance, today, the population of urban residents is reported to be approximately 54% of the 7.6 global population, but by 2030, those living in urban areas and cities will reach approximately 68%. This rapid urbanization is prompting a surge in demand for both products and services, with monetary transactions being at the core. This is further emphasized in view of the direct impacts on the economic performance of urban areas. These transactions, as noted by Courbe et al. (2016), have been catalyzed by the emergence of newer, safer, and more efficient and faster monetary systems that have been enabled by the availability of advanced technological applications. Lyons et al. (2017) note that besides an increase in infrastructural development focusing on the financial sector, financial institutions and corporations have introduced innovative ways to ensure that the increasing urban population is able to access and use their financial systems for both profitability and efficiency.

These financial transactions are not only riding on financial institutions but also driven by the surge of technological application in cities, more so through the smart cities concept, that have captured the attention of large information and communication technology (ICT) corporations. To maximize on the potentials created by the smart city concept, despite it is still in its infancy stage, ICT corporations have been seen to provide different types of tech-inspired products, which in turn are stirring transaction-geared systems in positive ways. For instance, such technologies such as ridesharing in the likes of UBER and AirBnB in the hospitality industry have disrupted the economic activities in cities and increased transactions to unprecedented high numbers.

With profitability prospects in mind, companies such as MasterCard, Paypal, and mobile service providers in different countries are actively working to gain the trust of national and regional institutional bodies to drive the future toward a cashless system. This promises a number of benefits including efficiency, safety, increased financial inclusion, and the formalization of industries and merchants and benefits that have substantially been achieved in some developed and developing economies. According to Rogoff (2015), by moving toward a cashless economy, countries are assured of increased tax returns and reduced illegal activities, differing with the current case of cash. Lee further adds that cashless systems have the potential to increase the traceability of payments, and this ensures that the different forms of shadow economy that have existed in different economies would be reduced. This, according to Nasr et al. (2018), would be facilitated by the increased inclusion of larger groups of people into formalized financial systems.

While the said benefits are prompting positive economic performances, there are a number of notable challenges that surround the increase in transactions especially related to cashless systems in urban areas. In this regard, issues such as privacy, security, and oversight become paramount and need to be weighed against the advantages of the systems. It is then understood that overlooking these has the potential to delay or hamper the global uptake of cashless systems in cities, and this would have far reaching impact on the tech giants and startups that are gearing to rely on such systems. On the same, as shared by Cohen et al. (2020), such systems have the premise to lead to a reallocation of resources, where the formal economy would be more favored than the informal sector, which constitute a large part of the economy in developing and less developed economies, hence increasing tax revenues, transparency, and accountability in various levels.

To lead to its actualization, the exploitation of advanced technologies such as blockchain technology, quantum cryptography, 5G, and others are pursued to aid in overcoming some of those challenges related to security and privacy of transactions (Allam, 2018c, Allam, 2019a, Allam, 2020b, 2020c; Allam and Dhunny, 2019; Allam and Newman, 2018b; Allam and Jones, 2019; Shahab and Allam). In instances where such have been used for the formulation of contracts, technologies such as blockchain are observed to show potential to increase transparency and trustworthiness, qualities that are sought in monetary transactions. As shared by Elisa et al. (2018), these technologies allow for decentralization of services such that transactions do not require the interventions of third parties and are securely disturbed across networks both in a verifiable and immutable way. Combining these different technologies in actualizing the cashless system can render it even more feasible, as each of those is fashioned to achieve specific role within the digital realm. For instance, 5G, though being seen to expose users to issues of privacy and security breaches, has the potential to accelerate the capability of Internet of things (IoT) by reducing energy consumption while at the same time increasing on communication quality (Yan, 2019). In addition, quantum cryptography promises enhanced security of future

Internet (Zhou et al., 2018), whereas blockchain technologies allow for decentralization of systems and distribution of information via networks. The utilization of these technologies, coupled with others, in an efficient manner can ensure they complement each other and, in the long run, render a secure, fast, efficient, and reliable platform conducive for a future cashless society.

CITIES AND TRANSACTIONS

The increase in transactions is being influenced not only by the increasing population and the associated rise in urbanization but also by the ever-increasing number of IoT devices in cities. As the smart cities concept gains traction, ICT corporations are also observed to increase their investments, R&D, and other activities to ensure that they produce high-quality and on-demand products that can allow them to share and, where possible, to dominate the digital market (Allam, 2017, Allam, 2018a, 2018b, Allam, 2019b, Allam, 2020a; Allam and Newman, 2018a; Allam and Jones, 2020; Allam and Jones, 2019; Allam and Allam, 2020). Such activities as highlighted by Statista Research Department (2016) have prompted the number of IoT devices to increase from approximately 15.5 billion devices in 2015 to 26.66 billion devices in 2019. Going forward, Manyika et al. (2015) estimate that the activities in the digital market will prompt the numbers to increase to approximately 43 billion devices by 2022 and over 75 billion devices by 2025. Here, the main impetus for these companies to continue increasing their production is the expected return from this market, which according to Market Watch (2019) is expected to reach a high of USD 2108.2 billion in 2023 from a previous recorded high of USD 679.4 billion in 2016. Another report by Manyika et al. (2015) predicts that this IoT market (representing over 75 billion projected devices) has the potential to grow to between USD 3.9 trillion to USD 11.1 trillion by 2025. Despite the variation in estimates, the constant supports a lucrative economic frontier, which is expected to continue attracting even more players. Such increase in both the market share and number of IoT devices translates to an exponential increase in transactions as devices communicate with each other (also a form of transaction), whether financial, contractual, and others.

The exponential increase in the number of IoT devices also translates to an increase in the functions that such are designed to perform. Today, these are ubiquitous in different sectors such as health, transport, education, and security sector, where data are sourced in different forms, such as through wearable devices, smart cameras, smart locks, drones, and sensors among others (Fig. 8.2).

They are also popular in communication, especial across social media platforms, data centers, operational quarters, and others. These are also in use in security sectors with smart sensors and cameras being very popular.

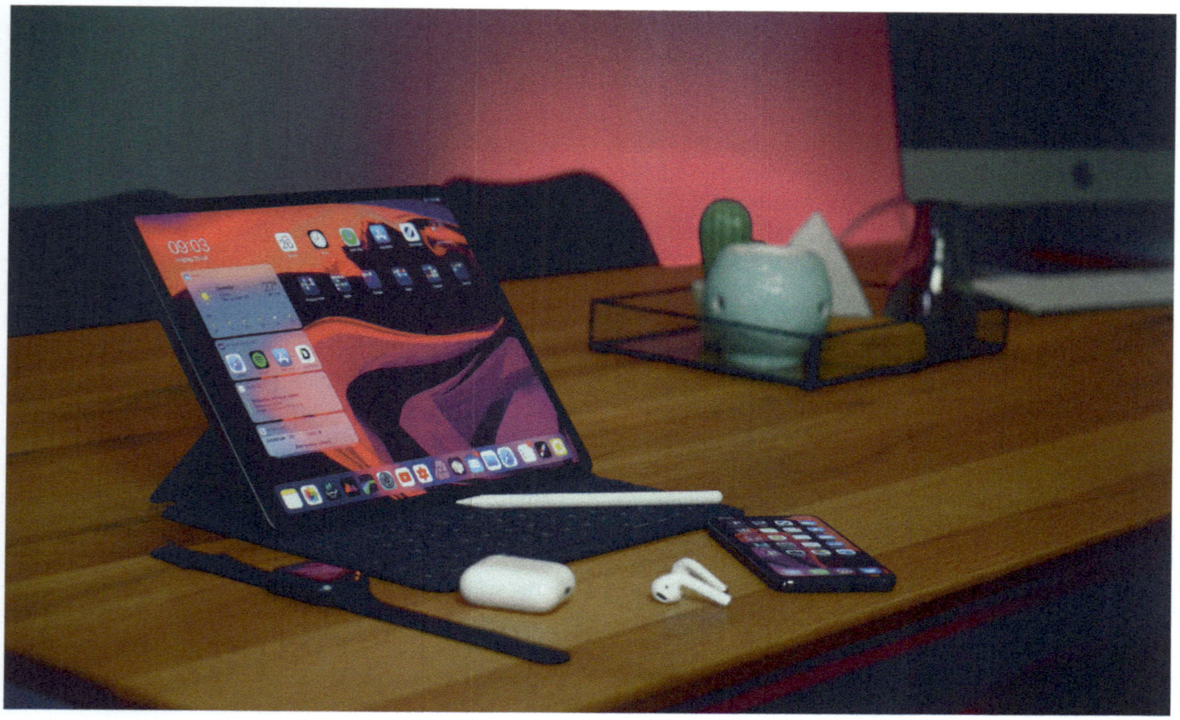

FIG. 8.2 Common smart devices.

The apex of all these increases and widens the uses of said devices, leading to the creation of a lucrative market, especially one that has emerged from the transaction payments through these devices. Roy (2019) expresses that the increase in transaction payments based on these IoT devices is influenced by, among other things, the ability to enhance identity management and the uniform and efficient experience that the devices offer when financial transactions are performed in their platforms. On the same, Gill et al. (2019) note that the popularity of financial transactions via IoT devices is also increasing due to the fact that such have allowed for increased financial inclusion, rendering easier ways of conducting the said transactions. Their ability to integrate with different financial platforms and service providers makes them even more popular, and when that element is coupled with increasing online shopping platforms, and other e-commerce related businesses, the transactions thereof are vast.

To put the aforementioned into perspective, the use of IoT devices in banking and other financial institutions such as insurances will see financial transactions reach a total of USD 116.27 billion by year 2026, a growth rate of approximately 26.5% (Fortune Business Insight, 2019). Such transactions, as reported by Tata Consultancy Services (TCS, 2015), are stimulated by the budgetary investment by financial institutions, with some allocating even more than 30% of their budgets to IoT technologies, and following the positive outcome that such investments have had, the report notes that some institutions are willing to increase their spending to reach 34% this year (2020). Tanna (2019) expresses that such investments include financial institutions increasing their collaboration with tech companies to ensure quality and customized devices are produced that would improve not only payment experiences but also their potential to allow customers to access statement reports and notifications among other benefits. With such investments, it is expected that transaction costs have continued to reduce, and this has translated to a 64% adoption rate of financial IoT transactions globally (Shevchyk, 2019).

Besides the financial sector, IoT devices have also increased payment transactions in other diverse sectors, more so those that rely on the automation dimension that is enabled by some of the smart IoT devices. For instance, it is not unusual to find automated hypermarkets such as Alibaba, Amazon, and other online shopping platforms that integrate different types of payment methods. These have become very popular in different countries, and their numbers keep on increasing as IoT platforms keep on increasing. In the transportation sector, availability of IoT technology has allowed for the introduction of autonomous vehicles in a number of cities. It has also made it possible for startups to emerge that concentrates on bike-sharing services in different urban areas across the globe, and all these are benefiting from availability of different payment options built from IoT platform. On the increase in payment options, McKee (2019) explains that this is happening due to the capacity of IoT to allow connected devices or endpoints to be used as a platform for purchasing and receiving payment. Due to this development, McKee (2019) argues that the growth rate of IoT-enabled transaction has been rising and will continue to grow at a compound annual rate of growth (CARG) of 125%.

As large corporations continue to compete to tap into this IoT-enabled market and hence continue to support the rationale of increasing IoT-enabled transaction, much progress is expected to ease fluidity of digital monetary exchange. In particular, their involvement is expected to help in reducing the time for monetary transactions in a secure and transparent fashion while encouraging the emergence of new startups focusing on offering digital solutions for urban challenges, and all these will ultimately benefit urban dwellers who will have more time at their disposal to enjoy the plethora of activities that cities have to offer.

PAYMENT GIANTS AND SMART CITIES

As the concept of smart cities gains ground across the globe and the importance of IoT networks is better understood by diverse sectors, as elaborated earlier, the increasing future impact of digital monetary transaction in cities is further underlined by the rush of different payment giants to position themselves into this arena. As noted by Sito (2019), such includes opening the "doors" and lifting of stringent local and regional regulations to allow clients, especially those based in overseas to link their accounts to international banks cards. This is evident in the case of conservative payment giants such as Alipay and WeChat Pay, both based in China (Liu, 2019). In other fronts, some have seen to enter into agreements and buying stakes from overseas local Fintech companies such as in the case of *VISA*, which is reported to have paid USD 200 million to Nigeria's Interswitch payment company for a 20% stake (PYMNT, 2019).

Payment giants that are seen to be repositioning themselves to better tap into the future digital market include MasterCard, VISA, American Express from North America, Alipay, TenPay and WeChat Pay from China, and Worldline from South Africa. Others include Paytm based in India, Apple Pay, and Amazon Pay among others. Currently, AliPay is observed to be among the largest payment platform with over 1.2 billion active users against 926 million (Szmigiera, 2020a) active users and 1.14 billion (Szmigiera, 2020b) users for MasterCard and VISA, respectively, and the decision to allow users from other regions to link their accounts with international bank cards means that it would continue to grow. This payment platform and WeChat Pay are observed to be pivoted by their mother companies; Alibaba and Tencent, both having an active stake in online businesses (CGAP, 2019). Following the introduction of their individual payment platforms, Badi et al. (2017) report that these two payment platforms have managed to attract unprecedented payment transaction volumes, and as the global population continue to embrace the concept of a cashless society, such transactions, irrespective of geographical location, will be massive. MasterCard, one of the most widespread payment platforms, has been instrumental in actualizing the vision of digital monetary transactions. In addition to its 926 million credit card holders across the globe, the payment giant has an ambitious program dabbed MasterCard Lab that focuses on bringing financial inclusion to over 500 million people who have had no opportunity to join formal financial platforms (Szmigiera, 2020a). They intend to achieve this by investing in agricultural sectors, microretail sectors, and education sectors. Others, such as VISA, as shared earlier are seen to be active in acquiring or partnering with local Fintech companies to ensure that they increase their market transactions and, in the course of doing this, they bring on board more clients into the digital monetary service arena.

While different payment giants across the globe may have different backgrounds, visions, and missions, they share a commonality in their bid to move the global financial and monetary services from the rigid cash-based system to a more flexible one. The emergence of digitally oriented urban fabrics, especially based on the smart cities concept, has played a critical role in actualizing this mantra as most stakeholders in these cities positively welcome such systems that support seamless transactions. The complexity of urban fabrics coupled with the demands by the increasing urban population is seen to be slowly becoming disconnected with the idea of a cash-based economy and is preferring digital transactions that offer numerous alternatives and flexibilities, including security. The proliferation of smart devices, especially smartphones, has been instrumental in advancing digital payment services, and as Merchant Savvy (2020) reports, these have allowed over 1 billion people to transact via different mobile payment apps worldwide. On this, it is expected that the spirited effort in bringing more people on board will see the number of mobile payment users rises to approximately 1.3 billion people globally. Such an increase in the number of users will push the mobile payment market size to over USD 3081 billion by 2024, from the USD 881 billion recorded in 2018 (Lewis, 2019). In addition to the proliferation of smart devices in cities, the availability of technologies such as blockchain technologies, quantum cryptography, and faster mobile Internet such as 4G, and now 5G, are becoming key elements not only in promoting the speed of transacting but also in increasing transparency, security, costs, and privacy.

Another key factor in pushing the transition from the cash to cashless-based payment system is to increase the collaboration between different payment giants. Though these payment giants have traditionally been seen as competitors, it is surprising that they are seen to have slowed down competition against each other and directed their competitive attention against the use of physical cash. For instance, as noted earlier, AliPay and WeChat Pay and others have allowed their customers to link their accounts with international banks so they can enjoy unlimited digital monetary transactions (FOMO Pay, 2020). Khanna and Martins (2018) of McKinsey argue that the success of the digital payments is gaining traction due to change in mind-set of global population that is seen to favor the digital payment. In such, the digital payment giants are poised to continue boosting their revenues and, hence, their spirited efforts to position their products in line with digital technologies. One of the strategies used for this repositioning is the forming of mergers between two or more payment companies, irrespective of geographies. For instance, the Payments Journal (2018) reported that the Japanese Rakuten Company invested $20 million to form a merger with Azimo, a UK-based payment service provider, and the purpose was to help them wage a spirited challenge against their rival PayPal. Another strategy that is seen to be popular in the recent past is that of giant e-commerce businesses and companies introducing their own digital payment platform, like the case of Alibaba with AliPay, Samsung with Samsung Pay, and Google introducing Google Pay, such that their clients are provided with an all-inclusive experience when purchasing their products. Such start-ups are also observed to have opened their "doors" so that their customers can link their conventional bank accounts with digital payment platforms, and this has seen the slow phasing out of hard currency to give way to digital ones functioning with e-wallets.

THE PAYMENT MARKET OF URBAN SERVICES

As shared in the sections earlier, the rapid urbanization rate is leading to increased pressures on resources and services, and such trends have resulted into numerous challenges, including resource scarcity, increasing vulnerabilities to climate change, increasing cases of informal settlements, and increasing numbers of informal economies among numerous others. These challenges are widely discoursed and documented in high level meetings, and varying economies are seen to undertake diverse measures, which include introducing a wide range of products to ensure that universally agreed recommendations, such as those proposed in the Sustainable Development Goals (SDGs) (UN Environment Program, 2015) and the New Urban Agenda (NUA) (United Nations, 2016) document, are adhered to. In particular, the products are seen to target an efficient delivery of services to urban dwellers coupled with the preservation of qualities pertaining to safety, privacy, resiliency, liveability, economic equality, and other such elements.

One such product that has become popular is the employment of digital solutions, especially those that abide to the smart cities concept. For instance, it is not unusual to find governments, especially in developed economies advocating and implementing the concept of mixed-use high-rise buildings incorporating digital solutions to ensure an optimal consumption of resources such as water, energy, and construction materials. The use of high-rise buildings ensures that available spaces are efficiently utilized to cater for the increasing urban population residential needs, while providing better options to access services such as entertainment and recreation, hotel, financial services, and shopping within the same building. Effective integration of such mixed services in each locality is facilitated by the availability of different digital solutions from the use of sensors and smart devices that monitor, control, and report on the demand, usage, and other aspects appertaining to available resources.

Another solution that is being taken to address the phenomenon is what is seen a rush in urban areas to formalize economies, an issue that is prevalent in most developing economies that are dominated by economic activities that are mostly unregulated. Dasgupta (2016) postulates that this is achieved through the creation of a conducive environment for informal sectors to manage and engage in individual transactions and for them to engage in commercial relations while supporting the value chain of subcontracted relationships. Such environments are achieved by streamlining the regulatory framework such that those in informal sectors are able to access tax breaks and able to register their business without encountering bottlenecks while also having access to different incentive packages that would allow them to compete with those already in formal sectors. McCaig (2015) shares that the formalization of economies allows governments to not only increase their revenue collection base but also address issues such as unemployment, which in part are to blame for the creation of informal settlements in developing, and in a majority of least developing, economies.

Creating a conducive environment has seen the rise of startups, especially those relying on modern technologies to offer avant-garde solutions to challenges posed by urbanization. On this, while large corporations are synonymous with large transactions, the governments' rush to integrate small businesses to formal arenas means even more transactions, which ultimately translates to increased governmental revenue, derived from the increased work opportunities that are created when the small business joins the formal mainstream. It is also tied to the increased, prompt, and voluntary tax submissions as those who join the formal sector are able to derive incentives in form of government protection and financial support so they can manage to compete with established business and large corporations in particular. While this is the case, Banks et al. (2020) acknowledge that in the global south, the informal sector represents a large consumer market that has little competition, but this could be corrected by formalization.

One of the strategies that has been observed to be popular with governments in this digital era in their bid to bring onboard the informal sector into the mainstream is the emphasis on the adoption of online services such as registration of businesses, application for licenses, payment of mandatory fees and taxes, to name a few. Such approaches have reduced bureaucracies, bottlenecks, and red tapes that crowd traditional business environments. O'Mahony et al. (2019) postulate that the availability of advanced technologies and the integration of such technologies in different devices, especially smart phones and other such mobile devices, have increased formal transactions. A report by the World Bank (Klapper et al., 2019) further showcases that in the recent past, due to ubiquitous digital technologies, a large number of informal business have gained access to financial institutions, and this has been enabled by the increased penetration of mobile devices. The report also acknowledges that financial inclusion has provided millions of such businesses a lifeline and, even more, allowed governments that leverage on digital technologies to increase their financial base from those businesses.

By having informal economies into formal financial systems, they are able to access financial support, which has been a hindrance for them to enter into formal markets, and large corporations have capitalized on such to increase their economies of scale, hence edging out any competition from such small-scale businesses (Bennett and Lewis, 2012). But, as is evident in different economies, the small-scale startups have valuable services to offer in all sectors. For instance, in the transport sector, these have revolutionized the taxi and car-sharing businesses by introducing innovative online services such as requesting for a ride and integrating digital payment methods among other smart services. In the art and creative sector, the availability of digital solutions has allowed remote communities to preserve and showcase their works and arts and, by so doing, has not only expounded their income base but has also served to place their economies in the global map, as art enthusiasts, travelers, and tourism are able to sample some of products and services that such economies can offer (Cotirlea, 2014; Genç, 2017; Hocaoğlu, 2017). There are numerous other such examples when it comes to showcasing how much the formalization of economies can transform an economy and solve emerging challenges experienced in the urban areas.

URBAN SOLUTIONS BY PAYMENT GIANTS

The contribution of technology today is apparent in various facets of the economies. As has been showcased earlier, technologies have brought a wide array of digital solutions especially in the urban areas and have eased the pressure brought about by population increase and urbanization. Technology has also been instrumental in shaping political and economic agendas that have been set, not only in local scenes but also in international spheres. For instance, in the discourse about climate change mitigation, financial inclusion, reduction of social and economic inequality, and other issues, the role of technology has been apparent. For instance, to actualize the SDGs advanced by the United Nations in 2015, Tjoa and Tjoa (2016) acknowledge that diverse technologies are required for every single of the 17 SDGs. In the case of the Paris Agreement, the role of technology is clearly outlined, and it is categorically noted that the goals outlined in the agreement would be rapidly accelerated through the integration of different technologies in varying processes of the agreement. On the local scene, sectors such as communication, transport, education, health, tourism, and others have benefited from an advancement in technology. All these transformations that the world is experiencing as a result of technological advancement are being taken seriously due to the highlighted potential in economic and social terms, and both large and small payment giants have been seen to contribute to this growth as it is evident that their efforts are directed toward creating products that would centrosome control on this growing market.

In the payment arena, the digital revolution sparked an innovative wave that has seen the emergence of companies such as PayPal, Alipay, TenPay, Samsung Pay, and WeChat Pay among many others. These have disrupted numerous industries, leading to the emergence of others. In Kenya, for instance, the mobile payment platform M-Pesa has become ubiquitous such that it is integrated in any sector where payment is required. In addition, these also sparked the emergence of online markets, especially online shopping platforms where sellers and buyers across the globe interact seamlessly at convenience and are able to pay and sell goods courtesy of these payment platforms. The payment services are not only popular with those trading on tangible products but also gain ground in the service industry. The popularity of these new startups has been seen to also prompt traditional international payment giants such as MasterCard and VISA to expand their trading limits by joining the digital industry. Their engagement in the digital platform, however, is different, as it clearly depicts how the payment industry have taken a detour to embrace the new technological wave. It also shows that competition in this industry is increasing and traditional financial approaches are becoming almost obsolete, especially if the target customer base comprises of those shifting from informal to formal economies and those who had been previously locked out of the financing realm by bureaucracies, bottleneck, and regulations that are synonymous with the traditional financial sector.

On this front, the traditional payment giants have been forced to propose innovative strategies allowing their old clients and those joining their customer base to experience the conveniences brought about by digital technologies. On this, MasterCard introduced programs such as Cities Possible, Priceless Cities, and an array of Smart City solutions such as the MasterCard Lab, MasterCard City Key (MasterCard, 2019), and MasterCard Engage (MasterCard, 2020) among others. On its part, VISA support program such as FastTrack was initiated in Dubai and is intended to help startups specializing in providing digital support to urban areas to increase their connections to support highly innovative solutions (Geronimo, 2018). It also has a product dubbed *Visa Global Transit Solutions* and *Visa Ready* that target to offer seamless commuting experience across the globe. Other payment giants such as Western Union have also been seen to offer innovative solutions, like the introduction of their mobile app: *WU App*, which is compatible with smart devices, hence allowing clients to transact from any place at any time (Western Union, 2020).

The digital solutions for cities offered by those payment giants, as shown earlier, are well defined, and there is an increasing shift from closed-loop to open-loop systems, meaning that companies are less keen on developing proprietary technologies to maintain their competitiveness. This is shown by how companies such as AliPay are now allowing their customers to link international bank accounts, allowing transactions from their AliPay accounts. Therefore, on this, it looks like the first traditional payment giant to engage the market in a meaningful fashion will benefit from consumer retention. The "meaningful fashion" here entails ensuring that clients are able to derive benefits, while at the same time, they are assured of their privacy and security.

On this, Elliott and Laker (2019) demonstrate that MasterCard has already initiated work toward shifting to open-loop system with pilot programs in transportation sector having been initiated in cities such as London, Vancouver, and Sydney. Here, like in the case of AliPay that has allowed its clients to link their international bank accounts, MasterCard allows clients to use a payment platform they are already accustomed to while paying for transit, and this has been seen to work considerably well. But while that is the case, Zamer (2018) establishes that there are some hurdles that MasterCard and other traditional payment giants have to overcome to win the confidence of clients. Such include transaction security, data protection, and the associated costs that clients must bear. Regarding data protection, it would be an underestimation to wish the threat away as ownership, access, and control of data have become one of the lucrative businesses in this modern era. On this, it then behooves the competing traditional payment giant that are gearing to take control of the increasing payment market by fully shifting to open loop system to demonstrate to clients of its better framework and to guarantee on both privacy and the security of transactions.

CONCLUSION

This chapter explored how COVID-19 provided an increasing pressure to shift from cash-based to cashless system and showcased how payment giants and ICT corporations have, for long, been active in providing the foundational structures for this transition. One challenge is that this disruption may see the emergence of new players, supporting that economic systems and players need to be proactive and early movers if they want to keep a competitive edge on the market.

REFERENCES

Allam Z. (2017) Building a Conceptual Framework for Smarting an Existing City in Mauritius: The Case of Port Louis. Journal of Biourbanism 4: 103–121.

Allam Z. (2018a) Contextualising the Smart City for Sustainability and Inclusivity. New Design Ideas 2: 124–127.

Allam Z. (2018b) Focus Group Findings for Smart Urban Regeneration. Journal of Urban Regeneration and Renewal.

Allam Z. (2018c) On Smart Contracts and Organisational Performance: A Review of Smart Contracts Through the Blockchain Technology. Review of Economic and Business Studies 11: 137–156.

Allam Z. (2019a) Achieving Neuroplasticity in Artificial Neural Networks Through Smart Cities. Smart Cities 2.

Allam Z. (2019b) The Emergence of Anti-Privacy and Control at the Nexus Between the Concepts of Safe City and Smart City. Smart Cities 2: 96–105.

Allam Z. (2020a) Privatization and Privacy in the Digital City. In: Allam Z (ed) Cities and the Digital Revolution: Aligning Technology And Humanity. Cham: Springer International Publishing, 85–106.

Allam Z. (2020b) Theology, Sustainability and Big Data. In: Allam Z (ed) Theology and Urban Sustainability. Cham: Springer International Publishing, 53–67.

Allam Z. (2020c) The Triple B: Big Data, Biotechnology, and Biomimicry. In: Allam Z (ed) Biotechnology and Future Cities: Towards Sustainability, Resilience and Living Urban Organisms. Cham: Springer International Publishing, 17–33.

Allam Z and Allam Z. (2020) Seeking Liveability Through the Singapore Model. Urban Governance and Smart City Planning. Emerald Publishing Limited, 45–76.

Allam Z and Dhunny ZA. (2019) On Big Data, Artificial Intelligence and Smart Cities. Cities 89: 80–91.

Allam Z and Jones DS. (2019) The Potential of Blockchain within Air Rights Development as a Prevention Measure against Urban Sprawl. Urban Science 3: 38.

Allam Z and Jones DS. (2020) On the Coronavirus (COVID-19) Outbreak and the Smart City Network: Universal Data Sharing Standards Coupled with Artificial Intelligence (AI) to Benefit Urban Health Monitoring and Management. Healthcare 8: 46.

Allam Z and Newman P. (2018a) Economically Incentivising Smart Urban Regeneration. Case Study of Port Louis, Mauritius. Smart Cities 1: 53–74.

Allam Z and Newman P. (2018b) Redefining the Smart City: Culture, Metabolism and Governance. Smart Cities 1.

Auer R, Cornelli G and Frost J. (2020) Covid-19, Cash, and the Future of Payments. BIS Bulletin. BIS.

Badi M, Dab S, Paoli P, et al. (2017) Global Payments 2017: Deepening the Customer Relationship. Boston Consulting Group.

Banks N, Lombard M and Mitlin D. (2020) Urban Informality as a Site of Critical Analysis. The Journal of Development Studies 56: 223–238.

Bennett D and Lewis C. (2012) Achieving Competitive Edge: Getting Ahead Through Technology and People Proceedings of the OMA-UK Sixth International Conference: Springer London.

CGAP. (2019) China: A Digital Payments Revolution. Available at: https://www.cgap.org/research/publication/china-digital-payments-revolution.

Chunshan M. (2020) On China, COVID-19, and Conspiracy Theories. Available at: https://thediplomat.com/2020/03/on-china-covid-19-and-conspiracy-theories/.

Cohen N, Rubinchik A and Shami L. (2020) Towards a cashless Economy: Economic and Socio-Political Implications. European Journal of Political Economy 61: 101820.

Cotirlea D. (2014) From Place Marketing to Place Branding Within the Nation Branding Process: a Literature Review.

Courbe J, Engel Mv, O'Hara C, et al. (2016) Financial Services Technology 2020 and Beyond: Embracing Distruption.

Crowder J, Laird R, McLaughlin J, et al. (2020) COVID-19: Its impact on Banking, Fintech, and Payment: FAQs. Available at: https://www.jdsupra.com/legalnews/covid-19-its-impact-on-banking-fintech-62463/.

Dasgupta M. (2016) Moving From Informal to Formal Sector and What it Means for Policymakers. Available at: https://blogs.worldbank.org/jobs/moving-informal-formal-sector-and-what-it-means-policymakers.

Elisa N, Yang L, Chao F, et al. (2018) A Framework of Blockchain-Based Secure and Privacy-Preserving E-government System. Wireless Networks.

Elliott J and Laker S. (2019) Is Now the Time for Open-Loop Transit in the United States? Available at: https://www.intelligenttransport.com/transport-articles/78096/open-loop-payments-united-states/.

FOMO Pay. (2020) Traditiona Banks Aware of Threat Posed by Fintech Giants WeChat Pay and Alipay. Available at: https://www.fomopay.com/2017/08/24/traditional-banks-aware-threat-posed-fintech-giants-wechat-pay-alipay/.

Fortune Business Insight. (2019) IoT in BFSI Market Size To Reach USD 116.27 Billion By 2026; Growing Utilization of IoT Solutions in the Banking Sector Will Support Growth. Available at: https://www.fortunebusinessinsights.com/press-release/internet-of-things-iot-in-bfsi-market-9467.

France-Presse A. (2020) Chinese Banks Disinfect Banknotes to Stop Spread of Coronavirus. Available at: https://www.theguardian.com/world/2020/feb/15/chinese-banks-disinfect-banknotes-to-stop-spread-of-coronavirus.

Gardner B. (2020) Dirty Banknotes May be Spreading the Coronavirus, WHO Suggests. Available at: https://www.telegraph.co.uk/news/2020/03/02/exclusive-dirty-banknotes-may-spreading-coronavirus-world-health/.

Genç R. (2017) The Impact of Augmented Reality (AR) Technology on Tourist Satisfaction. In: Jung T and Dieck MCt (eds) Augmentedd Reality and Virtual Reality, Progress in IS. Springer International Publishing, 109–116.

Geronimo A. (2018) Fast Track Growth: Visa Mentors Dubai Tech Startups. Available at: https://www.tahawultech.com/industry/financial-services/fast-track-growth-visa-mentors-dubai-tech-startups/.

Gill SS, Tuli S, Xu M, et al. (2019) Transformative Effects of IoT, Blockchain and Artificial Intelligence on Cloud Computing: Evolution, Vision, Trends and Open Challenges. Internet of things 8: 1–33.

Hocaoğlu D. (2017) Challenges in Promoting Cities Through Culture Within the New Global Economy. In: Association M (ed) Advertising and Branding: Concepts, Methodologies, Tools, and Applications. Hershey, PA: IGI Global, 1258–1279.

Khanna S and Martins H. (2018) Six Digital Growth Strategies for Banks. Available at: https://www.mckinsey.com/business-functions/mckinsey-digital/our-insights/six-digital-growth-strategies-for-banks.

Klapper L, Miller M and Hess J. (2019) Leveraging Digital Financial Solutions. Washington DC: International Bank for Reconstruction and Development/The World Bank.

Lee MJSRAHC. Can Tax Incentives for Electronic Payments Reduce the Shadow Economy? Korea's Attempt to Reduce Underreporting in Retail Businesses.

Lewis R. (2019) Global Mobile Payment Market to Exceed USD $3,081 Billion by 2024. Available at: https://abnews-wire.blogspot.com/2019/04/global-mobile-payment-market-to-exceed.html.

Liu A. (2019) An Analysis of the PBOC's New Mobile Payment Regulation. Available at: https://www.cato.org/cato-journal/winter-2019/analysis-pbocs-new-mobile-payment-regulation.

Lyons AC, Grable JE and Zeng T. (2017) Infrastructure, Urbanization and Demand for Bank and Non-Bank Loans of Households in The People's Republic of China. ADBI Working Paper 767. Tokyo, Japan: Asian Development Bank Institute.

Manyika J, Chui M, Bisson P, et al. (2015) The Internet of Things: Mapping the Value Beyond the Hype. McKinsey & Company.

Market Watch. (2019) In Terms of Value Internet of Things (IoT) Global Market Is Predicted To Witness CAGR of 17.56% and Expected to Attain USD 2,108.2 Billion by 2023. Available at: https://www.marketwatch.com/press-release/in-terms-of-value-internet-of-things-iot-global-market-is-predicted-to-witness-cagr-of-1756-and-expected-to-attain-usd-21082-billion-by-2023-2019-10-03.

MasterCard. (2019) Press Releases: Mastercard Showcases Next Steps in Advancing Urban Inclusion at United States Conference of Mayors in Honolulu. Available at: https://newsroom.mastercard.com/press-releases/mastercard-showcases-next-steps-in-advancing-urban-inclusion-at-united-states-conference-of-mayors-in-honolulu/.

MasterCard. (2020) Mastercard Engage. Available at: https://www.mastercard.us/en-us/issuers/products-and-solutions/grow-manage-your-business/mastercard-engage.html.

McCaig B. (2015) Why Developing Countries Should Create More Formal Jobs. Available at: https://www.weforum.org/agenda/2015/08/why-developing-countries-should-create-more-formal-jobs/.

McKee J. (2019) The Internet of Payment Has Arrived. Available at: https://www.forbes.com/sites/jordanmckee/2019/

10/09/the-internet-of-payments-has-arrived/#24e82f5e3e69.

Merchant Savvy. (2020) Amazing Stats Demonstrating the Unstoppable Rise of Mobile Payments Globally. Available at: https://www.merchantsavvy.co.uk/mobile-payment-stats-trends/.

Molten V and Webster G. (2020) Coronavirus Conspiracy Claims: What's Behind a Chinese Diplomat's COVID-19 Misdirection. Available at: https://fsi.stanford.edu/news/china-covid19-origin-narrative.

Nasr E, Helmy M and Ghlyazuddin A. (2018) Financial Inclusion Through Digital Financial Services and FinTech: The case of Egypt. Kuala Lumpur, Malaysia: Central Bank of Egypt/Digital Financial Services/AFI/Alliance for Financial Inclusion.

O'Mahony J, Simes NHR, Smith X, et al. (2019) Mobile Nation 2019: The 5G Future. Australia: Deloitte.

Payments Journal. (2018) The Digital Payment Industry is Still a Very Diverse Landscape. Available at: https://www.paymentsjournal.com/digital-payment-industry-diverse-landscape/.

PYMNT. (2019) Visa to Invest $200 in Nigerian FinTech Interswitch. Available at: https://www.pymnts.com/news/investment-tracker/2019/visa-to-invest-200m-in-nigerian-fintech-interswitch/.

Rogoff K. (2015) Costs and Benefits to Phasing out Paper Currency. 29: 445–456.

Roy M. (2019) IoT Swinging its Magic Wand in the Payments World. Available at: https://www.entrepreneur.com/article/333430.

Shahab S and Allam Z. Reducing Transaction Costs of Tradable Permit Schemes Using Blockchain Smart Contracts. Growth and Change n/a.

Shevchyk V. (2019) How IoT Changes Banks and FinTech Companies. Available at: https://readwrite.com/2019/10/14/how-iot-changes-banks-and-fintech-companies/.

Sito P. (2019) Alipay Launches International e-wallet, Giving Foreigners Access to Mobile Payment Platform in First for China. Available at: https://www.scmp.com/business/article/3036366/alipay-launches-international-e-wallet-giving-foreigners-access-electronic.

Statista Research Department. (2016) Internet of Things – Number of Connected Devices Worldwide 2015–2025. Available at: https://www.statista.com/statistics/471264/iot-number-of-connected-devices-worldwide/.

Szmigiera M. (2020a) Number of MasterCard Credit Cards Worldwide 2019. Available at: https://www.statista.com/statistics/618137/number-of-mastercard-credit-cards-worldwide-by-region/.

Szmigiera M. (2020b) Number of VISA Credit Cards in the U.S. and Worldwide 2016–2019. Available at: https://www.statista.com/statistics/618115/number-of-visa-credit-cards-worldwide-by-region/.

Tanna S. (2019) IoT in Banking and Financial Services Market is Estimated to Grow at a CAGR of 55.3% Over the Forecast Years (2019 – 2027), with Wearable Devices Being Increasingly Adopted by the Masses: Says Absolute Markets Insights. Available at: https://www.globenewswire.com/news-release/2019/03/06/1749109/0/en/IoT-in-Banking-and-Financial-Services-Market-is-Estimated-to-Grow-at-a-CAGR-of-55-3-Over-the-Forecast-Years-2019-2027-with-Wearable-Devices-being-Increasingly-Adopted-by-the-Masses.html.

TCS. (2015) Internet of Things: The Compete Reimaginative Force. TCS Global Trend Study. Bombay, India: Tata Consultancy Services.

The Financial. (2020) Banks Sterilizing Paper Money to Reduce the Rist of Covid-19 Transmission. Available at: https://www.finchannel.com/society/health-beauty/coronavirus-update/77825-banks-sterilizing-paper-money-to-reduce-the-risk-of-covid-19-transmission.

Thomas Y, Vogel G, Wunderli W, et al. (2008) Survival of Influenza Virus on Banknotes. Applied and Environmental Microbiology 74: 3002–3007.

Tjoa AM and Tjoa S. (2016) The Role of ICT to Achieve the UN Sustainable Development Goals (SDGs). In: Mata F and Pont A (eds) ICT for Promoting Human Development and Protecting the Environment. Cham, Switzland: Springer.

UN Environment Programme. (2015) Goal 11: Sustainable cities and communities. Available at: https://www.unenvironment.org/explore-topics/sustainable-development-goals/why-do-sustainable-development-goals-matter/goal-11.

United Nations. (2016) The New Urban Agenda *United Nations Conference on Housing and Sustainable Urban Development (Habitat III)*. Quito, Ecuador: United Nations, 66.

van Doremalen N, Bushmaker T, Morris DH, et al. (2020) Aerosol and Surface Stability of SARS-CoV-2 as Compared with SARS-CoV-1. New England Journal of Medicine 382: 1564–1567.

Western Union. (2020) Moving Money. Available at: https://corporate.westernunion.com/index.html.

WHO. (2020a) Coronavirus Disease 2019 (COVID-19): Situation Report – 92. Available at: https://www.who.int/docs/default-source/coronaviruse/situation-reports/20200420-sitrep-91-covid-19.pdf?sfvrsn=fcf0670b_4.

WHO. (2020b) Novel Coronavirus (2019-nCoV): Situation Report -11. Available at: https://www.who.int/docs/default-source/coronaviruse/situation-reports/20200131-sitrep-11-ncov.pdf?sfvrsn=de7c0f7_4.

WHO. (2020c) Report of the WHO-China Joint Mission on Coronavirus Disease 2019 (COVID-19). World Health Organisation, 1–40.

Wong L. (2020) Cashless Transactions Spike as COVID-19 Forces Public to Adapt. Available at: https://www.straitstimes.com/tech/cashless-transactions-spike-as-covid-19-forces-public-to-adapt.

Yan G. (2019) Simulation Analysis of Key Technology Optimization of 5G Mobile Communication Network Based on Internet of Things Technology. International Journal of Distributed Sensor Networks 15: 1–11.

Zamer KZ. (2018) Account Based Ticketing: The Benefits and Drivers for Transit Operators. Journal of Transportation Technologies 8: 331–342.

Zhou T, Shen J, Li X, et al. (2018) Quantum Cryptography for the Future Internet and the Security Analysis. Security and Communication Networks: 1–7.

CHAPTER 9

Oil, Health Equipment, and Trade: Revisiting Political Economy and International Relations During the COVID-19 Pandemic

INTRODUCTION

The COVID-19 pandemic took the world by surprise, as it started slowly in Wuhan, China, with the first known cases being only 41, by the time it became identified. However, in a space of 4 months, it had transformed from being just another type of coronavirus, to a "Public Emergency of Global Concern", to a global pandemic. In the course of writing this chapter, the coronavirus responsible for the COVID-19 had spread from Wuhan, the initial epicenter, to the whole of China, to its neighbors, and finally, to 210 countries and territories (Worldometer, 2020). The number of confirmed cases also increased from the 41 first known cases to over 3 million confirmed cases and over 210,000 casualties (Spotlight, 2020). During the same period, the epicenter for this virus had moved from China, to Europe and to the United States, and in each of those regions; large-scale devastation, deaths, and economic disruptions have been observed. However, on the impacts, no single country has been spared since even those with few confirmed cases have experienced one or more forms of disruptions, especially due to the widespread suspension of international and local transportation, thereby interrupting supply chains of different products and services, disruption of tourism industry, manufacturing sector, schooling systems, and others. Those disruptions also affected small-scale businesses, which in most countries have been offering lifelines to the majority of the population.

As the pandemic spread, the whole world was seen to be collaborating in fighting the virus. For instance, when the epicenter was in China, it received personal protective equipment (PPE) and medical supplies from the United States, its immediate trade and power competitor (U.S. Embassy in Georgia, 2020). Also, when the situation started to worsen in the United States, Russia, its longtime foe, sent a plane full of medical supplies to help them respond to the virus as reported by Seligman (2020). Besides sharing of health equipment, there have been numerous monetary aid flows between nations, organisations, and even individual contributions targeting regions and countries that were vulnerable and those that were overwhelmed by the disease. For instance, Cuba showed incredible generosity by sending medical personnel to different places such as Italy, South Africa, and other 12 nations that are understaffed in their hospitals (Petkova, 2020).

Despite the widespread togetherness and empathy toward those that were highly hit, when the pandemic started to become serious in almost every part of the world -with the number of confirmed cases and deaths starting to grow exponentially, countries started to close their borders and institute stringent measures. Others banned entry of foreigners, and permanent residents and citizens returning from countries affected by the virus were forced to quarantine for a minimum of 14 days. Other countries imposed nationwide lockdowns and curfews, only exempting essential service providers. In other instances, countries such as Russia (AFP, 2020), Germany (Hodgson, 2020), India (Suneja, 2020), and also those in the European regions (Euroean Commission, 2020) imposed strict requirements and regulations that were to guide the exportation of PPEs (Glöckle, 2020). Such actions were taken in each individual country, and region, as it became apparent that the world was experiencing a shortage of the PPEs and other medical supplies, despite the increasing number of people getting infected. The shortage of those PPEs was confirmed by the World Health Organization which was calling on countries with manufacturing capabilities to assist those struggling with to acquire those, so as to reduce exposure of health workers and

Surveying the Covid-19 Pandemic and Its Implications. https://doi.org/10.1016/B978-0-12-824313-8.00009-7

other frontline personnel fighting against COVID-19. In some cases, for instance, in Bangladesh (Mahmud, 2020), Italy (Aljazeera, 2020), and the United Kingdom (Express & Star, 2020), health workers had been reported to have paid the ultimate price of life after being infected while in hospital with lack of sufficient PPEs, being taunted as one of the reasons for medical personnel infection.

The shortages and strains globally were prompted by the widespread lockdown that countries had imposed, thus resulting to reduce the global supply of raw materials and from the shutting down of factories that produce those products. The shortages also came due to the restriction on international travels, both air and sea, where the little available resources could not reach different parts of the globe in time or would not reach at all. These disruptions in the production/manufacturing sectors and in the supply chain also prompted countries to retreat to formulate nationalist policies that put their interests first. For instance, in most economies, especially in developed countries, there is a notable rush to provide economic stimulus and family reliefs to caution businesses, thus allowing them to continue maintaining the service of employees even during those periods when operations were almost completely grounded. The family reliefs were advanced to caution citizens and permanent residents from the harsh economic realities that COVID-19 had exposed the global population. On this, the United States offered a $2 trillion stimulus package (Carney, 2020), whereas Germany, though it is the green light from its parliament, offered a 750 billion euros ($810 billion) to mitigate the disruptions brought by the pandemic (Reuters, 2020a). In the United Kingdom, Morales et al. (2020) report that the government had announced over 65.5 billion pounds ($80.06 billion) to support the self-employed. Similar measures have been advanced in different other countries, which adds to the protectionism shown through border restrictions and banning of flights and exportation of medical supplies. In the United States, President Donald Trump went further to ban immigration to the United States (Zere, 2020) to protect Americans against competition for the few jobs available where almost 30 million had filed unemployment claims by April 30, 2020 (Jones, 2020).

Those forms of protectionism, though justified, show how this pandemic has exposed economies, including developed ones. In the less developed economies, the situation was tougher and as reported by United Nations World Food Programme, by the end of this year, the number of the hungry would double to 265 million people (Anthem, 2020), and such would be brought by the numerous impacts of COVID-19 in those economies. Therefore, even as nations look inwardly, there is need for such with capacity to assist to consider doing so as the pandemic shook every social structures as well as the economic foundations of vulnerable economies.

TRADE DISRUPTIONS ON THE GLOBAL SUPPLY CHAIN

Since globalization, the world's engines had been running smoothly and had never been halted, even in times of turmoil in some parts of the globe. But the unexpected has happened for the first time, where COVID-19 pandemic was seen to have prompted the grinding halt of not a few but all of the world's engines. The unavoidable lockdowns and stringent border restrictions and travel suspensions just being a few of the underlying factors that made the running of the world engines untenable. The other factors are the morbidity levels across the globe that the disease caused and the unimaginable fear on the humanity and governments, including the most powerful ones, like in the west and in the north.

The challenges that the world faced started in China, where the coronavirus started slowly, but within days, it spread widely and in unprecedented levels warranting the closure of all economic activities, including manufacturing sectors and industries. The disruptions in China immediately had ripple effects on all other parts of the world, especially noting that China has, for a long time, been the world's manufacturing capital. The disruptions came just when the consumer demand for different products in other countries from different parts of the world was on a high and rising as depicted in a "United Nations Conference on Trade and Development (UNCTAD)" report showing that exports in 2019 grew by 9.7% in 2018, with China being the world's leading merchandise trader of the year (UNCTAD, 2020). On this, developed economies alone exported goods worth US$ 8777 billion, whereas least developed economies also exported US$193 billion worth of goods (WTO, 2019). During the same period, it is noted that due to favorable trade, the total gross domestic product (GDP) for the entire globe rose to US$ 135.178 trillion (WTO, 2019). This figure represents a 26% growth increase in the GDP from 2008 to 2018, where there has been no disruption. Surprisingly, export of pharmaceuticals has been the second best performing (a 4.2% yearly rise since 2008) after the professional and management consultancy sectors. The United States was the largest exporter globally, spending over US$ 2.5 trillion in 2018 (WTO, 2019).

When the coronavirus broke in China, other countries tried to step up and fill the market gap that it left, but this was also short lived, especially to the speed at which the coronavirus spread from China to the rest of the world, especially to Europe, which is exporter of manufactured goods, especially pharmaceuticals, as shown by Workman (2020). The spread of the virus prompted lockdowns, border restrictions, and travel bans, meaning that even available products would become hard to export to different parts of the world. On the same, demand for different products reduced significantly, with that of medical supplies and PPEs shooting to an all-time high, as scarcity, hoarding, and export restrictions all playing a part. Even after China overcame the virus, and resumed its production, it was becoming difficult to ship manufactured goods, first, because of the travel restrictions, and second, because of the deteriorating economic landscapes in different economies, with a substantial number of people losing their jobs globally. According to a report by the China's National Bureau of Statistics, the recovery of the country's production (Purchasing Manager's Index of 50.8 points) has been far much better compared with the recovery in demand for the products (CNBS, 2020). This could be explained by the fact that apart from China, most of major exporters like the United States were still experiencing unprecedented challenges of COVID-19 and were yet to lift lockdown restrictions, leaving alone opening their borders or suspending travel bans.

The disruption in the supply chain also placed tremendous pressures on existing products on the market, with some facing an exponentially demand that could not be met, while the demand for others experienced an unimaginable plunge. Those that experienced an increase demand include pharmaceuticals, PPEs, ventilators, and other products required in the health sectors, especially with the ranging impacts of coronavirus. According to a WHO modeling, every month, there is need for 89 million medical masks, 76 million examination gloves, and at least 1.6 million goggles (WHO, 2020). In most economies, there were report of exceeding shortages, prompting the WHO to urge those with manufacturing capacity to help in producing these items in large quantities (WHO, 2020). In other countries such as the United States, it was reported that the government was prompted to force, through an executive order, major companies such as General Motors (GM) to produce ventilators to help bridge the gap that the increasing confirmed cases for coronavirus created (Haynes, 2020). The motor company was later joined by other companies such as Ford and Tesla in helping the government by mass producing the urgently needed ventilators and other medical supplies. In Europe, the carmakers joined to help build ventilators whose demand was skyrocketing, but with very little supply available (Kinch et al., 2020). Globally, Parker (2020) estimated that over 880,000 extra ventilators were required to satisfy the global hospital demand, with 75,000 of those required in the United States; hence, the interventions by those companies could not have come at a better time.

In other places, such as in the oil-producing countries, including the United States, the impacts of COVID-19 on different economic sectors such as transport and manufacturing saw the demand for oil and oil products plummeting in rates not experienced in recent history. This prompted a slump in the oil prices, as far as 55% in the Organization of the Petroleum Exporting Countries (OPEC) (Turak, 2020), with the prices in the United States for the first time in history going below US$0 (Suleymanova, 2020). The fall in prices even prompted the OPEC to contemplate reducing their production capacity to void the losses and overproduction. This move was, however, not welcome by all partners, especially by Russia, which rejected such calls (Faucon and Said, 2020). In the succeeding section, more on the impacts of the trade disruption will be discussed, especially the consequences that ensued.

THE OIL MARKET AND THE UNCERTAINTIES IT RAISED

While countries rushed to institute nationwide lockdowns and impose restriction on the transport sectors, leaving only a few essential service providers to operate, their actions led to an immediate effect on the energy sector. In many economies, including China, the United States, and a large number of European economies, the demand for energy plummeted rapidly, causing a subsequent crash in the oil markets as introduced earlier. With this, for the first time in history, the pressure in the oil market demanded a reduction in production to check on the losses prompted by the reduced oil prices and also by the reduced demand. According to theInternational Energy Agency (IEA), in the month of April alone, the demand for oil across the globe fell by an average of 29 million barrels per down, compared with demand for the same last year (IEA, 2020). This reduction was the lowest that has been witnessed since 1995. The price of crude oil in April was also reduced to a historical low of negative USD-37, meaning that the producers were forced to pay buyers for them to take the oil away as nobody wanted to hold onto oil (Ambrose, 2020). Following these unprecedented times, the OPEC and its allies reached an agreement after lengthy parlays to recommend a reduction in production of approximately 9.7 million barrels per day (mb/d) beginning as of May 1 (Stevens, 2020), which is also the largest cut in production in history. In the agreement, the deal was that each member would reduce their normal daily production, such that, when accumulated, the total reduction would amount to 9.7 million barrels per day. For instance, Mexico agreed to lower its daily production by 400,000 bpd, to be maintained for 2 months (May 1—June 30) (Stillman et al., 2020). Thereafter, each of the 23 countries that were part of the meeting would taper their production, to ensure that the daily production would not be over 7.7 mb/d, as compared with a similar period last year. This would last from July 1 to December 31. As from January 2020 to April 2022, the production is expected to maintain a reduction rate of 5.8 mb/d when another meeting will be held to review the situation market situation (OPEC, 2020).

In the non-OPEC countries, their accumulated total of oil production reduction is expected to drop by 5.2 million b/d between May and June. Also, between July and December, due to some increase in demand as some states, countries, and even region will have gradually started opening up their economies and hence, increase the demand for oil to certain levels, the reduction in these non-OPEC countries will improve to reach 2.3 million b/d (EIA, 2020). But such projection will depend on whether the situation of COVID-19 pandemic will have improved, especially in the United States, which is currently the most affected country globally. These reductions in production were necessary, especially noting that in the United States, the prices of crude oil had plunged from a high of $18 per barrel to a low of -$38 in just hours after there was an oversupply prompted by lack of storage facilities (Ngai et al., 2020). In Canada, this was seen to have fell by approximately 74.07% in a span of only 1 month from US$12.84 per barrel (Sönnichsen, 2020a) to US$6.51 per barrel (Sönnichsen, 2020b) between March 2020 and April 2020.

Since the discovery of oil, and the subsequent demand for it in different economic sectors across the globe, oil has always been a highly valued commodity, with oil-producing countries enjoying very healthy economic growth over the years. In particular, most of the countries in the Gulf region can attribute their high economic growth to their oil endowment. But, the unexpected COVID-19 outbreak and the subsequent rapid spread of the coronavirus threw into disarray those economies, as their economic lifeline was threatened by the low demand for oil. The most challenging part on this is the uncertainty as to how long the COVID-19 crisis was to last and how far down will this have plunged the oil market. As has been discussed earlier, oil-producing nations braced themselves for further drops in demand and prepared to continue lowering their production till 2022 (EIA, 2020). This projection could be somehow pegged on the fact that health experts and agencies have warned that the earliest a vaccine for the virus could be made available is late 2021 (Cullen, 2020). And with such, it means that it would be long before countries resume to their previous normal or at least adopt to "a new normal," which cannot be predicted how it will treat the oil market.

For now, oil posed as one of the sectors that had supported the economy is on its knee in many economies, forcing governments to consider bailout plans for it. For instance, Lefebvre (2020) reported that in the United States, President Trump was planning as to how to bail the industry, before it completely collapses. According to experts, the recovery of this market is dependent on how long the industries that rely on it will be grounded and how they will also recover post-COVID-19 (Rechtsteiner, 2020). And, by the look at how the OPEC and its allies crafted their recommendations, it may take a substantial amount of time before the industry regains its previous economic metrics. The situation would even worsen if the recession that has been projected to succeed the COVID-19 crisis will actualize. On this, from a historical perspective, recessions have always had bad impact on the oil and energy market (Mahalik and Mallick, 2014), and the coming one would be no different. Furthermore if different nations, regions, and economies were to decide to transition out of oil-dependent economies by embracing renewable energy, this would mark a positive outlook toward a new global political economic landscape. But it would be a setback to the oil-producing countries, which will also be recovering from both the impacts of COVID-19, which have substantially affected them, and also from the recession.

THE TRADE POLITICS OF HEALTH EQUIPMENT IN A TIME OF SUDDEN SCARCITY

As the spread of COVID-19 reached (by the time of writing) to over 212 countries and territories, and the number of those infected continues to increase from the current figure of 3.3 million, and the deaths reaching almost 250,000 globally, the scarcity of medical supplies continues to remain one of the stumbling blocks (WHO, 2020). At the beginning, this shortage was attributable to the reduction in the manufacturing activities, more so in China after it instituted a statewide lockdown and restricted any forms of activities except for the supply of essential supplies (Bradsher and Alderman, 2020). Later on, as from the end of March 2020, the country's manufacturing sector gradually returned, reaching an operation capacity of almost 80% by mid-April 2020 (CNBS, 2020). But, even as they started to produce the much needed medical supplies, they faced the unprecedented challenge in the supply chain as travel across and within most countries had been suspended or banned. Though the country has a robust and excellent link to almost all parts of the globe due to air and shipping routes, moving the manufactured good became a sudden challenge.

As those challenges were being experienced, on local scenes, there was mounting pressure on existing stocks of health equipment, especially as the number of those needing hospitalization continues to swell. In some countries, to supplement the diminishing stocks they had, the local manufacturing sectors were put to maximum operational capacities, but still their efforts seemed not to suffice to satisfy increasing demand. For instance, in the United States, 3M and the Prestige Ameritech companies (Martineau, 2020), the largest producers of N95 masks, together with other local small competitors, initiated their full operation capacities to meet the demand for over 300 million N95 masks that the health sector had estimated would be required in March, but their effort only allowed them to produce a maximum of 50 million masks (Leary and Hufford, 2020). This was computed even after President Trump had invoked the Defense Production Act (DPA) to force the 3M Company to increase their production capacity and to stop exporting any mask outside of America (Heilweil, 2020). In Europe, the same scenario of shortage was live and hurting (Tsang, 2020), and the potential companies such as Innovatec GmBH & Co.KG based in Germany and Bavaria-based Sandler AG and others that could fill the gap were only managed to do this after June or August (Burger, 2020). However, even after their input, the global requirement for respirators was not expected to be met. For instance, it is estimated that Europe needs at least 10 million N95 masks every day, which translates to more than 3.8 billion masks a year, and this could change if the number of infections were to increase (Burger, 2020). Local companies were not anticipating a pandemic, or such a surge in demand was insufficiently prepared to meet this demand.

Amid those supply shortages, governments, besides that of the United States, have set to force companies prioritize production of medical supplies and, in other cases, have seized the control of shipment and supply of those products to ensure that they remain within the boundaries of the country. For instance, in the United States, the control of production, supply, and shipment of these vital supplies was now under the Federal Emergency Management Agency (FEMA) (Kanno-Youngs and Nicas, 2020). It was accused of using Korean War-era production tactics where the government would force companies to prioritize government orders over any other clients (Kanno-Youngs and Nicas, 2020). In the United Kingdom, though in soft tone, Prime Minister Boris Johnson urged car makers in the country to prioritize manufacturing of ventilators and other supplies that could ease the pressure in the medical sphere (Faulconbridge et al., 2020). In Czech Republic, the government adopted the same approach taken by the Russian, Indian, and German governments by banning the exportation of medical supplies (Stickings, 2020). Furthermore, the Czech government was also gearing to control and regulate the sale of those supplies locally, to ensure that it could supply health workers and medical fraternities whenever and wherever required (Žurovec, 2020).

In other cases, governments have even been accused of applying underhand tactics to ensure they have supplies in their country. For instance, the US government was accused by the local government of Berlin of "piracy" for redirecting over 200,000 masks en route to Germany to be used locally (BBC, 2020a). These had been exported by the 3M Company, but the government "confiscated" the shipment and returned it to the United States. Germany also lost over 6 million masks in a Kenyan airport in March in unclear circumstances (Simsek, 2020). In South Korea, anyone implicated of hoarding masks or any other medical items in high demand in hospital was assured of a 2 years jail term or fines/penalties reaching up to $42,000 (Choi, 2020). In Indonesia, the security officers were forced to conduct a wide search after it became clear that people had purchased and stockpiled masks, with an aim of hoarding them until prices were favorable. In one warehouse, they were able to seize a consignment of 600,000 masks and arrested the owners who are facing jail terms of hefty penalties for their actions (Williams, 2020).

These and many other actions and strategies that governments across the globe have undertaken to ensure that they secure every available medical supplies in their countries only exemplify that medical supplies have now been branded as high-value commodities and are guarded with every ounce of energy and force. Such moves, coupled with border restrictions and banning of foreign citizens, and the counteraccusations on responsibility of governments on stopping or escalating the spread of coronavirus could pose serious security threats. Such scenarios are uncommon and could only be traced back to situations witnessed during the World War II (WW2) and will be expounded further in the next section.

THE BIGGEST GLOBAL DIPLOMATIC CHALLENGE SINCE WORLD WAR II

With the increased pressure on trade, which has prompted governments to take unprecedented and drastic actions such as those discussed earlier, all aimed at safeguarding local health, social, and economic stabilities, there have been little relative global government-led action of meaningful significance. In particular, it has been noted that each government has formulated and implemented their own unique policies and measures without regard of what their neighbors, trade partners, or competitors are doing or which policies they have in place. The surprising aspect from the approaches that each government has taken is that all are meant to address a common enemy, which, as argued by Guy (2020), could be defeated in a much easier way if there was global coordination and unity. To the contrary, the solitary approach by governments has been seen to arouse local, regional, and international disagreements and disharmonies that are a threat to global security. For instance, before the emergence of coronavirus in Wuhan, China, the United States and China were engaged in trade wars, which led to US banning products from China and imposing heavy taxes on others (AP, 2019; BBC, 2019). But the rivalry between these global economic giants was awakened by the emergence of coronavirus, with the United States accusing China of hiding information, thus affecting US preparedness (Sevastopulo and Manson, 2020). The disharmony escalated with the United States halting its funding to the World Health Organization (WHO) and accusing of the latter of collaborating with China in misinforming the world about the emergence of the virus (Smith, 2020).

With no endpoint as to when the COVID-19 crisis may end, plus the numerous challenges such as the shortages in the health sector, the widespread job loss, the social tension as people get tired of staying at home, and other issues, there are fears that more drastic actions may be inevitable. On this, it would not be surprising to see people, groups, or even governments use excessive force in a bid to demand some compliance on a number of pressing concerns. In fact, even such has started in China, where locals have been reported in a number of occasions to have violently attacked minority groups (mostly Africans) by ejecting them from their apartments and preventing them from accessing restaurants, food store, and other basic facilities (Davidson, 2020). In the Heilongjiang province, China, there also looms heightened discord between local government and the Russian government due to suspension of the Suifenhe land port over the coronavirus cases reported to be from Chinese nationals returning from Russia (Wu, 2020). Suspending the port meant curtailing movement of trade within the border towns between the two countries; for this reason, the Russian side threatened to deport the Chinese citizens (Qi and Sheng, 2020). While these examples exemplify the delicate situations that were live in different parts of the world, an urgent global solution and guideline were required on different issues.

One of the bodies that is taking leadership on this front, especially on global collaboration on the health sector, is the WHO, but its soar relationship with the United States, which is also its major financier, is proving a difficult situation. On the same, its reputation was questioned when its Director-General publicly accused Taiwan of racism and personal attacks on him (Hioe, 2020), where Taiwan launched a scathing counterattack accusing the WHO chief's accusation as "imaginary and irresponsible" (BBC, 2020b). Others who would be expected to have provided leadership included the United States, being a superpower and the largest economy, but their solitary approach to fighting the coronavirus, including suspending flights, banning noncitizens, and banning exportation of medical supplies from its land showed the contrary (Fuchs, 2020; Reuters, 2020b; Zere, 2020). The European Union fell short when it launched strict export regulation on health supplies, amid scarcity in other areas, especially to vulnerable nations (Euroean Commission, 2020). Therefore, it is incumbent upon a global unbiased organization, to take charge and ensure that the geopolitical tensions being witnessed do not escalate to events or situations that would jeopardize global peace. And on this, the UN body was rightly constituted for such a noble cause, especially noting that it was formed to ensure that world peace is maintained (UN). While it is true that the UN Secretary General has invariably called for global unity to find a lasting solution, the powerful arm of this body, the UN Security Council, has conspicuously been missing on the front line, especially to ensure that peace will not be threatened (Gladstone, 2020).

With the current reluctant approach to this global crisis by the UN Security Council, there are fears that the deepening crisis escalating to conflicts may arise. To put this into perspective, as noted earlier, the United States had already withdrawn its funding to the WHO, and previously, it had also halted its financial support to UNESCO, another UN body. If the COVID-19 crisis continues, hence causing more economic, social, and even political strains, there are possibilities that other key financiers of these international bodies may also follow the lead by the United States and withdraw their financial support, and instead, redirect the funding internally to support different sectors locally. With such a scenario, that would leave the UN with limited resources; thus, it would not be in a position to undertake its responsibility or even safeguard the strides it has already made in different spheres globally. Unfortunately, the actions of halting financial support for such bodies in times of the COVID-19 pandemic impact not only on the health sector but also on other related sectors. This will also act as a dangerous international precedence in world diplomacy and international relations. On this, it is worth noting that, besides the coronavirus, the world is still under serious threats from other sever threats such as climate change and hunger. And, already, the World Food Programme have indicated that by the end of the year, following the emergence of coronavirus, those facing acute hunger globally would double to reaching over 265 million people (Anthem, 2020). Similarly, in respect to climate change, if history was to repeat itself, it would be disastrous as the gains already achieved, especially in regard to Paris Agreement, and others would be watered down as nations try to restore their economies.

REFERENCES

AFP. (2020) Russia Bans Export of Masks, Hazmat Suits to Fight Coronavirus. Available at: https://www.themoscowtimes.com/2020/03/04/russia-bans-export-of-masks-hazmat-suits-to-fight-coronavirus-a69516.

Aljazeera. (2020) One Hundered Italian Doctors Have Died of Coronavirus. Available at: https://www.aljazeera.com/news/2020/04/italian-doctors-died-coronavirus-200409211435347.html.

Ambrose J. (2020) Oil Prices Dip Below Zero as Producers Forced to Pay to Dispose of Excess. Available at: https://www.theguardian.com/world/2020/apr/20/oil-prices-sink-to-20-year-low-as-un-sounds-alarm-on-to-covid-19-relief-fund.

Anthem P. (2020) Risk of Hunger Pandemic as COVID-19 Set to Almost Double Acute Hunger by End of 2020. Available at: https://insight.wfp.org/covid-19-will-almost-double-people-in-acute-hunger-by-end-of-2020-59df0c4a8072.

AP. (2019) Trump's 15% Tariffs on $112 Billion in Chinese Goods Take Effect Available at: https://www.cnbc.com/2019/09/01/trumps-15percent-tariffs-on-112-billion-in-chinese-goods-take-effect.html.

BBC. (2019) Trump Escalates Trade War With More China Tariffs. Available at: https://www.bbc.com/news/business-49199559.

BBC. (2020a) Coronavirus: US Accused of 'Piracy' Over mask 'Confiscation'. Available at: https://www.bbc.com/news/world-52161995.

BBC. (2020b) Coronavirus: WHO Chief and Taiwan in Row Over 'Racist' Comments. Available at: https://www.bbc.com/news/world-asia-52230833.

Bradsher K and Alderman L. (2020) The World Needs Masks. China Makes Them, but Has Been Hoarding Them. Available at: https://www.nytimes.com/2020/03/13/business/masks-china-coronavirus.html.

Burger L. (2020) Europe's Scramble for Face Masks Prompts Longer Term Rethink. Available at: https://www.usnews.com/news/world/articles/2020-04-16/europes-scramble-for-face-masks-prompts-longer-term-rethink.

Carney J. (2020) Senate Unanimously Passes $2T Coronavirus Stimulus Package. Available at: https://thehill.com/homenews/senate/489590-senate-passes-2-trillion-coronavirus-stimulus-package.

Choi D. (2020) Face Mask and Hand Sanitizer Hoarders Face $42,108 Fine and Up to 2 Years in Prison Under New South Korean Law amid coronavirus spread. Available at: https://markets.businessinsider.com/news/stocks/face-mask-hand-sanitizer-hoarders-south-korea-2020-2-1028874053.

CNBS. (2020) Decline of Major Economic Indicators Significantly Narrowed Down in March. Available at: http://www.stats.gov.cn/english/PressRelease/202004/t20200417_1739339.html.

Cullen S. (2020) Coronavirus Vaccine Won't Be Ready Until End of 2021 Under "Most Optimistic" Scenario – European Expert. Available at: https://edition.cnn.com/world/live-news/coronavirus-pandemic-04-28-20-intl/h_599d6dcfa0dc6c66d271aa7c4c81e835.

Davidson H. (2020) Chineseofficial: Claims of Racial Targeting Are 'Reasonable Concerns'. Available at: https://www.theguardian.com/world/2020/apr/13/chinese-official-claims-racial-targeting-reasonable-concerns.

EIA. (2020) Short-Term Energy Outlook. Available at: https://www.eia.gov/outlooks/steo/report/global_oil.php.

Euroean Commission. (2020) Commission Publishes Guidance on Export Requirements for Personal Protective Equipment. Available at: https://trade.ec.europa.eu/doclib/press/index.cfm?id=2123.

Express & Star. (2020) The NHS Workers Who Have Died During the Coronavirus Pandemic. Available at: https://www.expressandstar.com/news/uk-news/2020/04/23/the-nhs-workers-who-have-died-during-the-coronavirus-pandemic/.

Faucon B and Said S. (2020) Russia Blocks OPEC Response to Coronavirus. Available at: https://www.wsj.com/articles/russia-blocks-opec-response-to-coronavirus-11580992799.

Faulconbridge G, Holton K and Pitas C. (2020) Make us Ventilators to Fight coronavirus, UK Asks Ford and Rolls Royce. Available at: https://www.reuters.com/article/us-health-coronavirus-britain/make-us-ventilators-to-fight-coronavirus-uk-asks-ford-and-rolls-royce-idUSKBN21317A.

Fuchs MH. (2020) The US-China Coronavirus Blame Game is Undermining Diplomacy. Available at: https://www.

theguardian.com/commentisfree/2020/mar/31/us-china-coronavirus-diplomacy.

Gladstone R. (2020) U.N. Security Council 'Missing In Action' in Coronavirus Fight. Available at: https://www.nytimes.com/2020/04/02/world/americas/coronavirus-united-nations-guterres.html.

Glöckle C. (2020) Export Restrictions Under Scrutiny — the Legal Dimensions of Export Restrictions on Personal Protective Equipment. Available at: https://www.ejiltalk.org/export-restrictions-under-scrutiny-the-legal-dimensions-of-export-restrictions-on-personal-protective-equipment/.

Guy K. (2020) Coronavirus Shows We Are Not at all Prepared for the Security Threat of Climate Change. Available at: https://theconversation.com/coronavirus-shows-we-are-not-at-all-prepared-for-the-security-threat-of-climate-change-136029.

Haynes D. (2020) Trump invokes Defense Production Act to Force GM to Make Ventilators. Available at: https://www.upi.com/Top_News/US/2020/03/27/Trump-invokes-Defense-Production-Act-to-force-GM-to-make-ventilators/2851585339926/.

Heilweil R. (2020) Trump Ordered More N95 Masks. 3M Says His Tactics Could Make the Shortage Worse. Available at: https://www.vox.com/recode/2020/4/1/21196941/coronavirus-n95-mask-respirator-shortage-trump.

Hioe B. (2020) Who Director-General Accuses Taiwan of Campaign Against Him Involving "Racism" Against Africans. Available at: https://newbloommag.net/2020/04/09/tedros-racism-comments/.

Hodgson C. (2020) Export Bans Blocked Signed Contracts to Buy PPE, MPs Told. Available at: ft.com/content/8c0a29fc-a523-4901-a190-fe5a2dcc8faa.

IEA. (2020) Oil Market Report -April 2020. Available at: https://www.iea.org/reports/oil-market-report-april-2020.

Jones C. (2020) Jobless Claims Climb to 30 Million in Six Weeks as COVID-19 Layoffs Continue to Rise. Available at: https://www.usatoday.com/story/money/2020/04/30/unemployment-benefits-3-8-million-file-jobless-claims-amid-pandemic/3046759001/.

Kanno-Youngs Z and Nicas J. (2020) 'Swept Up by FEMA': Complicated Medical Supply System Sows Confusion. Available at: https://www.nytimes.com/2020/04/06/us/politics/coronavirus-fema-medical-supplies.html.

Kinch D, Villa A, Holman J, et al. (2020) Carmakers in Europe, US Switch to Ventilator Production, Taking Further Toll on Metals Demand. Available at: https://www.spglobal.com/platts/en/market-insights/latest-news/petrochemicals/032420-carmakers-in-europe-us-switch-to-ventilator-production-taking-further-toll-on-metals-demand.

Leary A and Hufford A. (2020) Trump Administration Orders 167 Million Face Masks From 3M for Coronavirus Pandemic. Available at: https://www.wsj.com/articles/trump-administration-orders-167-million-face-masks-from-3m-11586209922.

Lefebvre B. (2020) Available at: https://www.politico.com/news/2020/04/21/trump-pledges-financial-aid-to-oil-industry-198112.

Mahalik MK and Mallick H. (2014) Energy Consumption, Economic Growth and Financial Development: Exploring the Empirical Linkages for India. The Journal of Developing Areas 48: 139-159.

Mahmud F. (2020) Hundreds of Doctors in Bangladesh Infected With Coronavirus. Available at: http://web.archive.org/web/20200425044259/https://www.aljazeera.com/news/2020/04/hundreds-doctors-bangladesh-infected-coronavirus-200423080515266.html.

Martineau P. (2020) The 'Surreal' Frenzy Inside the US' Biggest Mask Maker. Available at: https://www.wired.com/story/surreal-frenzy-inside-us-biggest-mask-maker/.

Morales A, Meakin L and Atkinson A. (2020) U.K. Virus Aid Package Beats Financial Crisis Stimulus. Available at: https://www.bloomberg.com/news/articles/2020-03-26/u-k-s-sunak-pledges-coronavirus-support-for-self-employed.

Ngai C, Raimonde O and Longley A. (2020) Oil Plunges Below Zero for First Time in Unprecedented Wipeout. Available at: https://www.bloomberg.com/news/articles/2020-04-19/oil-drops-to-18-year-low-on-global-demand-crunch-storage-woes.

OPEC. (2020) The 10th (Extraordinary) OPEC and non-OPEC Ministerial Meeting Concludes. Available at: https://www.opec.org/opec_web/en/press_room/5891.htm.

Parker T. (2020) 880,000 More Ventilators Needed to Cope With Coronavirus Outbreak, Says Analyst. Available at: https://www.nsmedicaldevices.com/analysis/coronavirus-ventilators-global-demand/.

Petkova M. (2020) Cuba Has a History of Sending Medical Teams to Nations in Crisis. Available at: https://www.aljazeera.com/indepth/features/cuba-history-sending-medical-teams-nations-crisis-200331112744040.html.

Qi W and Sheng Y. (2020) China, Russia Appear to be in Discord Over Whether to Re-open Land Poart Amid Pandemic. Available at: https://www.globaltimes.cn/content/1185193.shtml.

Rechtsteiner RO. (2020) Oil Prices Could Remain Depressed for at Least a Year. Here's Why. Available at: https://www.weforum.org/agenda/2020/04/oil-prices-could-remain-depressed-for-at-least-a-year-heres-why/.

Reuters. (2020a) Factbox: Germany's Anti-Coronavirus Stimulus Package. Available at: https://www.reuters.com/article/us-health-coronavirus-germany-measures-f/factbox-germanys-anti-coronavirus-stimulus-package-idUSKBN21C26Y.

Reuters. (2020b) Portugal to Treat Migrants as Residents During Coronavirus Crisis. Available at: https://www.reuters.com/article/us-health-coronavirus-portugal/portugal-to-treat-migrants-as-residents-during-coronavirus-crisis-idUSKBN21F0N7.

Seligman L. (2020) Russia Sends Plane With Medical Supplies to US for Coronavirus Response. Available at: https://www.politico.eu/article/coronavirus-russia-sends-plane-with-medical-supplies-to-us-for-response/.

Sevastopulo D and Manson K. (2020) Donald Trump Threatens to Freeze Funding for WHO. Available at: https://www.ft.com/content/193453e3-479f-4fef-9234-d0f9f14c5a6e.

Simsek A. (2020) German Shipment of 6 Million Masks Lost in Kenya. Available at: https://www.aa.com.tr/en/africa/german-shipment-of-6-million-masks-lost-in-kenya-/1777508.

Smith D. (2020) Trump Halts World Health Organisation Funding Over Coronavirus 'Failure'. Available at: https://

www.theguardian.com/world/2020/apr/14/coronavirus-trump-halts-funding-to-world-health-organization.

Sönnichsen N. (2020a) Western Canadian Select (WCS) Crude Oil Monthly Price 2019–2020. Available at: https://www.statista.com/statistics/729770/western-canadian-select-monthly-crude-oil-price/.

Sönnichsen N. (2020b) Western Canadian Select (WCS) Crude Oil Weekly Prices December 2019–April 2020. Available at: https://www.statista.com/statistics/466200/western-canadian-select-weekly-price/.

Spotlight. (2020) Global Death Toll From Coronavirus Tops 200,000, 813 Recovered. Available at: https://www.spotlightnepal.com/2020/04/26/global-death-toll-coronavirus-tops-200000-813000-recovered/.

Stevens P. (2020) OPEC and Allies Finalize Record Oil Production Cut After Days of Discussion. Available at: https://www.cnbc.com/2020/04/12/opec-and-allies-finalize-record-oil-production-cut-after-days-of-discussion.html.

Stickings T. (2020) Countries Around the World Hoard Medical Supplies to Tackle Coronavirus: Germany and Russia Ban Exports, South Korea Stockpiles Masks and India limits Paracetamol Sales. Available at: https://www.dailymail.co.uk/news/article-8073633/Countries-world-hoard-medical-supplies-tackle-coronavirus.html.

Stillman A, Blas J, Smith G, et al. (2020) Mexico Reaches Deal with U.S. to Cut Oil Production Allowing for OPEC+ Output Cuts. Available at: https://time.com/5818938/opec-oil-deal-coronavirus-mexico/.

Suleymanova R. (2020) Crash! US Crude Futures Turn Negative for First Time in History. Available at: https://www.aljazeera.com/ajimpact/crash-crude-futures-turn-negative-time-history-200420183431731.html.

Suneja K. (2020) Government Bans Exports of Certain Masks, Ventilators, Raw Material for Masks, Coveralls. Available at: https://economictimes.indiatimes.com/news/economy/foreign-trade/government-bans-exports-of-certain-masks-ventilators-raw-material-for-masks-coveralls/articleshow/74718029.cms.

Tsang A. (2020) E.U. Seeks Solidarity as Nations Restrict Medical Exports. Available at: https://www.nytimes.com/2020/03/07/business/eu-exports-medical-equipment.html.

Turak N. (2020) Oil Prices May Now be at a Bottom After Historic OPEC Deal, US Energy Secretary Says. Available at: https://www.cnbc.com/2020/04/15/oil-prices-may-now-be-at-a-bottom-after-historic-opec-deal-us-energy-secretary-says.html.

U.S. Embassy in Georgia. (2020) Coronavirus Aid From U.S. Groups Arrives in China. Available at: https://ge.usembassy.gov/coronavirus-aid-from-u-s-groups-arrives-in-china-february-6/.

UN. Maintain International Peace and Security. Available at: https://www.un.org/en/sections/what-we-do/maintain-international-peace-and-security/index.html.

UNCTAD. (2020) Total Merchandise Trade. Available at: https://stats.unctad.org/handbook/MerchandiseTrade/Total.html.

WHO. (2020) Shortage of Personal Protective Equipment Endangering Health Workers Worldwide. Available at: https://www.who.int/news-room/detail/03-03-2020-shortage-of-personal-protective-equipment-endangering-health-workers-worldwide.

Williams T-A. (2020) Police Seize 600,000 Face Masks From Indonesian Warehouse After Country's First Coronavirus Case Sparks Panic Buying and Soaring Prices. Available at: https://www.dailymail.co.uk/news/article-8073145/Police-seize-600-000-face-masks-Indonesian-warehouse-countrys-coronavirus-case.html.

Workman D. (2020) Drugs and Medicine Exports by Country. Available at: http://www.worldstopexports.com/drugs-medicine-exports-country/.

Worldometer. (2020) Report Coronavirus Cases. Available at: https://www.worldometers.info/coronavirus/.

WTO. (2019) World Trade Statistical Review. Geneva, Switzerland: World Trade Organisation.

Wu H. (2020) Remote Chinese City Hit by Coronavirus After Weeks of Feeling Safe. Available at: https://www.reuters.com/article/us-health-coronavirus-china-border/remote-chinese-city-hit-by-coronavirus-after-weeks-of-feeling-safe-idUSKCN21Y0J2.

Zere AT. (2020) Trump's Travel Ban: Thousands of Lives in Limbo. Available at: https://www.aljazeera.com/indepth/opinion/trump-travel-ban-thousands-lives-limbo-200213123339756.html.

Žurovec M. (2020) Respirator Prices Will be Regulated Due to Coronavirus. Available at: https://www.mfcr.cz/cs/aktualne/tiskove-zpravy/2020/ceny-respiratoru-budou-kvuli-koronaviru-37782.

CHAPTER 10

Underlining the Role of Data Science and Technology in Supporting Supply Chains, Political Stability and Health Networks During Pandemics

INTRODUCTION

In a period of just 4 months, the global landscape had been overturned by the coronavirus, which was not seen as a threat in the initial stages when reports from started trickling from Wuhan, China. In fact, for almost 2 weeks after it was reported on December 31, 2019, it had only affected 41 people and had not spread to any other regions, or outside the city of Wuhan. For this reason, even the World Health Organization hesitated to identify it as a Public Health Emergency of International Concern (PHEIC) (WHO, 2020c) and as global pandemic (Branswell, 2020). But when it started to spread, first to neighboring regions, and to more parts of the China, and finally, to regions far and wide, it caused unprecedented panic and fears. Worse still, the number of infections started to increase exponentially, with substantial numbers of deaths in different parts of the world. By the end of 4 months, the disease, which was later renamed to COVID-19, had infected over 3 million people and killed over 215,000, with most of the deaths witnessed in the most developed regions and countries (Sullivan et al., 2020). Worse still, it had sparked fear and panic on governments prompting them to institute some measures with far-reaching impacts on societies, economies, the political sphere, and also the environment.

For the first time in history, numerous countries had instituted lockdowns in their countries (Barry and Jordans, 2020; Bermingham, 2020), imposed border restrictions, banned noncitizens or permanent residents from their countries, and grounded transportation networks. There have been also total suspension of flights, on both domestically and internationally (Pham, 2020), and unprecedented use of security forces in different countries to impose those measures. Economies across the globe have been halted, with only a few sectors, more so those providing essential services allowed to perform. The measures have also been accused of disrupting of supply chain (Cohen, 2020; OECD, 2020; Shwartz, 2020), thus prompting wide-scale scarcity of basic things including medical supplies that have been in great demand in different parts of the globe.

Socially, the emergence of COVID-19 brought unprecedented pains, fears, agony, and disarray as people, in their thousands, and millions are hospitalized, others separated with their loved ones forever. In worse-case scenarios, in areas with high daily death rates, deaths from hospitals were buried in mass graves with relatives void of the opportunity to say good bye. The devastation has been even worse on those who traveled outside their countries, and with lockdowns and restricted transportation, people have had to remain displaced until such measures are eased or lifted. The measures that have been imposed in different countries have also seen unprecedented impacts on livability, especially in urban areas where people are forced to remain indoors, with limited supplies (Nkengasong and Mankoula, 2020; Wearden and Jolly, 2020), with no social interactions, and with pressures from loss of jobs and source of their livelihoods. Such have prompted social strives, where in different parts of the globe such as in India, the United States, and Germany, residents of some towns called for lifting of lockdowns and other restrictions. Such issues were arising when the United Nations' World Food Programme had warned that the effects of COVID-19 would result into increase in the

Surveying the Covid-19 Pandemic and Its Implications. https://doi.org/10.1016/B978-0-12-824313-8.00010-3

number of acute hunger, affecting more than 265 million people globally (Anthem, 2020).

Politically, as the COVID-19 situation escalated, more political tensions were built. For instance, countries have been seen trading accusations as to the responsibility that each has played in escalating the situation. Others such as China have been accused by countries such as the United States, Germany, the United kingdom, Spain, and even France of having mishandled the situation and failing to share conclusive information and data in time to allow others to prepare (Bronstad, 2020; Pleasance, 2020). On other occasions, the United States has been blamed for instituting measures such as banning European travelers into the United States, also for banning exportation of medical supplies and other issues (Larsen and Gramer, 2020). In fact, with no immediate end on sight for this pandemic, there were fears that the tension may even escalate to dangerous heights, warranting interventions of international bodies.

While the emergence of COVID-19 had severely impaired the global systems, it however, exposed the importance and power of modern technologies in helping address events such as pandemics. For instance, in the first stages of the outbreak of this virus, when the Chinese scientists and authorities and the WHO were trying to identify the virus (WHO, 2020d), and whether it could have impacts beyond Wuhan, a tech startup named BlueDot was able to detect that the world was facing an outbreak, which may end up having global impact. Using real-time data from different sources such as airlines ticketing and numerous news outlets, it made the prediction 9 days earlier, before the WHO made the announcement (Allam et al., 2020; Bowles, 2020). On the same, Allam et al. (2020) highlighted that there was also another startup named Metabiota that correctly predicted that the outbreak would spread to the neighboring regions in a matter of time, and a week later, the prediction came true as Japan, Thailand, Singapore, and others that had been noted as potential target for the outbreak confirmed their first cases. Besides those, even when countries went on lockdown, the use of technology became even more apparent, as devices such as drones, robots, sensors, smart helmets, and thermal detectors were widely used for different purposes such as delivery, identifying potential coronavirus virus cases and other purposes (WHO, 2020b). Technologies such as artificial intelligence (AI), machine learning, natural language processing, and big data have also been instrumental in some countries in implementing quarantines, in search for vaccines and drugs and in helping reduce further spread of the virus.

After such success on the use technology, it is incumbent upon different stakeholders in the global sphere to invest more resources in ensuring widespread of the same in different sectors; as going forward, the global systems will require a concerted effort to restore. For instance, in the economic front, there are signs that the world may be headed for a recession and that would have far-reaching impacts not only on the economies (Africa Renewal, 2020; Statista, 2020a, 2020b; Stephanie and Gerstel, 2020; Wang, 2020; Wearden and Jolly, 2020) but also on the environment. On this, with the use of technologies in sectors such as agriculture, manufacturing, energy production, and building and construction, it would be possible not only to revive the economies but also to void impacts on the environments. By ensuring continuity of the strides already made in different sectors, more so the environmental, the world may escape the dangers posed by climate change and others that are related to environmental sustainability (Allam and Jones, 2019). With that background, this chapter will concentrate on discussing the role of technology and data science in supporting supply chains, economies, and political sustainabilities.

MANAGING PANDEMICS WITH DATA SCIENCE AND TECHNOLOGY

The occasional occurrence of pandemics in the world is not unusual from a historical perspective. Since time immemorial, humans have had to contend with these, but, fortunately, most of those remained local, especially due to a number of factors. First, the global population has been played a significant part in the spread of pandemics, and in earlier days, population were relatively smaller and people were sparsely distributed. Secondly, the interaction between different groups of people from different countries and regions was limited as transportation infrastructures were not well developed, until recently. Also, urbanization was not as pronounced as it is today, and this played a key role in preventing widespread. Today, things are extremely different, as the population has already increased to 7.6 billion people, and it is projected to reach a high of 8.5 billion by 2030 and to 9.7 billion by 2050 (UN, 2019). Furthermore, technological advancement is at all-time high, and this has made interactions, communication, transportation, and research among other things more robust and efficient. These modern facts have made it possible for pandemics to be widespread and devastating. Therefore, in the case of infectious diseases like the COVID-19, it is not surprising that they spread quite fast and impact numerous people and sectors in a short period of time. For instance, by the time of writing this chapter, the coronavirus had spread to over 212 countries, infecting over 3 million people and killed over 215 people. It had also started to spark some political and economic tensions, besides impacting greatly the social aspects in every part of the globe.

The technological advancement, however, cannot be overlooked on the lens of facilitating spread, but its greatest strength has been in controlling and preventing further spread and devastations. For instance, during the Spanish flu outbreak (1918–20), where technology was rudimentary, over 50 million people lost their lives (Martini et al., 2019). However, as technology continued to advanced, including in the medical fields, the succeeding pandemic such as the 2002–03 severe acute respiratory syndrome (SARS) spread was effectively contained, and it only spread into 26 countries and only infected 8000 people over that period. Even other outbreaks such as the middle east respiratory syndrome (MERS) (CDC, 2019), Ebola (Wojda et al., 2015), Zika (Kazmi et al., 2020), and influenza like the swine flu (Aris-Brosou et al., 2017) that have broken out did not have devastating impacts as compared with the Spanish flu. In fact, even the HIV that emerged in the 1970s, and is still present to date, has well been managed due to availability of technologies (The, 2017). Despite that, these have had some significant impacts on social and economic frontiers, which cannot be overlooked and which demand even further advancement in the medical field to help with the identification of outbreaks before they spread.

One of the most novel ways of ensuring that future outbreaks can be contained is widespread application of data computation and analysis (Allam and Jones, 2020), which already, as discussed in the previous section, was instrumental in making predictions about the outbreak and spread of COVID-19 by BlueDot and Metabiota. In other fields such as climate change, the application of predictive technologies has been widely used, and these have had significant impacts in helping promote discourses on climate sustainability, emissions reduction, and the need to adopt alternative energy production (Allam, 2020a, 2020b). While the use of technology is being promoted, it is not meant to debase the role of other players in the medical world, but such would supplement the efforts, by making the work of investigators, pharmacists, researchers, and others even more pronounced and with far-reaching outcomes. It would also help in hastening processes, making decisions, collecting data, and reducing human errors in interpretation of said data, thus reducing misdiagnosis and other such issues that have occasionally been witnessed in the medical field (Allam et al., 2019). Such benefits are made even more robust by the availability of diverse data sources, data collecting technologies, and different data sharing platforms. For instance, with the increase of Internet infrastructures, now supporting even 5G in some regions (O'Mahony et al., 2019), and with the availability of numerous smart, mobile devices such as phones, drone, wearable technologies, and cameras, data generation and sharing is becoming pronounced. Similarly, the increase in number of social media platforms (Cinnamon et al., 2016), increased online news outlets, and mobile Apps among others are helping in generating unprecedented amounts of data (Allam, 2020b). The use of such Apps has earlier been used, especially during the 2010 Haiti earthquake and the cholera outbreak in the same country where health professionals collaborated with telecom companies such as Digicel (largest telecompany in the country) to track the movement of people. This allowed for optimal resource management and also in deployment efforts of those offering different forms of assistance (Bengtsson et al., 2011; Lu et al., 2012).

Even in the current pandemic, there is evidence of widespread use of technologies, besides what BlueDot and Metabiota did. In different parts of the globe, governments, telecoms, and startups have been seen to develop different Apps and online tools such as trackers that have helped in tracking and mapping the spread of the disease (Porterfield, 2020; Voa Student Union, 2020; Wakefield, 2020b). For instance, in South Korea, it is reported that they developed a platform that allowed security and health personnel effectively impose quarantine and would warn them whenever individuals were flaunting such measures (Park, 2020). Computation technologies were also widely used in China to combat the spread of COVID-19 (Chaturvedi, 2020), and even as it continued to spread in other countries, we have seen rival tech companies such as Apple and Google collaborating to make tracking tools to aid in effective mapping and tracking of the spread of the virus (Apple, 2020). By tapping on these technologies, there are possibilities of enriching the available database such that even in the future, it would be easier to address emergencies of whatever nature. On this, the most promising thing with the use of data computation technologies is that data from different spheres could be collated and analyzed to reach an informed conclusion. This is how BlueDot company made the prediction through the use of a wide expertise network as it hosts a rich expertise base comprising of meteorologists, software developers, data scientists, ecologists, geographers, epidemiologists, veterinarians, and others, thus allowing them to make informed conclusion, which are inspired by insights from the diverse backgrounds (BlueDot, 2020a, 2020b). Going further, even post-COVID-19, the role of computation technologies will continue, especially in reevaluating the policy responses, and hence help different stakeholders to identify areas of weakness and how such could be strengthened in case of similar future major disruptive events.

HEALTH DIGITAL INFRASTRUCTURES AND DATA CRUNCHING

Following the numerous technological interventions initiated to combat the COVID-19 pandemic, it is now evident that technology, especially related to data storage, data processing and sharing is part of the backbone of the health industry. This has been given the impetus by the happening in the technological sphere where much effort has been made in improving data collection methodologies, with the use of smart devices gaining traction. In regard to data storage, developments have been made significantly, where research is being performed to see whether it could be possible to store such in human genomes or proteins such that, in the future, unlimited amounts of data could be stored. In regard to data processing, as noted earlier, the medical field would benefit even further through the upcoming advancements in AI-driven tools, the advancement in machine learning technologies, and also the improvement in big data technologies. With these technologies, it will be possible to process vast amount of data, in real time and from diverse sources as noted earlier; hence, the insights and conclusion drawn from such will have far-reaching impacts.

This far, in the medical field, with such technologies, there is evidence that it is now possible to perform noninvasive surgeries that reduce fatalities and also reduce healing time for patients, and such have proven beneficial (Elrod, 2014), especially during this period of COVID-19. Others such as the 3D printing are gaining traction, especially in address complex medical issues, especially those requiring implantation of biomedical devices. According to Javaid and Haleem (2020), 4D printing is offering the possibility to have relatively smaller implant devices at the comfort of patients. In the case of COVID-19, already, with the available data, researchers have estimated and predicted the various case scenarios that different countries would face, especially in terms of fatality and recoveries, and infection, hence allowing all involved parties to prepare (Giordano et al., 2020; Tokars et al., 2004). For instance, in the United States, using such computation, it was estimated that country may have an approximate death toll of 200,000 and have millions affected. And already, the number of infections in the country has clocked over 1 million (Cole et al., 2020).

When those technologies and many others are complemented by data computation, the medical field can be made to benefit even further, and already, market of those devices and the number of companies investing in the medical fields are increasing. In particular, with the notable achievements and recognition that data processing startups have gained over this period of COVID-19 following the correct predictions made, the market for smart devices will continue to grow even further. On this, before the emergence of the pandemic, it had been projected that the number of Internet of things (IoT)–supported devices in the health industry would reach a total of 30 billion devices by 2020 and 75 billion devices by 2025 (Digital Information World, 2020), thus pushing the device market to US$534.3 billion (Fortune Business Insight, 2019). Mordo Intelligence (2019) undervalues the market and argues that it will increase to a high of US$172.46 billion by 2025 from a high of US$55.5 billion report in 2019. But in both predictions, it is true that the growth in the market is relatively high, at a compounded annual growth rate (CAGR) of more than 20% each year. Mordo Intelligence (2019) credits such increase in number to factors such as the improvement in accuracy and connectivity that such devices have made possible in the healthcare sector and also the emergence of big data in healthcare such that any amount of data that such could generate would be stored and processed without fear of lack of storage.

With the world focusing on statistical modeling for data gathering from the increasing COVID-19 cases, and solutions driven from processing that data, it means that solutions derived may also be technologically driven. In fact, even as governments, scientists, agencies, individuals, and other stakeholders intensify the search for a vaccine and drug for this disease, already, as noted earlier, technological processes have managed to assist in reducing the spread of the virus. For instance, the example cited in the previous section about the use of mobile platforms in the Republic of South Korea to enforce quarantine is proof that technology holds a sizable share in bringing to an end the coronavirus menace and that of future pandemics. It is worth noting that using technology, the Chinese authorities managed to identify the coronavirus genome sequence and posted the same on a public database where it could be accessed by all accredited researchers (ECDC, 2020). Within no time, labs across the world had access to this, and they managed to clone it (Scott et al., 2020). Through such public platforms, those labs shared information and data on all the experiments that failed, helping reduce repetition, and they are also helping researchers on areas to focus (Ramiah, 2020). In other cases, through statistical modeling, organizations, including the WHO and others, have been able to develop dashboards that are helping to track the spread of coronavirus, and these are providing people with real-time updates on what is happening across the globe (WHO, 2020a). Similarly, using these modeling, especially those that are AI driven, China managed to diagnose thousands of coronavirus cases, as these could read through thousands of CT scans in a record time with an accuracy level of over 96% (Ramiah, 2020). This helped reduce time and also ease the pressure on the radiologists who were already overwhelmed due to the fast rates at which cases were being confirmed and hospitalized. An article posted in the University of Copenhagen website (UoC, 2020) explains that AI will, in such cases, go ahead to predict the patients who may urgently be in need of ventilators, depending on severity of their case.

AI-based machine learning and natural language processing have also been employed in health facilities in other countries with huge success rates (Wright, 2020), thus providing hope in the fight against the spread of the virus, and finally, finding a cure for the disease. But its most promising use, in respect to fighting the COVID-19 pandemic, is its ability to crawl through the data pertaining to the 15,000 approved drugs already on the market and make predictions from over 8 million possible pairs or over 10.5 billion triple-drug combinations. But with AI-powered technologies, researchers predict that possible combination of drugs; whether a part or triple that could go to human trials would take only few weeks. And, already, companies such as Healx (Earley, 2020), Exscientia (Exscientia, 2020), Scipher Medicine (Wakefield, 2020a), and others are also in advanced stages of proposing possible drugs that could be repurposed and be tried as cures for COVID-19.

Outside the hospital environment, as noted in the previous chapters, giant corporations such as Apple, Google, Alibaba, Tencent, and others have been seen to develop Apps and platforms that provide data sharing platforms, and such have helped in mapping areas where cases were spreading faster and where people could get help and get tested. All the data collected from these platforms and numerous others that are actively being used elsewhere across the globe would remain its usefulness, even post-COVID-19, but this will require a superior statistical modeling tools to manage the increasing magnitude of such data. In this case, therefore, it will not be farfetched to employ the services of AI-driven technologies such as machine learning, natural language processing, and others such as big data that have already proven capable of delivering quality statistical results in real time and with high levels of reliability.

THETECHNOLOGICAL BACKBONE AND GLOBAL STABILITY

During the period where C0VID-19 has engulfed the world and brought almost everything at a standstill, the role of data processing and sharing is not only being hailed in the health sector but also seen to be critical in other spheres such as the economy, society, and the environment. In the economic sector, there is much that the emergence of the coronavirus has prompted, especially with restriction on movements, grounding of transportation and lockdowns. Firsts, as noted by the International Labour Organization (ILO, 2020), these measures meant to assist the health sector have transformed the way a majority of people work. On this, a portion of the workforce has managed to continue working from home via teleworking, or through other means. But a majority of the population, especially those in the informal sector, have had their routines greatly disrupted, with a majority globally already filling for unemployment claims. For instance, in the United States, in about 6 weeks, from March to April 2020, over 30 million people filled unemployment claims (Jones, 2020), higher than the December 2008 recession where 11.1 million people filed similar claims (Department of Labor, 2009). Such happenings have increased economic pressures on families, forcing them toward seeking family relief, and other social support systems to see them through the period of aforementioned restrictions. With the disruptions in the labor market, Mahler et al. (2020) used data processing to showcase that the estimation on issues such as global poverty will tilt upward, whereas, in the absence of the coronavirus, this year (2020), the global poverty rate would have followed the projected historical trend that showed that it could decrease. But now, with the available data from over 166 countries on those locked down, those losing their jobs and the disruption on other economic areas, it shows that the pandemic will push the poverty by around 0.5% higher from 2019 rate, and 0.8% higher from what had been predicted earlier (Mahler et al., 2020). Data processing has also been used during this period to predict that the current health crisis could lead to a recession, where some experts argue that already, the recession has already started in the United States (Stewart, 2020).

The disruptions in the economic sectors have not only prompted challenges on the economic front butalso raised concerns on the security sector, especially with countries seen to short-circuit and ban the exportation of health equipment of other countries. These have raised fears of lack of transparency, thus affecting global collaboration on the fight against the virus. In particular, the issue of data on infections, deaths, and medical supplies has sparked political tensions between different countries, even prompting accusations on independent bodies such as the WHO (Sevastopulo and Manson, 2020). The need for transparency on data sharing on COVID-19 has thus been emphasized by different global organizations like the United Nations (UN), World Bank, and others (The World Bank, 2020). According to The World Bank (2020), data transparency not only would help in reducing political tension and win over the coronavirus but is also prerequisite in weathering down the economic shocks affecting the global economy, especially by helping enhancing trust in governments, hence promoting investments especially post-COVID-19.

In a bid to ensure that the issue of transparency, especially on the origin and the outbreak of the virus, is established, countries such as the United States have been seen to establish fact-finding committees, whereas others such as Germany, Sweden, and Australia are considering doing the same in due course (Amaro, 2020). The need for reverse engineering as reported in an article posted in Nature Medicine (Oppmann, 2020) is warranted by the lack of collaboration, especially by the Chinese, whom the European Union (EU) chief, Ursula von der Leyen, said need to be involved in the investigation of the origin of the virus, so that more understanding on the origins can be uncovered, leading to better preparations for future pandemics (Amaro, 2020). The first such reverse engineering was performed by researchers at Peter Doherty Institute for Infection and Immunity in collaboration with Royal Melbourne Hospital and University of Melbourne where a copy of virus was grown in the lab from samples from an infected patient (Reuters, 2020). The need for participation of as many parties as possible is to elucidate the real origin of the virus, and issues that have raised numerous theories, where the United States claimed that it may have originated from a virology laboratory in Wuhan, China (Stanway, 2020; Borger, 2020; Law, 2020). China strongly rejected this theory and is also backed by the WHO, which warned against blaming individual countries for the virus outbreak and spread since this would jeopardize the steps already in place to stop its spread (Pérez-Peña and McNeil, 2020).

The availability of diverse institutions, governments, and laboratories and hospitals participating in the fact finding about the coronavirus does not only offer hope and possibilities of gathering data across a diversity array of networks and regions, but also their findings would facilitate efforts of finding a cure for the virus. The identification of the genome sequencing of the virus, for instance, is a positive in the search for vaccines, and drugs, especially noting that these genome sequences are deposited in the public databases, where all researchers can access them. The same are also submitted to the "Global Initiative on Sharing All Influenza Data" (GISAID) platform. As noted earlier, despite the controversies that are associated with the source of the virus, knowing the actual source would not only hasten in the development of the vaccine and cure but also help in winning back confidence of numerous stakeholders, whom, to this far, have shown dissatisfaction on how the whole issue of the pandemic has been managed. Winning the confidence of everyone will help in further collaboration efforts in eliminating the virus, unlike the scenario where individual country is seen to be looking inwardly and applying their own policies, trials, and test, and treating information from other countries with suspicion.

DATA-DRIVEN CITIES AND NETWORKS FOR FUTURE RESILIENCE

While the exploding demand for data-driven solutions at this particular period is all geared toward overcoming the spread and impacts of the coronavirus, this may spark and reignite the need for smart cities concepts, which peaked in 2015 (Allam and Newman, 2018; Allam, 2018). In the current dispensations, most of the digital solutions that cities across the world have been observed to be concentrating on is the health sector with the aim of containing any incidence of coronavirus, especially to prevent further spread (Allam et al., 2020; Allam and Jones, 2020). On this front, numerous devices and technologies, such as state-of-the-art thermal imaging sensors, smart helmets with sensors, use of drones, robots, and mobile phone applications have been in use in this period to help in screening and providing contactless diagnosis against the virus. Even postcoronavirus, such technologies will still remain relevant, as they also will be part of numerous other IoT devices that are seen to be increasing, as the demand for smart solutions increases. On this, even before the emergence of coronavirus, the demand for smart cities, as expressed by Mordor Intelligence (2018), was growing, and this had catalyzed the demand for IoT devices, which, by 2019, were only 26.66 billion devices and had been projected to reach a high of 75.44 billion devices by 2025, as the application of smart cities concept continued. Besides this, the global market for the IoT solutions had reached a high of over US$212 billion by 2019, and the projections were that it would cross US$1.6 trillion by 2025 (Liu, 2019). According to Horwitz (2019) from Cisco, currently, the number of IoT-connected devices globally is over 31 billion, and she also predicts that they would increase to over 75 billion devices by 2025, especially due to improvement in areas such as Internet connectivity where many cities will have the 5G services by then. As those devices increase, the smart cities market will also continue to grow, and as Smart Cities Association (2020) report showcases, it will improve from the 2019 $622 billion valuation to over US$ 3.48 billion valuation by 2016.

On the above, though the outbreak of COVID-19 may have somehow halted the attention on application of the smart cities concepts that different cities were piously pursuing, its management is seen to be prompting new legislations aimed at enhancing tech solutions to contain the spread, and most of these will survive postvirus. Their enactment, therefore, does not only address the virus, but in the future, they will also add to the existing ones on urban livability, and ultimately, they will lead to better urban and policy decisions. In particular, those policies have formulated to guide in restricting movements, instituting guidelines, and containing the transport sectors, and others will have a positive bearing in the future in ensuring issues such as traffic congestion, supply of basic services, and provision of securities and other issues are maintained. This will be based on the increasing data that different cities are generating those measures that have been placed to contain COVID-19. For instance, Das (Philip James) explains how the University of Newcastle is using smart technologies to track the adherence to social distancing measures in Newcastle, and after analyzing the massive data (capturing over 1.8 billion individual events), the conclusion is that the sensors being used were able to give real-time data on how people were responding and also identified areas and issues prompting bottlenecks. On this, as noted by Allam and Jones (2020), one of the issues that has appeared prominently in the course of containing the spread of COVID-19 is the nationalistic approach, in decision-making where each country has been observed to look inward, with little regard to the plight of its neighbors. Such an approach would be counterproductive in a smart cities concept, as the devices installed need to communicate with others within the network to ensure synchronization of data and information, hence reading to informed decisions and insight drawn after data analysis.

With lockdowns, it has been evident that urban livelihood was to be negatively impacted, and in no time, this came to pass, with citizens in a number of cities in different countries protesting. This situation in cities is largely blamed on the haphazardly formulated policies that were mechanically enacted with little consideration of the negative impact that they would draw on locals. In most cities, despite the high population and density, government was seen to delay in implementing measures that would allow them to manage early detection, which would eventually help to reduce the number of local transmissions that prompted the lockdown. However, the blame is not all on government, for it also took time before it was established that the virus could be transmitted from one person to the other. Therefore, in most cities, the lockdown came when local transmission had already spread. But while that is the case, local governments had the capacity to learn, especially by analyzing data of cities such as Wuhan, which was affected first, and see how cases were spreading quickly and thus prepare effectively, especially by formulating restrictions measures that are more flexible, while being effective, for locals. Such would have sufficed, as most urban cities are characterized of high-density and high-rise buildings, where during total lockdown, people would feel trapped, where Grant (2020) supports that the planning of such leaves only a little or no open spaces where people could move out for recreation. But with prior planning, as was observed in France, people had opportunities to walk out, albeit under very strict conditions. But while things have been complicated by lockdowns, one take-home after the COVID-19 is the need for intelligent urban planning principles, and this could be achieved by promoting decentralization, of some services, especially those that could be done achieved remotely as advised by Shenker (2020). Already, this has been happening in this era of COVID-19, where some people have been able to work from home via live telecommunicating. There has also been a widespread use of digital transactions such as use of mobile money transactions, which could help in decentralizing the financial services.

While the future postcovid is still uncertain, there are clear indications that the technological revolutions that were brought about to address it will remain as a legacy. There will be calls, soon enough, for communities, cities, and regions will use this momentum to craft more resilient fabrics while keeping in mind societal and economic equity in the process.

REFERENCES

Africa Renewal. (2020) ECA Estimates Billions Worth of Losses in Africa Due to COVID-19 impact. Available at: https://www.un.org/africarenewal/news/coronavirus/eca-estimates-billions-worth-losses-africa-due-covid-19-impact.

Allam MZ. (2018) Redefining the Smart City: Culture, Metabolism and Governance. Case Study of Port Louis, Mauritius. School of Design and Built Environment. Perth, Australia: Curtin University.

Allam Z. (2020a) Biotechnology to Render Future Cities as Living and Intelligent Organisms. In: Allam Z (ed) Biotechnology and Future Cities: Towards Sustainability, Resilience and Living Urban Organisms. Cham: Springer International Publishing, 1–15.

Allam Z. (2020b) Data as the New Driving Gears of Urbanization. In: Allam Z (ed) Cities and the Digital Revolution: Aligning Technology and Humanity. Cham: Springer International Publishing, 1–29.

Allam Z, Dey G and Jones DS. (2020) Artificial Intelligence (AI) Provided Early Detection of the Coronavirus (COVID-19) in China and Will Influence Future Urban Health Policy Internationally. AI 1: 156–165.

Allam Z and Jones D. (2019) Climate Change and Economic Resilience through Urban and Cultural Heritage: The Case of Emerging Small Island Developing States Economies. Economies 7.

Allam Z and Jones DS. (2020b) On the Coronavirus (COVID-19) Outbreak and the Smart City Network: Universal Data Sharing Standards Coupled with Artificial Intelligence (AI) to Benefit Urban Health Monitoring and Management. Healthcare 8: 46.

Allam Z and Newman P. (2018) Redefining the Smart City: Culture, Metabolism and Governance. Smart Cities 1.

Allam Z, Tegally H and Thondoo M. (2019) Redefining the Use of Big Data in Urban Health for Increased Liveability in Smart Cities. Smart Cities 2: 259-268.

Amaro S. (2020) EU Chief Backs Investigation into Coronavirus Origin and Says China Should be Involved. Available at: https://www.cnbc.com/2020/05/01/coronavirus-eu-chief-backs-investigation-with-china-into-origin.html.

Anthem P. (2020) Risk of Hunger Pandemic as COVID-19 Set to Almost Double Acute Hunger by End of 2020. Available at: https://insight.wfp.org/covid-19-will-almost-double-people-in-acute-hunger-by-end-of-2020-59df0c4a8072.

Apple. (2020) Apple and Google Partner on COVID-19 Contact Tracing Technology. Available at: https://www.apple.com/ke/newsroom/2020/04/apple-and-google-partner-on-covid-19-contact-tracing-technology/.

Aris-Brosou S, Ibeh N and Noël J. (2017) Viral Outbreaks Involve Destabilized Evolutionary Networks: Evidence from Ebola, Influenza and Zika. Scientific Reports 7: 11881.

Barry C and Jordans F. (2020) Virus death tolls soar in US, Italy, Iran as global lockdown intensifies. Available at: https://www.timesofisrael.com/virus-death-tolls-soar-in-us-italy-iran-as-global-lockdown-intensifies/.

Bengtsson L, Lu X, Thorson A, et al. (2011) Improved Response to Disasters and Outbreaks by Tracking Population Movements with Mobile Phone Network Data: A Post-Earthquake Geospatial Study in Haiti. PLoS Medicine 8: e1001083.

Bermingham F. (2020) Coronavirus: World faces 'Similar Economic Shocks' to China as the Global Lockdowns Escalate. Available at: https://www.scmp.com/economy/china-economy/article/3075414/coronavirus-world-faces-similar-economic-shocks-china-global.

BlueDot. (2020a) Better Public Health Surveillance for Infectious Diseases. Available at: https://bluedot.global/products/explorer/.

BlueDot. (2020b) BlueDot Protects People Around the World From Infectious Diseases With Human and Artificial Intelligence. Available at: https://bluedot.global/about/.

Borger J. (2020) Mike Pompeo: "Enormous Evidence" Coronavirus Came From Chinese Lab. Available at: https://www.theguardian.com/world/2020/may/03/mike-pompeo-donald-trump-coronavirus-chinese-laboratory.

Bowles J. (2020) How Canadian AI Start-up BlueDot Spotted Coronavirus Before Anyone Else Had a Clue. Available at: https://diginomica.com/how-canadian-ai-start-bluedot-spotted-coronavirus-anyone-else-had-clue.

Branswell H. (2020) WHO Says Coronavirus Is Not Yet a Pandemic but Urges Countries to Prepare. Available at: https://www.scientificamerican.com/article/who-says-coronavirus-is-not-yet-a-pandemic-but-urges-countries-to-prepare/.

Bronstad A. (2020) Class Action Filed Against China Over COVID-19 Outbreak. Available at: https://www.law.com/dailybusinessreview/2020/03/13/class-action-filed-against-china-over-covid-19-outbreak/?slreturn&=20200321022722.

CDC. (2019) Middle East Respiratory Syndrome (MERS). Available at: https://www.cdc.gov/coronavirus/mers/index.html.

Chaturvedi A. (2020) The China way: Use of technology to combat COVID-19. Available at: https://www.geospatialworld.net/article/the-sino-approach-use-of-technology-to-combat-covid-19/.

Cinnamon J, Jones SK and Adger WN. (2016) Evidence and Future Potential of Mobile Phone Data for Disease Disaster Management. Geoforum 75: 253–264.

Cohen A. (2020) Oil Markets Brace for WHO's Global Health Emergency Declaration. Available at: https://www.forbes.com/sites/arielcohen/2020/01/30/oil-markets-brace-for-whos-global-health-emergency-declaration/#4edef1357058.

Cole D, Bohn K and Bash D. (2020) US Could See Millions Of Coronavirus Cases and 100,000 or More Deaths, Fauci

Says. Available at: https://edition.cnn.com/2020/03/29/politics/coronavirus-deaths-cases-anthony-fauci-cnntv/index.html.

Das R. (Philip James) This Is How Smart City Technology Can be Used to Tell if Social Distancing Is Working. Available at: https://www.weforum.org/agenda/2020/04/smart-cities-technology-coronavirus-covid19/.

Department of Labor. (2009) TED: Unemployment in December 2008. Available at: https://www.bls.gov/opub/ted/2009/jan/wk2/art02.htm?view_full.

Digital Information World. (2020) IoT in Healthcare Expectations for 2020. Available at: https://www.digitalinformationworld.com/2020/02/iot-in-healthcare-expectations-for-2020.html.

Earley K. (2020) Healx Will Use AI to Seek Combination Therapies to Treat Covid-19. Available at: https://www.siliconrepublic.com/start-ups/treatments-combination-therapies-covid-19-healx.

ECDC. (2020) Event Background COVID-19. Available at: https://www.ecdc.europa.eu/en/novel-coronavirus/event-background-2019.

Elrod CS. (2014) Chapter 5 – Musculoskeletal System. In: Paz JC and West MP (eds) Acute Care Handbook for Physical Therapists (Fourth Edition). St. Louis: W.B. Saunders, 85-122.

Exscientia. (2020) Partnerships: Exscientia Announces Joint Initiative to Identify COVID-19 Drugs With Diamond Light Source and Scripps Research. Available at: https://www.exscientia.ai/news-insights/exscientia-announces-joint-initiative-to-identify-covid-19.

Fortune Business Insight. (2019) IoT in BFSI Market Size To Reach USD 116.27 Billion By 2026; Growing Utilization of IoT Solutions in the Banking Sector will Support Growth. Available at: https://www.fortunebusinessinsights.com/press-release/internet-of-things-iot-in-bfsi-market-9467.

Giordano G, Blanchini F, Bruno R, et al. (2020) Modelling the COVID-19 Epidemic and Implementation of Population-Wide Interventions in Italy. Nature Medicine.

Grant JL. (2020) What Cities Can Learn From Lockdown About Planning for Life After the Coronavirus Pandemic. Available at: https://www.journalpioneer.com/opinion/national-perspectives/what-cities-can-learn-from-lockdown-about-planning-for-life-after-the-coronavirus-pandemic-443138/.

Horwitz L. (2019) The Future of IoT Miniguide: The Burgeoning IoT Market Continues. Available at: https://www.cisco.com/c/en/us/solutions/internet-of-things/future-of-iot.html.

ILO. (2020) COVID-19 Impact on the Collection of Labour Market Statistics. Available at: https://ilostat.ilo.org/topics/covid-19/covid-19-impact-on-labour-market-statistics/.

Javaid M and Haleem A. (2020) Significant Advancements of 4D Printing in the Field of Orthopaedics. Journal of Clinical Orthopaedics and Trauma.

Jones C. (2020) Jobless Claims Climb to 30 Million in Six Weeks as COVID-19 Layoffs Continue to Rise. Available at: https://www.usatoday.com/story/money/2020/04/30/unemployment-benefits-3-8-million-file-jobless-claims-amid-pandemic/3046759001/.

Kazmi SS, Ali W, Bibi N, et al. (2020) A Review on Zika Virus Outbreak, Epidemiology, Transmission and Infection Dynamics. Journal of Biological Research 27: 5.

Larsen MS and Gramer R. (2020) China Casts Itself as Global Savior While U.S. and EU Focus on Virus at Home. Available at: https://foreignpolicy.com/2020/03/19/china-us-eu-coronavirus-great-power-competition/.

Law V. (2020) Coronavirus Origin: Few Leads, Many Theories in Hunt for Source. Available at: https://www.aljazeera.com/news/2020/04/coronavirus-spreads-leads-theories-origin-200407073509327.html.

Liu S. (2019) Global IoT Market Size 2017–2025. Available at: https://www.statista.com/statistics/976313/global-iot-market-size/.

Lu X, Bengtsson L and Holme P. (2012) Predictability of Population Displacement After the 2010 Haiti Earthquake. Proceedings of the National Academy of Sciences of the United States of America 109: 11576–11581.

Mahler DG, Lakner C, Aguilar AC, et al. (2020) The Impact of COVID-19 (Coronavirus) on Global Poverty: Why Sub-Saharan Africa Might be the Region Hardest Hit. Available at: https://blogs.worldbank.org/opendata/impact-covid-19-coronavirus-global-poverty-why-sub-saharan-africa-might-be-region-hardest.

Martini M, Gazzaniga V, Bragazzi NL, et al. (2019) The Spanish Influenza Pandemic: a Lesson From History 100 Years After 1918. Journal of Preventive Medicine and Hygiene 60: E64–E67.

Mordo Intelligence. (2019) Available at: https://www.mordorintelligence.com/industry-reports/internet-of-things-in-healthcare-market.

Mordor Intelligence. (2018) Smart Cities Market Size, Share – Segmented by Solution (Smart Mobility Management, Smart Public Safety, Smart Healthcare, Smart Buildings), and Geography – Growth, Trends and Forecast (2019–2024). Available at: https://www.mordorintelligence.com/industry-reports/smart-cities-market.

Nkengasong JN and Mankoula W. (2020) Looming Threat of COVID-19 Infection in Africa: Act Collectively, and Fast. The Lancet 395: 841-842.

O'Mahony J, Simes NHR, Smith X, et al. (2019) Mobile Nation 2019: The 5G Future. Australia: Deloitte.

OECD. (2020) Coronavirus: The World Economy at Risk. OECD.

Oppmann P. (2020) Cuba Is Going Under Lockdown Over Coronavirus Concerns. Available at: https://edition.cnn.com/world/live-news/coronavirus-outbreak-03-24-20-intl-hnk/h_7b694d17a78f2c02d7c76570e1726508.

Park JG. (2020) COVID-19: How a Phone App Is Assisting South Korea Enforce Self-Quarantine Measures. Available at: https://www.sbs.com.au/language/english/covid-19-how-a-phone-app-is-assisting-south-korea-enforce-self-quarantine-measures.

Pérez-Peña R and McNeil DG. (2020) W.H.O., Now Trump's Scapegoat, Warned About Coronavirus Early and Often. Available at: https://www.nytimes.com/2020/04/16/health/WHO-Trump-coronavirus.html.

Pham S. (2020) Airlines Around the World Are Suspending Flights to China as the Coronavirus Spreads. Available at: https://edition.cnn.com/2020/01/29/business/british-airways-coronavirus/index.html.

Pleasance C. (2020) Angela Merkel Becomes Latest World Leader to Hint China Has Mislead the World Over Coronavirus and Urges Beijing to be "More Transparent". Available at: https://www.dailymail.co.uk/news/article-8237283/Angela-Merkel-hints-China-mislead-world-coronavirus.html.

Porterfield C. (2020) Surge of Smartphone Apps Promise Coronavirus Tracking, But Raise Privacy Concerns. Available at: https://www.forbes.com/sites/carlieporterfield/2020/04/01/surge-of-smartphone-apps-promise-coronavirus-tracking-but-raise-privacy-concerns/#7c9191a72681.

Ramiah D. (2020) 10 Ways Technology is Helping to Fight the Coronavirus. Available at: https://www.cn.undp.org/content/china/en/home/ourperspective/ourperspectivearticles/2020/10-ways-technology-is-helping-to-fight-the-coronavirus.html.

Reuters. (2020) Australia Scientists to Share Lab-Grown Coronavirus to Hasten Vaccine Efforts. Available at: https://www.reuters.com/article/us-china-health-australia/australia-scientists-to-share-lab-grown-coronavirus-to-hasten-vaccine-efforts-idUSKBN1ZR2YD.

Scott S, Timms P and Florance L. (2020) Australian Lab First Outside of China to Copy Coronavirus, Helping Vaccine Push. Available at: https://www.abc.net.au/news/2020-01-29/wuhan-coronavirus-created-in-australian-lab-outside-of-china/11906390.

Sevastopulo D and Manson K. (2020) Donald Trump Threatens to Freeze Funding for WHO. Available at: https://www.ft.com/content/193453e3-479f-4fef-9234-d0f9f14c5a6e.

Shenker J. (2020) Cities After Coronavirus: How Covid-19 Could Radically Alter Urban Life. Available at: https://www.theguardian.com/world/2020/mar/26/life-after-coronavirus-pandemic-change-world.

Shwartz ND. (2020) Coronavirus Recession Looms, Its Course 'Unrecognizable'. Available at: https://www.nytimes.com/2020/03/21/business/economy/coronavirus-recession.html.

Smart Cities Association. (2020) Global smart cities market to reach a whopping $3.5 trillion by 2026. Available at: https://www.smartcitiesassociation.org/index.php/media-corner/news/1-global-smart-cities-market-to-reach-a-whopping-3-5-trillion-by-2026.

Stanway D. (2020) China Lab Rejects COVID-19 Conspiracy Claims, But Virus Origins Still a Mystery. Available at: https://www.reuters.com/article/us-health-coronavirus-china-lab/china-lab-rejects-covid-19-conspiracy-claims-but-virus-origins-still-a-mystery-idUSKCN22A0MM.

Statista. (2020a) Coronavirus (C0VID-19) Impact on GDP Growth in France 2020. Available at: https://www.statista.com/statistics/1103142/impact-coronavirus-gdp-france/.

Statista. (2020b) Forecasted Impact of Coronavirus (COVID-19) on GDP in Italy Q1-Q2 2020. Available at: https://www.statista.com/statistics/1101019/forecasted-impact-of-coronavirus-covid-19-on-gdp-in-italy/.

Stephanie S and Gerstel D. (2020) The Global Economic Impacts of COVID-19. Available at: https://www.csis.org/analysis/global-economic-impacts-covid-19.

Stewart E. (2020) The Coronavirus Recession is Already Here. Available at: https://www.vox.com/policy-and-politics/2020/3/21/21188541/coronavirus-news-recession-economy-unemployment-stock-market-jobs-gdp.

Sullivan H, Rawlinson K, Gayle D, et al. (2020) Known Global Covid-19 Deaths Pass 215,000 – as it Happened. Available at: https://www.theguardian.com/world/live/2020/apr/28/coronavirus-live-news-trump-says-china-could-have-stopped-virus-as-global-cases-pass-3-million.

The L. (2017) The global HIV/AIDS epidemic- progress and challenges. The Lancet 390: 333.

The World Bank. (2020) Transparency is Key to Weathering Shocks, Investing in Growth, and Enhancing Trust in Government. Available at: https://www.worldbank.org/en/news/press-release/2020/04/09/transparency-is-key-to-weathering-shocks-investing-in-growth-and-enhancing-trust-in-government.

Tokars JI, Richards C, Andrus M, et al. (2004) The Changing Face of Surveillance for Health Care—Associated Infections. Clinical Infectious Diseases 39: 1347–1352.

UN. (2019) World Population Prospects 2019. Washington, D. C: United Nations.

UoC. (2020) Artificial Intelligence to Predict Corona-Patients' Risk of Needing Ventilators. Available at: https://news.ku.dk/all_news/2020/04/artificial-intelligence-to-predict-corona-patients-risk-of-needing-ventilators/.

Voa Student Union. (2020) Phone Apps in China Track Coronavirus. Available at: https://www.voanews.com/student-union/phone-apps-china-track-coronavirus.

Wakefield J. (2020a) Coronavirus: AI Steps up in Battle Against COVID-19. Available at: https://www.bbc.com/news/technology-52120747.

Wakefield J. (2020b) Coronavirus: Tracking App Aims for One Million Downloads. Available at: https://www.bbc.com/news/technology-52033210.

Wang O. (2020) China May Adjust 2020 GDP Growth Target Due to Coronavirus, Goverment Policy Adviser Says. Available at: https://www.scmp.com/economy/china-economy/article/3051200/china-may-adjust-2020-gdp-growth-target-due-coronavirus.

Wearden G and Jolly J. (2020) IMF: Global Economy Faces Worst Recession Since the Great Depression. Available at: https://www.theguardian.com/business/live/2020/apr/14/stock-markets-china-trade-global-recession-imf-forecasts-covid-19-business-live.

WHO. (2020a) Coronavirus Disease 2019 (COVID-19): Situation Report – 85. Available at: https://www.who.int/docs/default-source/coronaviruse/situation-reports/20200414-sitrep-85-covid-19.pdf?sfvrsn&=7b8629bb_4.

WHO. (2020b) Novel Coronavirus (2019-nCoV): Situation Report- 2. Available at: https://www.who.int/docs/default-source/coronaviruse/situation-reports/20200122-sitrep-2-2019-ncov.pdf?sfvrsn&=4d5bcbca_2.

WHO. (2020c) Statement on the Meeting of the International Health Regulations (2005) Emergency Committee

Regarding the Outbreak of Novel Coronavirus (2019-nCoV). Available at: https://www.who.int/news-room/detail/23-01-2020-statement-on-the-meeting-of-the-international-health-regulations-(2005)-emergency-committee-regarding-the-outbreak-of-novel-coronavirus-(2019-ncov).

WHO. (2020d) *WHO Timeline - COVID-19*. Available at: https://www.who.int/news-room/detail/08-04-2020-who-timeline—covid-19.

Wojda TR, Valenza PL, Cornejo K, et al. (2015) The Ebola Outbreak of 2014–2015: From Coordinated Multilateral Action to Effective Disease Containment, Vaccine Development, and Beyond. Journal of Global Infectious Diseases 7: 127–138.

Wright D. (2020) AI Becomes An Ally in the Fight Against COVID-19. Available at: https://www.forbes.com/sites/servicenow/2020/04/17/ai-becomes-an-ally-in-the-fight-against-covid-19/#14ae98533f5f.

Index

Note: Page numbers followed by "f" indicate figures.